[redacted]

RELIEVING PAIN *Naturally*

SYLVIA GOLDFARB, PhD
ROBERTA W. WADDELL

Foreword by Dr. Jeffrey Perry, DO

SQUAREONE
PUBLISHERS

The therapeutic procedures in this book are based on the training, personal experiences, and research of the authors. Because each person and situation is unique, the author and publisher urge the reader to check with a qualified health professional before using any procedure where there is any question to appropriateness.

The publisher does not advocate the use of any particular diet or health treatment, but believes the information presented in this book should be available to the public.

Because there is always some risk involved, the author and publisher are not responsible for any adverse effects or consequences resulting from the use of any of the suggestions, preparations, or procedures described in this book. Please do not use the book if you are unwilling to assume the risk. Feel free to consult with a physician or other qualified health professional. It is a sign of wisdom, not cowardice, to seek a second or third opinion.

Cover Designer: Jacqueline Michelus
Typesetters: Gary A. Rosenberg & Theresa Wiscovitch

Square One Publishers
115 Herricks Road
Garden City Park, NY 11040
(516) 535-2010
www.squareonepublishers.com

Library of Congress Cataloging-in-Publication Data

Goldfarb, Sylvia.
Relieving pain naturally : a complete guide to drug-free pain management / Sylvia Goldfarb, Roberta W. Waddell.
p. cm.
Includes bibliographical references and index.
ISBN 0-7570-0079-7
1. Chronic pain--Alternative treatment. I. Waddell, Roberta W. II. Title.
RB127.G654 2005
616'.0472—dc22
2004022717

Printed in the United States of America

10 9 8 7 6 5 4 3 2 1

Contents

PART 1
Conditions

PART 2
Treatments

*"Where nature creates pain,
toxic substances have accumulated
and want to be eliminated."*

PHILLIPUS AUREOLUS PARACELCUS
(1493–1541)

Acknowledgments

Many people helped in the creation of this book. I am especially grateful to the following.

Dr. Edward M. Wagner, ND, longtime friend and co-author of my first two books for always taking time from his busy schedule to answer my questions about nutrition and supplements. Dr. Randy Coleman, ND, for his expertise regarding various types of bodywork. Larry Segal, DC, who helped answer my questions about chiropractic. Ed Snapp of Futures Unlimited for all the information about his innovative method of treating post-polio syndrome. Keep up the good work, Ed. Genevieve Renzi for her help in explaining various aspects of physical therapy. Geraldine DePaula, MD, for information about aromatherapy. Marshall H. Sager, DO, DABMA, FAAMA, and President of The American Academy of Medical Acupuncture for helping me understand the healing benefits of acupuncture. Lavar Tiller, personal trainer, for his help with my research, especially the benefits of exercise. The staff at The Center For Human Integration for enlightening me about the various methods of energy healing. Roberta Waddell, editor of my first three books, and my co-author. You really helped make the book better, Bobby.

SG

I first want to thank my natural and extended family, especially daughter Karen Waddell and cousin Elizabeth Karaman, whose support and encouragement were incalculable. I could never have done it without their help.

Thanks go to our publisher, Rudy Shur, for recognizing how this book was filling a gap, for trusting me in taking on the project, and for the sharp attention to details—his sensible suggestions and tweaks add much to the book's usefulness. Many thanks for everything go to my co-author, Sylvia Goldfarb, but most particular thanks go to her for jumpstarting the project by unstintingly and excellently researching and writing the initial versions for most of the chapters while I had to work (my thanks to Norman Goldfind for keeping me busy editing during this time). Thanks also to editor Wendy Sleppin. It's always good to have another pair of eyes reviewing a project, and hers were certainly keen. Thanks, Wendy.

A large number of surrounding people helped with the preparation of this book. I am extremely grateful to the doctors and health practitioners who reviewed chapters for accuracy, most notably Dr. Jeffrey Perry, who wrote the Foreword, and whose original idea it was to collaborate on a pain book. Thanks also to Drs. Robert Porzio and Avery Ferentz (too-soon deceased and very much missed), his widow, Satu Ferentz, and Dr. Linda Merkin, who all helped to make applied kinesiology easy to understand; to Jacques Depardieu who provided his enlightened approach to acupuncture, and traditional Chinese medicine (TCM) in general; to Dr. Pavel Yutsis, John Taggert of *The Family Health News,* and Ed McCabe, who each helped unscramble some of the more arcane aspects of the oxygen therapies; and to Drs. Emily Kane and Cathy Rogers for their valuable input on compresses, packs, poultices, hydrotherapy, and other naturopathic therapies.

Many thanks to Suzan Walter of the American Holistic Health Association, who time after time led me to other important organizations and people. I am most grateful to all the associations, doctors, and practitioners who helped me get their listings and studies right, and who supplied interesting case histories for their section of the book. And my thanks go to the government: Our tax dollars at work in a very good way with the people at the National Library of Medicine, who deserve special praise for the high quality of their help in the months I spent working with them and searching *PubMed.gov* for appropriate clinical studies—they truly make the ten minutes allowed each caller count.

On the technical end, my thanks to Mischa Beitz who used his considerable computer skills to keep the work flowing time after time. I am also grateful to Gary and Carol Rosenberg for all the technical and editorial questions they answered, and for their just plain support.

Finally, I want to acknowledge the brilliant Eugene Schwartz, my good friend for the final thirty years of his life, my boss for the last ten of those, and ultimately my facilitator, whose simple, unadorned statement, "You're my editor," got me started professionally on the word path I should have been on all along. Gene, wherever you are, please know that I never cease thanking you for giving me my future.

RWW

Foreword

From the pain of a hangnail on your finger or toe—a suppposedly minor misery that can end up dominating your day—to the devastating, acute pain of a herniated disc pressing on a nerve, or the more results-oriented pangs of childbirth, pain is with us in some form all of our lives. And no one seems exempt from it. You could say that pain is one of the bonds that links humans, and in fact all sentient beings.

My own relationship with pain began when I was a medical student on late night rounds in a hospital around Thanksgiving. One of the patients was a very old, comatose woman with severe contractures. It was my unpleasant job to draw blood from this frail, gnarled lady for no apparent purpose other than to perhaps make her chart feel better, certainly not her.

At that moment, I knew I had to figure out a way to improve patients' overall well-being. I vowed that, while I would always strive to provide the most up-to-date medical care, I would *never* forget that a significant goal of treatment was to minimize pain and suffering. And, to this day, that is still my goal, as it should be for all people entrusted with healing others.

Despite all the advances in medicine, however, and even though we have learned more and more about pain over the last few years, the study of pain has lagged behind—and this is in spite of the fact that *everyone* has some form of pain at one time or another.

In medical schools, there are many courses—cardiology, gastroenterology, nuclear medicine, psychology, surgery, and so forth—but what is astounding is that there is *no* course in pain itself. It is especially astounding because, when you enter a hospital setting as a medical student, you are immediately impressed, and dismayed (as I was), by the immense amount of pain and suffering. And impressed too by the fact that, even though you can save a life, there is still a great deal of pain and suffering which is less than optimally addressed.

In my work with patients at the Spine Center of the Hospital For Joint Diseases in New York, or The Center for Women's Health in Darien, CT, I have seen many different manifestations of pain, and my colleagues and I have used a wide variety of treatment modalities to alleviate pain. But, regardless of which methods we may employ, we all agree that the key to any effective treatment of pain is *proper diagnosis.*

When I see a patient for treatment, I first set out to pinpoint the correct diagnosis. If, for example, a patient presents with severe back pain, it is my job to make sure that pain is from a herniated disc and is not, instead, a potentially lethal abdominal aortic aneurysm. This is particularly important with back pain because the majority of it is non-specific.

Diagnosis isn't always possible, however, and sometimes there isn't any diagnosis that "modern medicine" can find and treat. I once had a patient who said she was suffering so much, she was going to kill herself. The MRI found *nothing* and the patient, who still complained of the pain, was, of course, disappointed, wondering how she could be treated if the doctors couldn't find the problem. In such a case, people often conclude that the patient is a malingerer, or that it's all in her head, but it's not. She really is suffering but, unfortunately, we can't find the exact cause. The next step then, after ruling out what this patient doesn't have, is to narrow down the alternative treatments that are available to her, treatments such as those discussed in this book for both diagnosed, specific sources of pain and the more general, undiagnosed ones.

Although many of these treatment suggestions may lead to a doctor or therapist, I always try to empower my patients to cooperate in their own healing, to practice self-help, by saying, "You're here for rehab and we're a big team," (I go through the long litany of treatment options) "but the captain of the team is *you.*" And throughout treatment, I reinforce this idea with the patient by reminding them that they are the most important person in the room.

There are some cases where orthodox treatments, including medication and surgery, are indicated. If masking allows a person in pain to accomplish things—an ibuprofen before exercising, for example—it's okay. Or, if a patient has progressive sciatica and disc herniation, with increasing weakness and loss of bladder control, that patient is going to need surgery. But, in less drastic cases of a herniated disc, where the neurological exam is normal and the patient is not neurologically compromised, has excellent muscles and reflexes, and can do anything he or she wants, I respond to the question, "How soon do I have to have surgery," by saying, "The good news is, the surgery is *elective* and there are alternative ways to approach the problem that don't involve surgery."

This book focuses on those ways, highlighting the more physical and immediate alternative methods of pain relief, and presenting them in a format that gives you easy, instant access to them.

As is commonly noted, medicine is both an art and a science. We could therefore say that the purpose of this book is to empower you to maximize this synergy for yourself in your own life and thereby improve the overall quality of your own health and well-being.

Dr. Jeffrey Perry, DO
Hospital For Joint Diseases, Spine Center
New York, New York

Preface

Several things came together to provide the impetus for this book. One of us, then the editor at a direct mail alternative health publishing house, was approached some time ago by a pain control specialist who suggested doing a book together on the subject. Although that project never materialized, the idea was set in motion and was further implemented by the author's own decades-long travails and travels in the realms of pain control seeking relief from her own persistent back pain.

This book, our effort to help you and others like you who may be hurting, is the end result. It is our aim to provide you with the most up-to-date information available for diagnosing and treating your pain. While we also inform you about mainstream methods to alleviate or eliminate unrelenting pain, and talk about treatments for acute and short-term pain, the primary focus of our book is on those least-invasive, non-drug-related treatments that have been proven safe and effective for relief from long-term, chronic pain.

The format we have chosen is intended to give you quick and easy access to the information you are seeking. In the first half of this two-part book, we have alphabetically listed individual conditions. For each of these, we present a summary of the problem, give its symptoms and causes, discuss diagnoses, conventional treatments and the problems with conventional treatments, then progress to a discussion of the appropriate alternative natural treatments for the condition, quoting doctors throughout. We give details on precisely what remedies to use, in what form, how often, and for how long, breaking them down by age, weight, and sex wherever appropriate. For additional information on treatments, we refer you back to the specific treatment section that applies. In the second part, you will find the treatments listed from A to Z. Here we give a summary of each treatment, its history, and its advantages. We list what conditions respond well to the treatment, explain—in a user-friendly, easy-to-follow style—how to use or make the treatment, and what, if any, warnings and contraindications there might be. To illustrate these topics, we have included case histories in the book.

To help you learn more about what we have discussed, there are lists of resources and references for each entry that include organizations, websites, and references specific to the particular condition or treatment. The lists are located at the back of the book. There are also general lists for these categories that you can access for further information, and all are relevant to chronic pain and natural health. Each entry in treatments has a section on successful clinical sudies for that modality, and unfamiliar treatments or arcane terms are defined as we write about them. To round this out, there is a comprehensive index allowing you instant access to the condition or treatment you are researching.

Since our book is basically an overview, it can serve as a reference guide to jump-start you onto a path of discovery and the eventual relief of your pain. You can use the book in several ways. It can be a quick, convenient access guide to a problem or treatment you are already familiar with, or it can be a resource guide to help you determine the cause of your pain and how you can alleviate it. Either way, we feel that by *Relieving Pain Naturally* you can stop hurting and start living.

Introduction

Pain is always unpleasant, but under certain circumstances it may be necessary. Yes, sometimes it is necessary—for instance, if you pick up something hot, the pain signals you to drop it before you do serious damage to your skin. This type of pain is called acute pain and is a natural response, a signal to your body that it has been injured or that something else is wrong.

Severe chest pain can warn you of an impending heart attack and can save your life by having you seek prompt medical attention. Acute pain can also result from injuries, burns, fractures, wounds, surgery, disease, or dental procedures. It can last for hours, days, or weeks and usually responds to medication, such as narcotics and/or analgesics (painkillers), which are useful in the short-term. In essence, these medications cover up symptoms and help you get over a crisis.

On the other hand, chronic pain can be constant or recurrent and can last for months, or even years. It becomes an unwelcome, twenty-four-hour-a-day companion. If you suffer from chronic pain, you should be aware that narcotics can be addictive, and anti-inflammatory drugs can cause problems if you use them for long periods. Ibuprofen, for example, can cause stomach ulcers, or other forms of internal bleeding, and kidney problems. Too much aspirin can also cause some bleeding problems and can lead to ringing in the ears, even hearing loss, sweating, visual problems, and rapid heartbeat. Acetaminophen is gentler on your stomach, but excessive use can cause liver damage, especially to those who use alcohol on a regular basis. The entire class of COX-2 inhibitors may be linked to potentially damaging side effects to the heart. This was the underlying reason why Vioxx was taken off the market.

Do you suffer from chronic pain and want to do something about it other than popping pills or just resting and applying heat or ice? Have you attempted to seek help outside mainstream medicine? Maybe you are so familiar with the early symptoms signaling the approach of your pain problem that you can often tell in advance when an attack is imminent. For example, you might be able to forecast when a migraine is about to descend on you. Do you have an arsenal ready to combat it? You probably do know ways to diminish its effect, but maybe you've also tried to research additional, alternative methods to relieve your pain and found yourself overwhelmed by the variety of information available. Those of you who are computer savvy and explore the Internet will find over a million websites dealing with alternative approaches to pain control. If you browse in a book store or library, you will notice that most pain books focus on a particular condition or a singular method of pain control, for example, magnet therapy, or a particular visualization technique.

Most practitioners only have expertise in their particular treatment so you might have to consult several until you find the one or two just right for your problem. This book, on the other hand, will give you conveniently accessible answers to your questions in one place, under one cover.

HOW TO USE THIS BOOK

The format we have chosen is intended to give you quick and easy access to the information you are seeking about alternative (and some conventional) methods that can be useful to relieve your pain. At the beginning of this two-part book, we have a Quick Help Chart, which is an alphabetical overview of both general pain conditions and specific conditions discussed in the book. It is accompanied by a summary of the best treatments for each condition. Within these summaries you will find the names of some treatments in boldface. While all the treatments mentioned can be effective, the boldfaced treatments may be most effective.

Part 1 of the book has an alphabetically listed entry for each of the individual conditions. In every entry, we summarize the problem, give its symptoms and causes, and discuss diagnoses—in keeping with the idea that a correct diagnosis of the problem is crucial to any pain treatment, we present several methods for pinpointing the root of the pain, including applied kinesiology (which also goes on to treat the diagnosed pain). We list conventional treatments for the condition, and the problems with some of these conventional treatments, then progress to a discussion of the appropriate alternative natural treatments for the condition, quoting doctors throughout. We give details on precisely what remedies to use, in what form, how often, and for how long, breaking them down by age, weight, and sex wherever appropriate. In the section on alternative natural treatments, we divide the therapies into those you can do yourself at home and those that require a healthcare professional or an advanced knowledge of the method. For additional information on suggested treatments, we refer you to the specific treatment entry that applies.

Part 2 of the book has entries on individual treatments, also listed from A to Z. We summarize each treatment method, and give its history and its advantages. We list what conditions respond well to the particular method, explain how to use or make it, and give whatever warnings or contraindications are applicable. In both parts of the book, we illustrate these topics with case histories.

To help you learn more about all the conditions and treatments, there are resources and references in the back of the book. They are listed by entry and include organizations, websites, and references specific to that particular entry's condition or treatment. An additional section on general resources for umbrella groups contains listings for pain-related alternative/holistic organizations, websites with information on treatments, and referrals to practitioners. Each treatment entry has an additional section on successful clinical studies for that modality, and any unfamiliar treatments or arcane terms are defined as they come up. To round this out, there is a comprehensive index allowing you instant access to the condition or treatment you are researching.

It is important to emphasize here that this book is intended for people who want to take an active role in their own health and not just leave the decision to others. It promotes alternative approaches over the use of painkillers and invasive methods (we include only two moderately invasive therapies, acupuncture and bee venom therapy, which the Chinese believe is the original root of acupuncture) because we believe that, in many cases, these methods can more effectively get to and treat the core of the problem, and can lead to long-lasting relief. It is interesting to note that, before they became part of the standard orthodox treatment lexicon, many methods were first called alternative, as for example, Sister Kenny's hot packs and physical therapy for polio instead of the bulky braces that had been standard treatment. Her methods replaced braces and became the mainstream treatment for polio.

Painkiller medicines, as we said, basically give relief by masking symptoms which invariably return when the effects of the medication wear off, in turn requiring the use of more painkillers, and leading, in a downward spiral, to the painkiller-addiction trap that many people fall into unawares when it's too late and they are confronted with another huge problem in addition to their original pain. We feel this vicious cycle can best be avoided by the use of alternative methods.

Additionally, in connection with conventional methods, be aware that researchers are working overtime to develop new drugs and new invasive procedures for pain eradication. That magical pill or new surgical procedure to banish pain forever is always just around the corner. The trouble is, however, there *are* no magic bullets, and as has too often happened in the past, that miracle drug or medical procedure can easily end up having unwanted, even disastrous side effects. For this reason, among others, caution is strongly advised when considering new drugs or treatments that are untested by time.

THE NATURE OF PAIN

Before delving into the solutions we have detailed for

THE COSTS OF CHRONIC PAIN

According to the National Chronic Pain Outreach Association (NCPOA), chronic pain affects one in ten Americans, and disables more people than cancer or heart disease. It costs the economy over $90 billion a year in medical costs, disability payments, and lost productivity, and yet it has received little attention from researchers until recently, and is consistently underfunded. It is also interesting to note that painkillers account for the largest percentage of prescribed medications in the United States.

you in the following pages, we feel it would be helpful to briefly discuss the nature of chronic and acute pain, a complex interaction of mind and body—even, according to some, a subjective experience. The old idea was that the intensity of the pain was directly related to the intensity of the injury. Still the theory for acute pain, and still taught in many medical schools, it is responsible for allopathic medicine's reliance on the idea that surgery or medicines can deal with the pain's origin and make it disappear. It doesn't take into account the pain that drags on, or the pain that is less visible yet still intense, the kind of pain that doesn't go away, even with medical intervention.

Pain pathways are very complex and can be rapid or slow. A pain signal can continue after an injury has supposedly healed, or even when an appendage has been amputated—a phenomenon known as phantom pain. Pain can get transmitted to the brain as something other than pain, or the brain can transmit a no-pain message back to the injured area. No matter what the injury, however, there is always continuous pain-to-brain-to-pain feedback.

Surgery can cut off the source of the pain, or drugs can numb it, but the pain can still manage to come back anyway, often initiating the aforementioned downward spiral of larger and larger doses of painkillers as the body develops more and more tolerance for them. The best alternative to this is to alter the attitude toward the pain—change how the body feels by changing how the brain reacts to the pain. And for this, it is important to know something about the physiology of pain.

THE PHYSIOLOGY OF PAIN

Pain begins in pain receptors, those nerve ends that lie along the body's periphery. Pain receptors react to a pain-causing occurrence—a cut, a burn, a scrape, or a blow, as from a fall, etc.—and immediately send the pain message through the body to the spinal cord where it continues on up to the brain.

As we said, there are basically two kinds of pain, acute and chronic. Both travel a similar *ascending* pathway, though at different rates of speed depending on which nerve fibers transmit the message, until they reach the brain, at which point they take separate routes.

Fast pain, the kind that feels like painful pressure and touch, is transmitted along large diameter, A-beta nerve fibers. *Slow pain,* is transmitted along two types of nerve fibers, A-delta and C, that are smaller in diameter. A-delta pain, although slower than A-beta, is the acute pain you feel when you get burned or cut. The more secondary dull, aching, burning, cramping, chronic pain, the type we are primarily concerned with in this book, is called slow pain. It is transmitted along the smaller and slower C-fiber nerves, one of two slower nerve fibers (the other being A-delta).

Although these pain messages travel similar nerve-fiber routes up to the brain, once there they diverge. The fast pain goes to the thalamus and the cortex (where most of the thought processes take place). If your thigh hits the sharp corner of a table, for example, your peripheral pain receptors in that area relay this fast pain message to a special area of the spinal cord, which recognizes it. The message is then relayed up the cord to the brain where the cortex prompts you to say "Ouch" and begin rubbing yourself. This acts to ameliorate the painful sensation.

The reason this works is because rubbing is a fast-pain sensation that gets rapidly transmitted over the large A-beta fibers, consequently cancelling out the sharp pain from bumping your thigh, which gets more slowly transmitted by the smaller A-delta nerve fibers. The end result is that the rubbing is all you feel, not the painful bumping encounter. It is this reaction in the body that helps to explain why a therapy like acupuncture, for example, works so well in lessening pain: the sufficient amount of stimulus received in (fast pain) acupuncture acts as a gate to close out the slower pain sensations.

The theory that there are gates on the bundles of spinal cord nerve fibers that can either open to transmit pain impulses to the brain, or close to cut them off, was first propounded in 1965 by Dr. Patrick Wall and Dr. Ronald Melzack, well-known researchers and authors in the field of pain-control studies. Their theory, since modified, has stimulated much of the current thinking on the subject of pain. Although the gate control theory is not able to explain several chronic pain problems, such as phantom limb pain, which require a greater understanding of brain mechanisms, it has become the overall standard for pain theories, helping those in the field to be more effective in their treatment of chronic pain.

Chronic pain moves along the slower pathway of the smaller C-fiber nerves and goes to the hypothalmus and the limbic structures (as do the smaller, slower A-delta nerve fibers). The hypothalmus is considered the central clearing house of the brain and, when it receives pain messages, it instructs the pituitary gland to release certain stress hormones. The limbic structures are where the emotions get processed and their involvement with pain messages helps to explain why your feelings can influence your pain.

Once a pain message has been received by any of these areas, the brain tries to block the message by sending a message back to the pain along the *descending* pathway, telling the body not to register pain until later, or even never. Not much is known about these descending tracts outside the fact that they are largely chemical and they function to shut the above-mentioned gates in the spinal cord to the ascending pain messages. These characteristics help to explain why such methods as biofeedback, self-hypnosis, guided imagery, and other therapies that rely primarily on the brain work so well to control pain.

In the pain-to-brain-to-pain transmission, neurotransmitters are an important link, acting to either kill the pain or produce it. In pain relief, serotonin and the group called endorphins and enkaphalins are important neurotransmitters that can be as powerful as morphine or heroin. Different people produce differing amounts of these neurotransmitters, which is why some people have a higher threshold of tolerance for pain than others. The athletes we regularly read about who perform heroic feats with broken or dislocated bones, or other severe injuries, may be able to do so because of their body's higher production of endorphins which literally override the pain-to-brain message.

We hope that knowing a little about the mechanisms of the pain process will help you to get the most out of this book. Our main purpose and focus in writing it has been to give you a comprehensive approach to dealing with your pain, preferably through alternative methods (for the reasons stated above), but also, when necessary, through safe and effective mainstream approaches as well. The information we present can help you assess your situation, learn about the many ways there are to manage your pain, and lead you to new options you may wish to try out, on your own or in conjunction with your pain control specialist.

We wish you luck in your quest for pain relief. Just remember: Even if we can't fully control what happens to us, we *can* control the way we deal with what happens to us.

Quick Help Chart

Below, in the left column, you will find an alphabetical listing of both general and specific pain conditions discussed in the book. To the right of each condition, you will find a summary of the best treatments for the condition. While all treatments mentioned can be effective to some degree, the treatments printed in boldface may be most effective.

Conditions	Treatments
Achilles Tendonitis	Acupuncture, Applied Kinesiology, Aromatherapy, **Castor Oil Packs**, Chiropractic, Exercise, Guided Imagery, **Heat/Cold Therapy**, Herbs, Homeopathy, Hydrotherapy, **Magnets**, Massage, Nutritional Therapy, Osteopathic Manipulation, **Physical Therapy**, Reflexology, Rolfing, Supplements.
Angina	Biofeedback, **Exercise**, Guided Imagery, Herbs, Homeopathy, Massage, **Meditation**, **Nutritional Therapy**, Qigong, Reflexology, Supplements, Tai Chi, Yoga.
Arm-Related Pain	*See* Bursitis, Carpal Tunnel Syndrome, Osteoarthritis, Rheumatoid Arthritis.
Arthritis	*See* Bursitis, Gout, Osteoarthritis, Rheumatoid Arthritis.
Back Pain	**Acupuncture**, **Applied Kinesiology**, Aromatherapy, Biofeedback, **Castor Oil Packs**, **Chiropractic**, Craniosacral Therapy, Cupping, **Exercise**, Guided Imagery, **Heat/Cold Therapy**, Herbs, Homeopathy, Hydrotherapy, Hypnosis, **Magnets**, **Massage**, Meditation, Nutritional Therapy, **Osteopathic Manipulation**, Oxygen Therapies, Physical Therapy, Qigong, Reflexology, Rolfing, Supplements, Tai Chi, Yoga. *See also* Rhematoid Arthritis, Osteoarthritis, Sciatica.
Bursitis	**Acupuncture**, **Applied Kinesiology**, Aromatherapy, Bee Venom Therapy, Compresses, Guided Imagery, **Heat/Cold Therapy**, Herbs, Homeopathy, Hydrotherapy, Nutritional Therapy, **Magnets**, Massage, Meditation, **Osteopathic Manipulation**, Physical Therapy, Reflexology, Rolfing, **Supplements**.
Carpal Tunnel Syndrome	**Acupuncture**, Applied Kinesiology, Chiropractic, Compresses, **Exercise**, Guided Imagery and Visualizations, **Heat/Cold Therapy**, Herbs, Homeopathy, Hydrotherapy, **Magnets**, Massage, Nutritional Therapy, Osteopathic Manipulation, **Physical Therapy**, Qigong, Reflexology, Rolfing, Supplements, Tai Chi, Yoga.
Cluster Headaches	Acupuncture, Applied Kinesiology, Aromatherapy, Biofeedback, Chiropractic, Compresses, Craniosacral Therapy, Cupping, Exercise, Guided Imagery, Heat/Cold Therapy, Herbs, Homeopathy, Hypnosis, Magnets, Massage, **Meditation**, Nutritional Therapy, Osteopathic Manipulation, **Oxygen Therapies**, Physical Therapy, Qigong, Reflexology, Supplements, Tai Chi, **Yoga**.

Conditions	Treatments
Crohn's Disease	Acupuncture, Applied Kinesiology, Aromatherapy, Biofeedback, **Castor Oil Packs**, Chiropractic, Craniosacral Therapy, Cupping, Exercise, Guided Imagery, **Herbs**, Homeopathy, Hypnosis, Massage, Meditation, Nutritional Therapy, Oxygen Therapies, Qigong, Reflexology, Supplements, Tai Chi, Yoga.
Dental Problems	Acupuncture, Applied Kinesiology, Aromatherapy, Castor Oil Packs, Chiropractic, Craniosacral Therapy, Guided Imagery, Heat/Cold Therapy, Herbs, Homeopathy, Magnets, Meditation, Nutritional Therapy, Osteopathic Manipulation, Physical Therapy, Reflexology, Rolfing, Supplements. *See also* Temporomandibular Joint (TMJ) Pain
Digestive-Related Pain	*See* Crohn's Disease, Diverticulitis, Irritable Bowel Syndrome (IBS), Ulcerative Colitis (IBD).
Diverticulitis	Acupuncture, Applied Kinesiology, Aromatherapy, Biofeedback, **Castor Oil Packs**, Chiropractic, Craniosacral Therapy, Cupping, Exercise, Guided Imagery, **Herbs**, Homeopathy, Hypnosis, Massage, Meditation, **Nutritional Therapy**, Qigong, Reflexology, Supplements, Tai Chi, Yoga.
Endometriosis	Acupuncture, Applied Kinesiology, Aromatherapy, Bee Venom Therapy, Biofeedback, **Castor Oil Packs**, Chiropractic, Craniosacral Therapy, Exercise, Guided Imagery, Heat/Cold Therapy, **Herbs**, Homeopathy, Massage, Meditation, Nutritional Therapy, Osteopathic Manipulation, Qigong, Reflexology, Supplements, Tai Chi, Yoga.
Face-Related Pain	*See* Temporomandibular Joint (TMJ) Pain, Trigeminal Neuralgia.
Fibromyalgia	**Acupuncture**, **Aerobic Exercise**, Aromatherapy, Bee Venom Therapy, Biofeedback, Guided Imagery, **Heat/Cold Therapy**, Herbs, Homeopathy, Hydrotherapy, Magnets, Meditation, **Nutritional Therapy**, Osteopathic Manipulation, **Oxygen Therapies**, Physical Therapy, Qigong, Reflexology, Rolfing, Supplements, Tai Chi, Yoga.
Foot-Related Pain	*See* Achilles Tendonitis, Neuroma, Peripheral Neuropathy, Reflex Sympathetic Dystrophy Syndrome (RSDS).
Frozen Shoulder	**Acupuncture**, Applied Kinesiology, **Chiropractic**, **Compresses**, **Exercise**, Heat/Cold Therapy, Hydrotherapy, Osteopathic Manipulation, Physical Therapy, Rolfing.
Gout	Acupuncture, Aromatherapy, Castor Oil Packs, Guided Imagery, Heat/Cold Therapy, Herbs, Homeopathy, Hydrotherapy, **Nutritional Therapy**, Qigong, Reflexology, Supplements, Tai Chi, Yoga.
Hand-Related Pain	*See* Carpal Tunnel Syndrome, Osteoarthritis, Rheumatoid Arthritis, Trigger Finger.
Headaches	*See* Cluster Headaches, Migraine Headaches, Premenstrual Syndrome (PMS), Tension Headaches.
Heart-Related Pain	*See* Angina.
Inflammatory Bowel Disease	*See* Crohn's Disease, Ulcerative Colitis.
Irritable Bowel Syndrome (IBS)	**Acupuncture**, Applied Kinesiology, Aromatherapy, Biofeedback, **Castor Oil Packs**, Chiropractic, Craniosacral Therapy, Cupping, Exercise, Guided Imagery, **Herbs**, Homeopathy, Hypnosis, Massage, Meditation, **Nutritional Therapy**, Qigong, Reflexology, Supplements, Tai Chi, Yoga.

Conditions	Treatments
Knee-Related Pain	*See* Osteoarthritis, Rheumatoid Arthritis.
Leg-Related Pain	*See* Osteoarthritis, Reflex Sympathetic Dystrophy Syndrome (RSDS), Rheumatoid Arthritis, Sciatica.
Migraine Headaches	**Acupuncture/Acupressure**, Applied Kinesiology, **Aromatherapy**, Bee Venom Therapy, Biofeedback, Chiropractic, Compresses, Craniosacral Therapy, Cupping, Exercise, Guided Imagery, Heat/Cold Therapy, Herbs, Homeopathy, Hydrotherapy, Hypnosis, **Magnets**, Massage, **Meditation**, Nutritional Therapy, Osteopathic Manipulation, **Oxygen Therapies**, Physical Therapy, Qigong, Reflexology, Supplements, Tai Chi, Yoga.
Neck-Related Pain	*See* Osteoarthritis, Rheumatoid Arthritis, Tension Headaches.
Neuroma	Acupuncture, Aromatherapy, Compresses, Guided Imagery, Heat/Cold Therapy, Herbs, Homeopathy, Hydrotherapy, Nutritional Therapy, Osteopathic Manipulation, Reflexology, Rolfing, Supplements.
Osteoarthritis (OA)	**Acupuncture**, **Applied Kinesiology**, Aromatherapy, **Bee Venom Therapy**, Castor Oil Packs, Chiropractic, Craniosacral Therapy, **Exercise**, Guided Imagery, **Heat/Cold Therapy**, Herbs, Homeopathy, Hydrotherapy, Magnets, **Massage**, **Nutritional Therapy**, **Osteopathic Manipulation**, Oxygen Therapies, Physical Therapy, Qigong, Reflexology, Rolfing, **Supplements**, Tai Chi, **Yoga**.
Pelvic Floor Tension Myalgia	**Acupuncture**, Applied Kinesiology, Aromatherapy, **Biofeedback**, Castor Oil Packs, Chiropractic, Craniosacral Therapy, Exercise, Guided Imagery, Heat/Cold Therapy, Hydrotherapy, Massage, Meditation, Osteopathic Manipulation, Qigong, **Reflexology**, Rolfing, Tai Chi, Yoga.
Peripheral Neuropathy	**Acupuncture**, Applied Kinesiology, Aromatherapy, Chiropractic, **Exercise**, Guided Imagery, Heat/Cold Therapy, **Herbs**, Homeopathy, Hydrotherapy, **Nutritional Therapy**, Osteopathic Manipulation, Oxygen Therapies, Reflexology, Supplements.
Phantom Pain	**Acupuncture**, Biofeedback, **Chiropractic**, Compresses, **Exercise, Heat/Cold Therapy**, Hydrotherapy, Hypnosis, Osteopathic Manipulation, **Physical Therapy**.
Plantar Fasciitis	Exercise, **Heat/Cold Therapy**, Hydrotherapy, Osteopathic Manipulation, **Physical Therapy**, **Stretching**.
Postherpetic Neuralgia	Aromatherapy, **Bee Venom Therapy**, Biofeedback, Craniosacral Therapy, Cupping, Guided Imagery, Heat/Cold Therapy, **Herbs**, Homeopathy, Hydrotherapy, **Massage**, Meditation, **Nutritional Therapy**, **Oxygen Therapies**, Qigong, Reflexology, Rolfing, Supplements, Tai Chi, **Yoga**.
Post-Polio Syndrome	Acupuncture, Applied Kinesiology, Aromatherapy, Castor Oil Packs, Chiropractic, Exercise, Guided Imagery, Heat/Cold Therapy, Herbs, Homeopathy, Hydrotherapy, **Magnets**, Massage, **Nutritional Therapy**, Osteopathic Manipulation, Oxygen Therapies, **Physical Therapy**, Qigong, Reflexology, Rolfing, Supplements, Tai Chi, Yoga.
Premenstrual Syndrome (PMS)	**Acupuncture**, Applied Kinesiology, Aromatherapy, Bee Venom Therapy, Biofeedback, **Castor Oil Packs**, Chiropractic, Craniosacral Therapy, Exercise, Guided Imagery, Heat/Cold Therapy, Herbs, Homeopathy, Massage, Meditation, Nutritional Therapy, Osteopathic Manipulation, Qigong, Reflexology, Supplements, Tai Chi, Yoga.

Conditions	Treatments
Reflex Sympathetic Dystrophy Syndrome (RSDS)	**Acupuncture**, Applied Kinesiology, Aromatherapy, Biofeedback, **Chiropractic**, Exercise, Guided Imagery, **Heat/Cold Therapy**, Herbs, Homeopathy, Hydrotherapy, Magnets, Nutritional Therapy, Osteopathic Manipulation, Oxygen Therapies, **Physical Therapy**, Reflexology, Rolfing, Supplements.
Rheumatoid Arthritis (RA)	**Acupuncture**, Applied Kinesiology, Aromatherapy, **Bee Venom Therapy**, Castor Oil Packs, Chiropractic, Craniosacral Therapy, Exercise, Guided Imagery, Heat/Cold Therapy, Herbs, Homeopathy, Hydrotherapy, Magnets, Massage, Nutritional Therapy, Osteopathic Manipulation, Oxygen Therapies, **Physical Therapy**, Qigong, Reflexology, Rolfing, Supplements, Tai Chi, **Yoga**.
Rotator Cuff Tendonitis	**Acupuncture**, Applied Kinesiology, Aromatherapy, **Castor Oil Packs**, Chiropractic, **Exercise**, Guided Imagery, Heat/Cold Therapy, Herbs, Homeopathy, Hydrotherapy, Magnets, Massage, Nutritional Therapy, Osteopathic Manipulation, Physical Therapy, Reflexology, Rolfing, Supplements.
Sciatica	**Acupuncture**, **Applied Kinesiology**, Aromatherapy, **Chiropractic**, Castor Oil Packs, Craniosacral Therapy, Cupping, **Exercise**, Guided Imagery, Herbs, Homeopathy, Hydrotherapy, Hypnosis, Magnets, **Massage**, Meditation, Nutritional Therapy, **Osteopathic Manipulation**, Physical Therapy, Qigong, Reflexology, Rolfing, Supplements, Tai Chi, **Yoga**.
Shoulder-Related Pain	*See* Bursitis, Frozen Shoulder, Osteoarthritis, Rhematoid Arthritis, Rotator Cuff Tendonitis.
Spinal Stenosis	**Aerobic Exercise**, **Physical Therapy**.
Sports-Related Pain	*See* Achilles Tendonitis, Back Pain, Bursitis, Plantar Fascia, Rotator Cuff Tendonitis, Sciatica, Tennis Elbow.
Tarsal Tunnel Syndrome	**Acupuncture**, Applied Kinesiology, Chiropractic, Compresses, Exercise, Guided Imagery and Visualizations, **Heat/Cold Therapy**, Herbs, Homeopathy, Hydrotherapy, **Magnets**, Massage, Nutritional Therapy, Osteopathic Manipulation, **Physical Therapy**, Qigong, Reflexology, Rolfing, Supplements, Tai Chi, Yoga.
Temporomandibular Joint (TMJ) Pain	Acupuncture, Applied Kinesiology, Aromatherapy, Biofeedback, Castor Oil Packs, Chiropractic, **Craniosacral Therapy**, Guided Imagery, Heat/Cold Therapy, Herbs, Homeopathy, Magnets, Meditation, Nutritional Therapy, Osteopathic Manipulation, Physical Therapy, Reflexology, Rolfing, Supplements. *See also* Dental Problems.
Tic Douloureux	*See* Temporomandibular Joint (TMJ) Pain, Trigeminal Neuralgia.
Tendonitis	*See* Achilles Tendonitis, Rotator Cuff Tendonitis.
Tennis Elbow	**Acupuncture**, Applied Kinesiology, Aromatherapy, Bee Venom Therapy, **Castor Oil Packs**, Exercise, Guided Imagery, Heat/Cold Therapy, Herbs, Homeopathy, **Magnets**, Nutritional Therapy, Osteopathic Manipulation, **Physical Therapy**, Reflexology, Rolfing, Supplements.
Tension Headaches	Acupuncture, Applied Kinesiology, Aromatherapy, Biofeedback, Chiropractic, Compresses, **Craniosacral Therapy**, Cupping, Exercise, Guided Imagery, Heat/Cold Therapy, Herbs, Homeopathy, Hydrotherapy, **Hypnosis**, Magnets, Massage, Meditation, Nutritional Therapy,

Conditions	Treatments
Tension Headaches (Continued)	Osteopathic Manipulation, **Oxygen Therapies**, Physical Therapy, Qigong, Reflexology, Supplements, Tai Chi, Yoga.
Thoracic Outlet Syndrome	**Exercise**, **Physical Therapy**.
Trigeminal Neuralgia	**Acupuncture**, Applied Kinesiology, Aromatherapy, Compresses, Cupping, Exercise, Guided Imagery, Heat/Cold Therapy, **Herbs**, Homeopathy, Meditation, Nutritional Therapy, **Osteopathic Manipulation**, Reflexology, Rolfing, Supplements.
Trigger Finger	**Acupuncture/Acupressure**, Applied Kinesiology, Aromatherapy, Castor Oil Packs, Chiropractic, **Exercise**, Guided Imagery, **Heat/Cold Therapy**, Herbs, Homeopathy, Hydrotherapy, **Magnets** Massage, Nutritional Therapy, Osteopathic Manipulation, **Physical Therapy**, Reflexology, Rolfing, Supplements.
Ulcerative Colitis (IBD)	Acupuncture, Applied Kinesiology, Aromatherapy, Biofeedback, **Castor Oil Packs**, Chiropractic, Craniosacral Therapy, Cupping, Exercise, Guided Imagery, **Herbs**, Homeopathy, Hypnosis, Massage, Meditation, Nutritional Therapy, Oxygen Therapies, Qigong, Reflexology, Supplements, Tai Chi, Yoga.

PART 1

Conditions

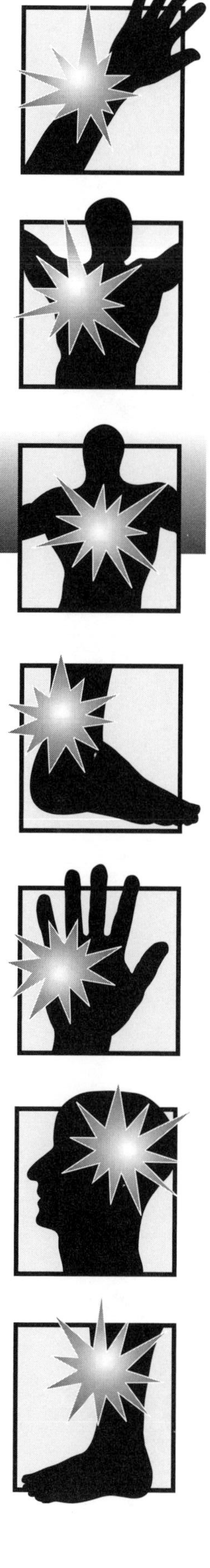

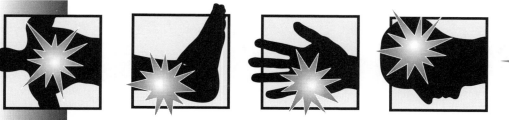

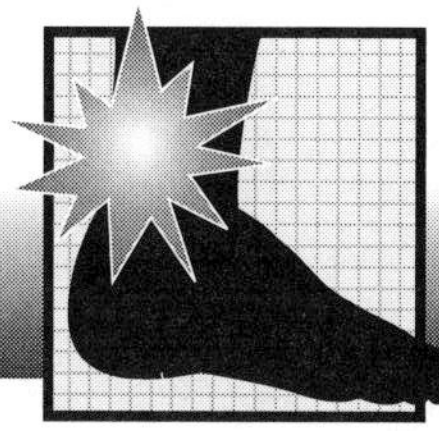

Achilles Tendonitis

This is an inflammation of the Achilles tendon, also called the heel cord. It is a prominent body feature at the back of the lower leg which attaches the two large calf muscles, the gastrocnemius and soleus, to the heel bone. Both of these muscles are needed to push off with the foot and rise up on the toes so we can walk. Achilles tendonitis is usually seen in young athletic types who engage in such sports as basketball and running. It can also occur later in life among those who are just starting to exercise because the muscles and tendon have lost their flexibility and cannot tolerate the new stress placed on them.

Symptoms

The heel experiences pain that worsens when walking or running. The skin over the tendon is swollen and warm, and the tendon is painful to touch.

Common Causes

Overdoing new exercise programs, especially if the muscles are not flexible enough to tolerate new stresses placed on them, is a frequent cause of this form of tendonitis. Other causes can include activities involving sudden stops and starts, such as baseball, football, running, and tennis, or it can be a result of wearing high heels and then switching to flat shoes or sneakers. Ballet dancers are also known to develop this problem.

A serious complication of Achilles tendonitis is a tearing of the tendon due to continued activity when it is inflamed. Do not try to work through the pain.

Diagnosing the Problem

When standing on your toes, there is a tenderness along the tendon, accompanied by pain. An MRI can show inflammation of the tendon, and x-rays can show any changes due to arthritis, which can contribute to tendonitis.

Conventional Treatments

- ❏ A flexible cast to immobilize the injured area and reduce swelling.
- ❏ Compressing the foot and ankle with an elastic bandage.
- ❏ Crutches to keep weight off the injured area.
- ❏ Elevating the foot above your heart as often as possible.
- ❏ Keeping weight off the affected foot as much as possible.
- ❏ Using ice packs for twenty minutes at a time every hour.
- ❏ Surgery, which involves removing the inflamed outer covering of the tendon and reattaching the torn tissues.

Surgery should be reserved for severe traumatic injuries, if the Achilles tendon is ruptured or torn away from the heel. The recovery period is several months.

SELF-HELP ALTERNATIVE TREATMENTS

The following techniques can be done at home. Although they may not work as fast as drugs or surgery, natural alternatives help the body heal itself. All herbs, homeopathic remedies, packs, and supplements discussed here are available in health food stores and, increasingly, in large drug and grocery stores, as well as on the Internet.

Aromatherapy

Aromatherapy can help relieve the pain of Achilles tendonitis, particularly the essential oils of clove bud, marjoram, rosemary, and pine. Add a few drops to vegetable oil and massage into the sore heel. Apply gently twice daily but do not use a vigorous massage over this (or any) swollen area. Essential oils are available in health food stores and stores specializing in aromatherapy products, which you can find in the yellow pages. (*See* AROMATHERAPY in PART 2 Treatment Section for additional information.)

Castor Oil Packs

Dip a piece of white flannel into some warm castor oil. Wring it out and place it over the affected heel. Cover with plastic and apply a heating pad for one hour. Do this twice daily. (*See* COMPRESSES, PACKS, and POULTICES in PART 2 Treatment Section for additional information.)

Diet

Tendonitis is inflammatory in nature so certain dietary modifications may be helpful.

Good Foods

All the foods listed below help to reduce inflammation.

- ❑ Foods that contain B vitamins, such as complex carbohydrates, fruits, nuts, seeds, vegetables, and whole grains.
- ❑ Fish, particularly wild salmon.
- ❑ Flaxseed meal.
- ❑ Fresh vegetables and fruits, preferably organically raised. Dark green vegetables contain antioxidants which help scavenge and neutralize the free radicals that are causing the inflammation.
- ❑ Garlic.

(*See* NUTRITIONAL THERAPY in PART 2 Treatment Section for additional information.)

Bad Foods

Avoid the following foods, which can all trigger an inflammatory reaction in your body.

- ❑ Alcohol.
- ❑ Processed foods and fast foods.
- ❑ Saturated fats, as found in meats and dairy products.
- ❑ Spicy foods.
- ❑ Sugary-type foods.
- ❑ White flour products, such as pasta and bread.

Heat Therapy/Cold Therapy

Applying cold to the painful tendon area in the foot reduces swelling, and heat helps increase blood flow once the swelling has gone down. (*See* HEAT THERAPY/COLD THERAPY in PART 2 Treatment Section for additional information.)

Herbal Remedies

- ❑ Black currant oil relieves pain and inflammation.
- ❑ Boswellia has anti-inflammatory properties and acts similarly to NSAIDs without the side effects of stomach irritation or ulceration.
- ❑ Cayenne ointment, applied topically, relieves pain.
- ❑ Coltsfoot and comfrey, used externally in soaks or poultices, reduce fluid retention. (Note: Comfrey taken internally has the potential to cause liver damage and should be used only under careful supervision.)
- ❑ Evening primrose oil relieves pain and inflammation.
- ❑ Ginger stimulates circulation.
- ❑ Hydrangea acts like cortisone.
- ❑ Watercress reduces fluid retention.
- ❑ White willow bark relieves inflammation and pain. Take 60–120 mg per day. Although its pain-relieving aspects are slower than aspirin, they last longer.
- ❑ Yucca is a precursor of synthetic cortisone. It enables your adrenal glands to produce and release their own cortisone into your system.

Take the above herbs as directed on label. They can also be used in teas and infusions. (*See* HERBAL REMEDIES in PART 2 Treatment Section for additional information.)

Homeopathic Remedies

You can self-treat with homeopathic remedies by selecting the one that most closely matches your symptoms. If you don't see improvement, try another, or a combination product. Follow the instructions on the label. If you do not have relief in a reasonable amount of time, consult a physician who specializes in homeopathic medicine.

- ❑ Arnica soothes inflammation. It is also available in cream and ointment form for external application.
- ❑ Calcarea phosphorica eases pain and stiffness.
- ❑ Hypericum eases nerve pain.
- ❑ Ruta graveolens helps ease stiffness and weakness.

Take the above remedies as indicated on label. Combination remedies sometimes work more effectively than single ones. (*See* HOMEOPATHY in PART 2 Treatment Section for additional information.)

Hydrotherapy

Running hot water over the painful tendon area while in the shower or soaking in a hot tub can help diminish the pain. (*See* HYDROTHERAPY in PART 2 Treatment Section for additional information.)

Magnet Therapy

Magnet therapy relieves pain, accelerates healing, and reduces inflammation. Placing magnets in the shoe of a foot affected by an Achilles tendon brings increased amounts of blood to the area, which, in turn, brings oxygen and other healing substances to reduce the pain. (*See* MAGNET THERAPY in PART 2 Treatment Section for additional information.)

Supplements

- ❑ Bromelain is a digestive enzyme if taken with meals, but it acts as an anti-inflammatory when taken on an empty stomach. Take 400 mg three times a day *between* meals.
- ❑ Flaxseed oil, 1–2 teaspoons daily.
- ❑ Magnesium citrate, 500 mg three times daily, acts as a muscle antispasmodic.
- ❑ Manganese, 25–100 mg twice a day during the acute phase. Then take 10–15 mg twice a day.
- ❑ Proteolytic enzymes taken between meals can reduce pain and swelling and help speed up the healing process. Take per instruction on label.
- ❑ Selenium, 100–200 mcg daily.
- ❑ Vitamin B_6 aids the normal function of nerve cells and helps reduce swelling because it has a natural ability to eliminate water retention. Dr. Edward M. Wagner, ND, recommends 200 mg three times a day. He says it is more effective to use the pyrodoxal #5 phosphate form of B_6 which has a higher assimilation rate than plain pyrodoxine.
- ❑ Vitamin B_{12}, sublingual, helps prevent nerve damage. Take 500 mcg twice daily. Note: For balance when taking individual Bs, be sure to supplement with a B-complex once daily, or a multivitamin containing Bs.
- ❑ Vitamin C (Ester-C), 1000 mg three times daily, is a general overall antioxidant.
- ❑ Vitamin E, 400 IU daily.

(*See* SUPPLEMENT THERAPY in PART 2 Treatment Section for additional information.)

ASSISTED ALTERNATIVE TREATMENTS

The following techniques may require specialized training or the aid of a healthcare professional.

Acupuncture and Acupressure

Acupuncture involves the insertion of extremely thin solid needles into specific points of your body to stimulate its own healing mechanism and improve blood flow to the affected areas. It also reduces inflammation, relieves pain, improves mobility, and there are rarely any risks or side effects. (*See* ACUPUNCTURE and ACUPRESSURE in PART 2 Treatment Section for additional information.)

Applied Kinesiology

Applied Kinesiology is excellent for reducing pain rapidly. The AK practitioner tests your muscles to determine the origin of your problem and then decides on the best course of action, choosing from a wide variety of therapeutic methods at her or his disposal. (*See* APPLIED KINESIOLOGY in PART 2 Treatment Section for additional information.)

Chiropractic

Chiropractic theory is based on the assumption that a properly aligned spine is essential for good health, and that any misalignment of the vertebrae in the spine causes pressure on the spinal nerves, leading to pain. The chiropractor makes spinal adjustments to move misaligned vertebrae to more normal positions which helps the nervous system to function properly. (*See* CHIROPRACTIC in PART 2 Treatment Section for additional information.)

Exercise and Stretching

Exercise and stretching can be helpful, but it must be carefully supervised in order not to further damage the affected area.

Gently flex and extend your foot twenty times, four times a day. Be sure to stop at any point you feel discomfort. (*See* EXERCISE, STRETCHING, and SPORTS in PART 2 Treatment Section for additional information.)

Guided Imagery

Guided imagery is a useful adjunct to help you manage your pain. In your mind, picture the painful heel as an object and bring in the appropriate tools to diminish the pain. (*See* GUIDED IMAGERY and VISUALIZATION in PART 2 Treatment Section for additional information.)

Massage

A massage helps bring blood to the affected area and relieve the pain. There are many kinds of massage therapies available and you can ask your practitioner to suggest the appropriate one for your Achilles tendonitis. (*See* MASSAGE in PART 2 Treatment Section for additional information.)

Osteopathic Manipulation

The goal of osteopathic manipulation in the treatment of Achilles tendonitis is to increase range of motion, decrease muscle tension, and improve blood circulation.

(*See* OSTEOPATHIC MANIPULATION in PART 2 Treatment Section for additional information.)

Physical Therapy

Physical therapy increases the range of motion in your joints and corrects and improves your body's natural healing mechanism. (*See* PHYSICAL THERAPY in PART 2 Treatment Section for additional information.)

Reflexology

Reflexology massage therapy can be performed on the part of the foot corresponding to the tendon area that is in pain. (*See* REFLEXOLOGY in PART 2 Treatment Section for additional information.)

Rolfing

Rolfing helps place your body in balance with gravity by releasing stress patterns that keep it out of alignment. It can have long-lasting effects in easing pain. (*See* ROLFING in PART 2 Treatment Section for additional information.)

PRACTICAL SUGGESTIONS

- ❏ An orthotic device may help reduce or eliminate pain.
- ❏ DMSO (dimethylsulfoxide), applied topically, may relieve pain.
- ❏ If you are just starting to exercise, be sure to stretch properly, then start out slowly and increase your activity gradually.
- ❏ Keep your body in a balanced alignment and change positions frequently.
- ❏ Keep your calf muscles strong and flexible. Have a knowledgeable practitioner suggest proper exercises.
- ❏ Once you are aware of the activity that produces your symptoms, stop doing it immediately. This is not a situation where you should work through the pain.
- ❏ Try not to overuse any one joint.
- ❏ Warm up and stretch before beginning any physical activities, such as running or sports.
- ❏ Wear shoes with low heels. If you have to wear high heels in your profession, be sure to do stretching exercises every night and morning.

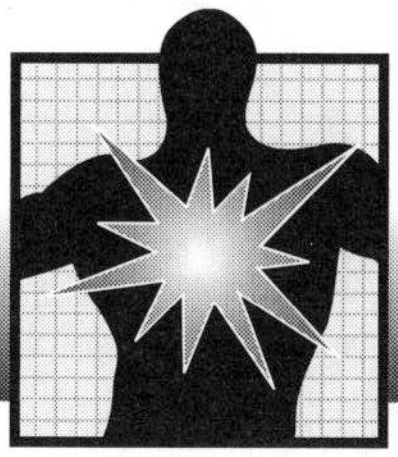

Angina

Angina is a symptom of myocardial ischemia which occurs when the heart muscle doesn't get enough blood to do its work. The myocardium is the heart muscle, and ischemia means lack of blood supply. Angina can be a warning sign that you are at risk for a heart attack. There are three types of angina: stable angina, unstable angina, and variant angina. Sometimes the pain is so mild that people think it is indigestion. For some, the pain is excruciating. If you are not sure, go to the nearest emergency room, especially if the attack lasts more than fifteen minutes.

Symptoms

Stable angina occurs during exercise. Unstable angina is not predictable and often occurs while at rest. It is more severe and can quickly lead to a heart attack. Pain may feel heavy, strangulating, or suffocating. Sometimes it starts under the breastbone on the left side and may radiate to the arm, jaw, left shoulder, neck, and throat. Variant angina can occur while at rest, or during exercise.

Cause

When fatty deposits accumulate in the arteries, they severely deplete the amount of blood and oxygen able to pass through the arteries, and the blood flow to the heart muscle gets lowered. The heart muscle then becomes weakened, and any increased load on it, such as physical exertion or emotional excitement, overburdens it, which leads to spasms and causes the pain known as angina.

Diagnosing the Problem

Angina is suspected when blood circulation to the heart is enough for normal needs, but insufficient when the heart's needs increase. For instance, pain may not occur while walking, but running can bring it on. If you experience chest pain while at rest, it could be unstable angina but, to be sure, a diagnosis must be made by a competent cardiologist.

Conventional Treatments

Angina can be treated with drugs or invasive techniques to improve the supply of blood to the heart. Some medications are intended for the heart muscle's blood supply or the heart's need for oxygen. Some help the blood vessels relax so their inside openings expand, improving blood flow and allowing more oxygen and nutrients to reach the heart muscle. The most frequently used drugs are:

- Aspirin. It makes blood less sticky and helps prevent clots.
- Beta blockers. They lower blood pressure and help reduce cardiac oxygen consumption by inhibiting the body's response to certain nerve impulses. This decreases the force and rate of the heart's contractions which reduces the amount of work the heart must perform and reduces its demand for oxygen. They also block the harmful effects of stress hormones on the heart.
- Calcium channel blockers. They relax the muscles surrounding the blood vessels. This helps widen the vessels, allowing more blood and oxygen to reach the heart.
- Nitrates, which expand the arteries to allow for greater blood flow. People with angina usually feel relief a few minutes after taking the medication.

Invasive techniques include:

- Angioplasty. When constricted blood flow is due to plaque formation, a catheter can be inserted into an artery in the arm or leg and guided to the obstructed coronary artery. Then a second catheter with a balloon tip is passed through the first catheter and is inflated at the site of the blockage. This compresses the plaque, thereby enlarging the inner diameter of the artery and allowing the blood to flow more easily. Then the physician deflates the balloon and withdraws both catheters.
- Coronary artery bypass surgery (CABG). A blood vessel, usually from a leg, is used to construct a detour around the blocked portion of a coronary artery. The surgeon attaches the ends of the blood vessel around each side of the blockage, which restores blood supply to the heart muscle.

Problems with Some Conventional Treatments

In general, all medication can do is control the symptoms of angina. It does not address its cause, which is a narrowing or blockage of the coronary arteries.

- Aspirin can cause bleeding. Even though low doses are used to treat angina, if you are taking aspirin, be sure to tell your doctor or dentist before any type of surgery is performed.

- ❑ Beta blockers can cause insomnia and fatigue. And sometimes they cause cholesterol levels to rise, which can lead to even more angina pain.
- ❑ Calcium channel blockers can lead to dizziness and lightheadedness.
- ❑ Nitrates can cause side effects, such as headaches and dizziness, and the body develops a tolerance for them when they are used for long periods of time.
- ❑ About 25 percent of those who have angioplasty experience a re-narrowing of the coronary artery. Then the procedure has to either be repeated or open heart surgery has to be considered.

SELF-HELP ALTERNATIVE TREATMENTS

The alternative treatments described below to help prevent an attack of angina in the future can all be done at home. (First, before embarking on any treatments, be sure you have been diagnosed with stable angina and not with unstable or variant angina.) All herbs, homeopathic remedies, and supplements discussed here are available in health food stores and, increasingly, in large drug and grocery stores, as well as on the Internet.

Diet

Making sure you have a wholesome, balanced diet is crucial to maintaining the health of your heart.

Good Foods

Overall, eat more fresh fruits, vegetables, and whole grains, such as oats, rice, and whole wheat. The following foods help the heart's blood flow so it requires less oxygen.

- ❑ Cantaloupe and cantaloupe juice help thin the blood and prevent angina attacks.
- ❑ Cod, mackerel, salmon, and tuna contain essential fatty acids that are critical for normal functioning of cells, muscles, nerves, and organs.
- ❑ Garlic and onions reduce serum cholesterol levels.
- ❑ Green tea helps keep cholesterol from clogging arteries.
- ❑ Kale is a good source of magnesium, which helps protect the arterial lining. Mustard greens, spinach, and turnip greens are also excellent sources of magnesium.
- ❑ Nuts (raw and unsalted) contain essential fatty acids. Walnuts are especially high in Omega 3s.
- ❑ Olive oil also contains essential fatty acids.

(*See* NUTRITIONAL THERAPY in PART 2 Treatment Section for additional information.)

Bad Foods

By avoiding the following foods in your diet, you can reduce the risk of angina.

- ❑ Alcohol.
- ❑ Animal fats.
- ❑ Black tea.
- ❑ Butter.
- ❑ Chocolate.
- ❑ Coffee.
- ❑ Fried foods.
- ❑ Hydrogenated oils.
- ❑ Processed and refined foods.

Other Substances to Avoid

Tobacco smoke. Stop smoking, and avoid second-hand smoke.

Herbal Remedies

- ❑ Alfalfa helps reduce blood cholesterol levels and plaque deposits on artery walls.
- ❑ Barberry is useful for cardiovascular disorders.
- ❑ Black cohosh is helpful with cardiac problems.
- ❑ Garlic helps the liver by preventing excess production of fat and cholesterol. It also lowers blood pressure and thins the blood.
- ❑ Ginger reduces cholesterol and blood pressure and helps prevent blood clots.
- ❑ Ginkgo biloba is an antioxidant and also improves blood flow in the body.
- ❑ Guggul reduces cholesterol.
- ❑ Hawthorn helps protect blood vessels from damage. It improves heart function and tolerance to exercise, strengthens the heart muscle, and aids in the excretion of excess salt and water. Take 60 mg of the extract three times a day.
- ❑ Lecithin acts as a fat emulsifier. Take 1 tablespoon of the granules three times daily.
- ❑ Turmeric helps prevent the formation of blood clots which could lead to a heart attack.

Take the above herbs as directed on label. They can also be used in teas and infusions. (*See* HERBAL REMEDIES in PART 2 Treatment Section for additional information.)

Homeopathic Remedies

The following remedies are for informational purposes only. Although you can self-treat with homeopathy for many conditions, do not attempt to do so if you suspect a heart attack. Seek emergency treatment immediately.

- ❑ Arsenicum album helps prevent angina attacks.
- ❑ Cactus grandiflorus can relieve pain during an acute attack of angina.
- ❑ Glonoine is a useful remedy for heart problems.
- ❑ Nux Vomica helps prevent angina attacks.

Combination remedies sometimes work more effectively than single ones. Take the above remedies according to instructions on the label. (*See* HOMEOPATHY in PART 2 Treatment Section for additional information.)

Supplements

- ❑ Arginine, an amino acid, stimulates blood-vessel dilation which improves your ability to exercise if you have angina. Take per label.
- ❑ Bromelain, per label, prevents excessive blood-platelet stickiness.
- ❑ Calcium aids the proper functioning of the cardiac muscle. Take 1500–2000 mg daily.
- ❑ Carnitine, an amino acid, improves your heart's functioning and reduces symptoms. Take 1 gram two to three times a day.
- ❑ Coenzyme Q_{10} helps the heart's energy-making mechanism so you have a greater ability to exercise without problems if you have angina. Take 150 mg a day.
- ❑ Fish oil reduces chest pain as well as the need for nitroglycerin. Take 3 grams three times a day.
- ❑ Magnesium helps relax the heart muscle and protects the arterial lining. Take 1000 mg daily in divided doses. Do not exceed 1000 mg. If you take a multivitamin, check the ingredients to see how much magnesium it contains and then subtract that amount from 1000. Do not take more than 300 mg if you have diseased kidneys.
- ❑ Vitamin E helps thin blood naturally. Take 400–800 IU daily.

(*See* SUPPLEMENT THERAPY in PART 2 Treatment Section for additional information.)

ASSISTED ALTERNATIVE TREATMENTS

The following techniques may require specialized training or the aid of a healthcare professional.

Exercise

Increased exercise can help ease symptoms of angina. You should consult a doctor before beginning an exercise plan. (*See* EXERCISE, STRETCHING, and SPORTS in PART 2 Treatment Section for additional information.)

Massage

A massage can relieve the painful symptoms of angina. There are many kinds of massage therapies available and you can ask your practitioner to suggest the appropriate one for your problem. Many conventional doctors are now extolling the benefits of massage. (*See* MASSAGE in PART 2 Treatment Section for additional information.)

Reflexology

Reflexology can send healing energy to the heart muscle. (*See* REFLEXOLOGY in PART 2 Treatment Section for additional information.)

Stress Management and Relaxation Techniques

Besides exertion, stress from emotional sources can precipitate an angina attack. Practicing some form of stress management, such as biofeedback, guided imagery and visualization techniques, meditation, yoga breathing exercises, or other types of relaxation for as little as fifteen minutes a day, can go a long way toward improving an angina condition. (*See* BIOFEEDBACK, GUIDED IMAGERY and VISUALIZATION, MEDITATION, and TAI CHI, QIGONG, and YOGA in PART 2 Treatment Section for additional information.)

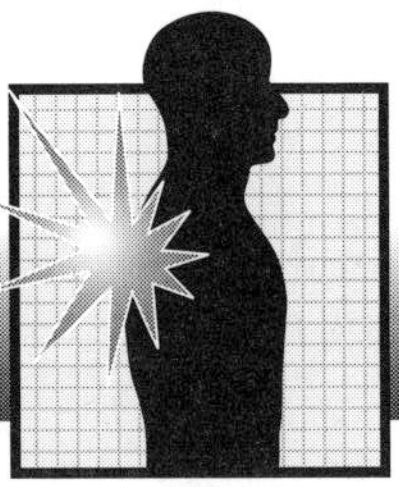

Back Pain

Back pain is the second most common medical complaint there is, superseded only by the common cold. Eight out of ten Americans develop back pain at some time in their lives, and they spend more than $26 billion annually to manage it. Dr. Jeffrey Perry of The Spine Center in New York says most people have what is called non-specific low-back pain (pain in the lumbar region of the back), but it can also manifest as cervical (neck) pain, or pain from herniated discs, the slippage of fluid from the cushioning discs that lie between the thirty-three S-curve-vertbrae of the spine. Don't go rushing for a disc operation, though, cautions Dr. Perry, because it is imperative to realize that one-third of the population has disc problems that are asymptomatic. You can have a herniated disc and not have any pain and, conversely, just because you have a disc herniation and pain, the ruptured disc may not be the cause of your pain. You could have the disc operation, he says, and still end up in pain afterwards, adding that a proper diagnosis is always key to effective pain management.

Back pain is a widespread condition that causes more loss of work time than any other ailment. It is not usually serious and can be prevented or treated, but sometimes it can indicate a serious problem. You should see a medical professional immediately if any of these symptoms occur: you have numbness or tingling in your arms and legs, or lose bladder or bowel control—these could indicate a spinal cord injury; you have a fever, which could be an infection; or you have a pain on one side, approximately at waist level—this could be a kidney infection.

Symptoms

Back pain can occur anywhere along the spine between the neck and hips, but the majority of it occurs in the lower back. This pain can be a persistent ache and/or stiffness, or it can be sharp and localized. It ranges from mild to severe and may be accompanied by muscle spasms.

Common Causes

There are so many possible causes of back pain that you have to wonder whether the back's central position, its fulcrum-like aspect in the body, makes it particularly vulnerable to injury, or whether it is because so many injuries to the body can cause radiating pain to the back. Like the chicken-or-egg question, we may never have the definitive answer, but here is an alphabetical listing of the principal reasons that pain either originates in, or radiates to, our backs.

- ❑ Degeneration of the joints, ligaments, muscles, or intervertebral discs.
- ❑ Exercising improperly before your muscles are warmed up.
- ❑ Getting up the wrong way from a bed or a seated position.
- ❑ Heavy lifting.
- ❑ Herniated disc(s).
- ❑ High heels.
- ❑ Inactivity.
- ❑ Injuries and accidents.
- ❑ Internal problems, such as diseases of the kidney, liver, ovary, or pancreas.
- ❑ Osteoarthritis.
- ❑ Osteoporosis.
- ❑ Overweight (if you are more than twenty pounds overweight, you greatly increase your risk of lower back pain).
- ❑ Poor posture.
- ❑ Pregnancy.
- ❑ Sedentary lifestyle.
- ❑ Sports that involve sudden stops and starts, twisting, jumping, and lifting, such as baseball, basketball, bowling, football, golf, tennis, and weightlifting.
- ❑ Stress.
- ❑ Strains, sprains, or overworking the ligaments and muscles surrounding the back.
- ❑ Vacuuming.
- ❑ Weak abdominal muscles (when your abdomen sags, it puts a greater load on your lower back).

Another cause could be Tension Myositis Syndrome (TMS), a term used by John Sarno, MD, a professor of clinical rehabilitation medicine at the New York University School of Medicine in New York City. Dr. Sarno has a theory that, in order to protect you from acting on, or being destroyed by, rage, your mind distracts you by creating back pain. He has written three books on this subject and says the syndrome mainly occurs in intelligent, talented people who are compulsive perfectionists, and who tend to put the needs of others before themselves.

Diagnosing the Problem

In order to determine the best course of treatment for you, and to rule out any serious pathology, there are several things your doctor can do. He or she might: check your reflexes; take an EMG (electromyogram) to measure whether your muscles or your nerves are the cause of the problem (treatment would vary according to the findings); give you an MRI (magnetic resonance imaging) to determine if there is any soft-tissue damage; or take x-rays to check for any structural damage.

Conventional Treatments

Western treatment of back pain is often ineffective, and sometimes back problems clear up spontaneously.

- ❑ Baclofen pump therapy. Baclofen is an antispasmodic pain controller which the implanted pump, a small titanium disc about three inches in diameter and one-inch thick, delivers on a long-term basis into the intrathecal spaces in the spine to help control severe spasticity. It is particularly useful for those who do not respond to oral doses of baclofen.
- ❑ Bed rest was formerly recommended, but some doctors now believe it takes two weeks to get back in shape for every week spent in bed.
- ❑ Botoxin injections. Botoxin is basically a poison but, in minute doses, it is used for muscle relaxation and helps with pain.
- ❑ Epidural steroid injections and nerve blocks (similar to epidural steroid injections) into the lumbar epidural space can relieve low back pain.
- ❑ Fentanyl patches or Lidoderm patches are easy to use, transdermal, non-invasive medications. Although their purpose is different from nitroglycerine patches, they are applied the same way and are considered cutting-edge conventional treatments.
- ❑ Muscle relaxants can help to calm spasms.
- ❑ Pain relievers, both over-the-counter and prescribed. NSAIDs are available without a prescription and include Aleve (naproxen), Advil, Motrin and Nuprin, (all forms of ibuprofen). Stronger painkillers requiring a prescription may include anti-inflammatories, such as prescription-strength ibuprofen, and possibly narcotic analgesics, such as Demerol, Oxycontin, and Tylenol with codeine.
- ❑ Physical therapy. Treatments help restore function, improve mobility, and relieve pain by using conservative methods that do not involve surgery. Performed by a professional physical therapist or a physiatrist (a doctor who specializes in physical medicine—physiatrists refer to themselves as "orthopedists without scalpels"), treatments include electrostimulation, hot and cold applications, massage, muscle-strengthening and stretching exercises, and ultrasound therapy. If you do not know a physiatrist, you have to be referred to a physical therapist by your regular doctor. (*See* PHYSICAL THERAPY in PART 2 Treatment Section for additional information.)
- ❑ Steroid injections can relieve pain quickly.
- ❑ Surgery is usually performed for instability of the spine, progressive weakness, correction of a malfunctioning part, or problems with bowel or bladder function.
- ❑ Transcutaneous electrical nerve stimulation (TENS units) is one of the treatments once considered alternative that is now mainstream. Pads connected to the unit by a wire are put over the painful area and a mild current is applied. The low amounts of electrical current sent to the nerves help to interrupt pain pathways.
- ❑ Trigger point therapy. A local anesthetic in a saline solution is injected directly into the muscle, enabling it to relax.

Problems with Some Conventional Treatments

- ❑ Epidural injections may have such side effects as headache, infection, and neurological problems.
- ❑ Muscle relaxants can cause sleepiness and impaired motor function.
- ❑ Narcotics can be addictive and sometimes cause severe constipation, plus they do nothing for the underlying cause of back pain.
- ❑ NSAIDs can cause gastrointestinal bleeding and stomach upset. Long-term use can lead to kidney problems.
- ❑ Steroid injections cannot be used for long-term relief. You should not receive more than three injections a year because of potential side effects. Too many of them can actually harm tissues and weaken bones.
- ❑ Surgery is not always successful, and problems often recur.

SELF-HELP ALTERNATIVE TREATMENTS

The following techniques can be done at home. Although they may not work as fast as drugs or surgery, natural alternatives help the body heal itself. All herbs, homeopathic remedies, packs, and supplements discussed here are available in health food stores and, increasingly, in large drug and grocery stores, as well as on the Internet.

Aromatherapy

Aromatherapy, particularly the essential oils of birch, black pepper, clary, coriander, ginger, horsebalm, hyssop, marjoram, peppermint, sage, rosemary, spike lavender, thyme, and wintergreen, can all help relieve muscle tightness and spasms. You can either put a few drops into a hot bath and soak, or add a few drops to vegetable oil and massage this into the affected area. Do not ingest essential oils or use them full strength as they are very powerful compounds. (*See* AROMATHERAPY in PART 2 Treatment Section for additional information.)

Castor Oil Packs

Dip a piece of white flannel into some warm castor oil. Wring it out and place it over the affected area of the back. Cover with plastic and apply a heating pad for one hour. Do this twice daily. (*See* COMPRESSES, PACKS, and POULTICES in PART 2 Treatment Section for additional information.)

Diet

Most back pain is inflammatory in nature so certain dietary modifications may be helpful.

Good Foods

Water. Many report relief within minutes if they drink two glasses of pure water as soon as the pain starts. Muscles are 75 percent water and your body needs a minimum of sixty-four ounces daily, in part to keep your muscles from cramping up. Dehydration caused by insufficient water intake can, therefore, be the cause of muscle-related aches and pains in the back. (*See* NUTRITIONAL THERAPY in PART 2 Treatment Section for additional information.)

Bad Foods

Meats and other animal protein products because they contain uric acid, which puts a strain on the kidneys. This can be a factor in back pain.

Other Substances to Avoid

Tobacco smoke. Smoking keeps oxygen and blood from getting to your back.

Exercise

Exercise can be very helpful in strengthening your back. Here are two highly effective exercises you can do.

1. Lie face down on the floor with your arms extended forward and your palms on the floor. Raise your left arm and right leg as high as is comfortable. Hold for ten seconds. Then return to the starting position and repeat with the right arm and left leg. Gradually work up to twenty repetitions.
2. A yoga posture called the cobra can relieve back pain. Lie face down with your arms at your sides. Anchor your heels under a chair and slowly raise your chest off the floor. Hold for two or three seconds and gradually work up to twenty repetitions.

Cycling, rowing, swimming, and walking are all beneficial exercises for your back. (*See* EXERCISE, STRETCHING, and SPORTS in PART 2 Treatment Section for additional information.)

Heat Therapy/Cold Therapy

Heat increases blood flow to the area in pain and cold reduces swelling. (*See* HEAT THERAPY/COLD THERAPY in PART 2 Treatment Section for additional information.)

Herbal Remedies

- ❑ Birch bark relieves inflammation. You can make a tea by placing a handful of leaves in two cups of boiling water and steeping them for ten minutes.
- ❑ Capsicum (red pepper) contains the pain-relieving chemical capsaicin. Used as a topical analgesic, it is available in commercial creams, or you can make some yourself by mashing some red pepper and mixing it with cold cream. Note: Keep your hands away from your eyes, and be sure to wash your hands thoroughly after applying it, as it can be extremely irritating to your eyes or other sensitive areas.
- ❑ Cardamom, rosemary, and sage all help relax muscles. You can make a tea of any of these by placing a handful of leaves in two cups of boiling water and steeping them for ten minutes.
- ❑ Valerian root, also a relaxant, is available as a tea. You might prefer taking it in capsule form, however, as many people think the tea tastes terrible. Take according to the label.
- ❑ Willow is a natural form of aspirin. You can make a tea by placing a handful of leaves in two cups of boiling water and steeping them for ten minutes.
- ❑ Yucca is an anti-inflammatory. Take according to the label.

Take the above herbs as directed on label. They can also be used in teas and infusions. (*See* HERBAL

REMEDIES in PART 2 Treatment Section for additional information.)

Homeopathic Remedies

You can self-treat with homeopathic remedies by selecting the one that most closely matches your symptoms. If you don't see improvement, try another, or a combination product. Follow the instructions on the label. If you do not have relief in a reasonable amount of time, consult a physician who specializes in homeopathic medicine.

- ❑ Aesculus relieves dull pain that worsens after walking or stooping.
- ❑ Arnica soothes muscles and aches and helps overcome severe pain. It is also available in a gel or ointment for external use.
- ❑ Bryonia helps when movement causes pain.
- ❑ Dulcanwa is useful for pain that is worse in damp or cold weather and is relieved by heat.
- ❑ Rhus toxicodendron aids morning stiffness.

Combination remedies sometimes work more effectively than single ones. (*See* HOMEOPATHY in PART 2 Treatment Section for additional information.)

Hydrotherapy

Use ice on the affected area for the first twenty-four to forty-eight hours. Then use moist heat for twenty-minute periods. (*See* HYDROTHERAPY in PART 2 Treatment Section for additional information.)

Magnet Therapy

Magnet therapy relieves pain, accelerates healing, and reduces inflammation. Magnets on and around the painful areas of the back can bring blood to the area which, in turn, brings oxygen and other healing substances to reduce the pain. Hold the magnets in place with a velcro strip, or tape them on. (*See* MAGNET THERAPY in PART 2 Treatment Section for additional information.)

Supplements

- ❑ Bromelain, 500 mg twice daily, acts as an anti-inflammatory.
- ❑ DL-phenylalanine (DLPA), 500 mg four times daily on an empty stomach, releases endorphins, the body's own natural painkillers. It can take up to seven days to be effective. After the pain is relieved, cut down on the dosage.
- ❑ Pantothene, 500 mg twice daily, acts as an anti-inflammatory.
- ❑ Vitamin B_1 (thiamine), 250 mg twice daily, acts as a muscle relaxant. Note: For balance, when taking individual Bs, be sure to supplement with a B-complex once daily, or a multivitamin containing Bs.
- ❑ Vitamin B_{12} sublingual, 1000 mcg twice daily, relieves nervous tension and helps relax your back.
- ❑ Vitamin C, 1000 mg three times daily, builds up collagen that strengthens and rebuilds back muscles.

(*See* SUPPLEMENT THERAPY in PART 2 Treatment Section for additional information.)

ASSISTED ALTERNATIVE TREATMENTS

The following techniques may require specialized training or the aid of a healthcare professional.

Acupuncture and Acupressure

Acupuncture is a powerful complementary therapy for back pain, with benefits to those who have not responded to bed rest, drugs, epidural injections, physiotherapy, or surgery. It also reduces the need for medication, and there are rarely any risks or side effects. (*See* ACUPUNCTURE and ACUPRESSURE in PART 2 Treatment Section for additional information.)

Applied Kinesiology

Applied Kinesiology is excellent for reducing pain rapidly. The AK practitioner tests your muscles to determine the origin of your problem and then decides on the best course of action, choosing from a wide variety of therapeutic methods at his or her disposal. (*See* APPLIED KINESIOLOGY in PART 2 Treatment Section for additional information.)

Chiropractic

Chiropractic theory is based on the assumption that a properly aligned spine is essential for good health, and that any misalignment of the vertebrae in the spine causes pressure on the spinal nerves, leading to pain. The chiropractor makes spinal adjustments to move misaligned vertebrae to more normal positions which helps the nervous system to function properly. (*See* CHIROPRACTIC in PART 2 Treatment Section for additional information.)

Craniosacral Therapy

A trained craniosacral practitioner can feel areas where healthy tissue function is restricted, usually due to physical or emotional trauma. The theory is that physical injuries and emotional traumas are stored or frozen in the body until they are released. (*See* CRANIOSACRAL THERAPY in PART 2 Treatment Section for additional information.)

Cupping

Cupping increases circulation, bringing blood to the cells. It helps promote energy flow, and can help to reduce back pain. (*See* CUPPING in PART 2 Treatment Section for additional information.)

Guided Imagery and Visualization

Guided imagery helps relieve stress and manage pain. Visualize your back as supple rather than stiff, and if muscle spasms are present, picture them as large waves gradually decreasing and receding. (*See* GUIDED IMAGERY and VISUALIZATION in PART 2 Treatment Section for additional information.)

Hypnosis

Hypnosis helps you relax, and relaxation alleviates stress which contributes to pain. (*See* HYPNOSIS in PART 2 Treatment Section for additional information.)

Massage

A massage can smooth out tight knots in the back and relieve the pain. There are many kinds of massage therapies available and you can ask your practitioner to suggest the appropriate one for your problem. Many conventional doctors are now extolling the benefits of massage. (*See* MASSAGE in PART 2 Treatment Section for additional information.)

Osteopathic Manipulation

The goal of osteopathic manipulation is to increase range of motion, decrease muscle tension, and improve blood circulation. (*See* OSTEOPATHIC MANIPULATION in PART 2 Treatment Section for additional information.)

Oxygen Therapy

Oxygen therapy enhances your body's ability to heal itself by encouraging its own natural production of oxygen. (*See* OXYGEN THERAPIES in PART 2 Treatment Section for additional information.)

Physical Therapy

Physical therapy aids back pain by correcting and improving your body's natural healing mechanism and increasing the range of motion in the joints. (*See* PHYSICAL THERAPY in PART 2 Treatment Section for additional information.)

Reflexology

Reflexology massage therapy can be performed on the part of the foot or hand corresponding to the area in the back that is in pain. (*See* REFLEXOLOGY in PART 2 Treatment Section for additional information.)

Rolfing

Rolfing can have long-lasting effects in easing back pain. (*See* ROLFING in PART 2 Treatment Section for additional information.)

Stress Management and Relaxation Techniques

Practicing some form of stress management, such as biofeedback, meditation, yoga breathing exercises, or other types of relaxation for as little as fifteen minutes a day can go a long way toward improving a painful back condition. (*See* BIOFEEDBACK, MEDITATION, and TAI CHI, QIGONG, and YOGA in PART 2 Treatment Section for additional information.)

ROLFING PAIN AWAY

John was a fireman and physical fitness addict in his thirties who worked out five days a week. He developed severe lower back pain which was diagnosed as compression of the lower back muscles that affected the fourth and fifth lumbar vertebrae.

When conservative therapy did not help, the orthopedic surgeons recommended their specialty. John was reluctant to go under the knife so, instead, he visited a Rolfer who had greatly helped some of his fellow workers. He had thirty- to sixty-minute treatments once a week for ten weeks, which elongated his lower back muscles.

Rolfing treatments are not pleasant, but they did the trick for John, and he had relief for the first time in five years. He never had to have the surgery, and still makes occasional visits to the Rolfer who is still keeping him pain-free in his work and his workouts.

Functional Restoration—Learning to Make Room for Back Pain

An estimated 70–80 percent of American adults experience back pain at some point in their lives, and a conservative estimate puts the cost of treatments at $26 billion a year. Listed in 1991 as the eighth leading reason for visits to doctors' offices, it is no wonder that back pain accounts for 2.5 percent of the total healthcare bill—a 30-percent increase since 1977.

A recent study at Duke University, published in the journal *SPINE*, found that, despite these staggering numbers, there was very little evidence that patients were better off for all the treatment. In fact, some doctors are now advocating that people who experience disabling pain for three or four months, and have only a 10–20 percent chance of improving in the next year, try something new: namely, learning how to live with the pain.

Programs called *functional restoration* are coming to the rescue for these people, with methods that include training in strength, flexibility, and endurance, plus counseling for anxiety, depression, and fear of re-injury.

One such center, established in the early 1980s, is The Productive Rehabilitation Institute of Dallas for Ergonomics (PRIDE). They claim a high success rate for their programs of one or two months, saying that, of the 3500 people disabled by back pain who completed their programs, well over 90 percent were able to return to work and lead productive lives. In a follow-up at one year, most of these people were still working at their jobs, with fewer than 2 percent, on average, getting more surgery or claiming new injuries to the treated areas. This approach could be an option for anyone with intractable pain that won't go away, despite treatments.

PRACTICAL SUGGESTIONS

- ❑ Lift properly, without bending at the waist. When you are lifting anything heavy, bend from your knees and keep your back straight. Hold the item close to your body.
- ❑ When you are carrying anything heavy, whether it is a baby or a briefcase, keep shifting it to the opposite side of your body.
- ❑ If you have to stand for long periods of time, place one foot on a stool and keep changing positions.
- ❑ If your work entails a lot of sitting, get a proper chair.
- ❑ Don't sit still for too long. Get up every half an hour or so and move around.
- ❑ Try to sit with your knees above your hips. It might help to keep your feet on a stool or a thick telephone book.
- ❑ If you have to move heavy items, push them rather than pull them.
- ❑ Sleep on a firm mattress.
- ❑ Do not rest a telephone between your shoulder and chin. If you have to be on the phone for long periods of time, use a headset or a speakerphone.
- ❑ Do not twist your back getting in and out of a car. Instead, turn your body to the side and put both feet on the ground to exit the car. Do the reverse getting into the car. Swing both legs in together to avoid twisting your back.

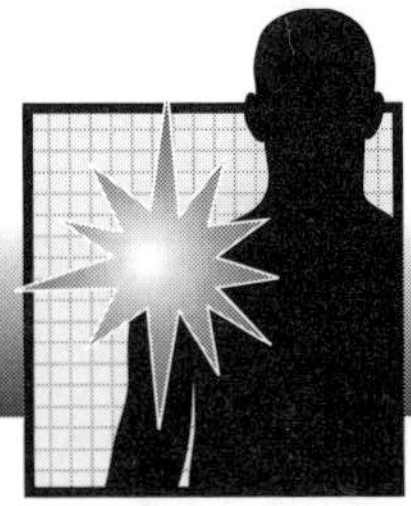

Bursitis

A bursa is a fluid-filled sac located between the bones, tendons, and muscles of the joints. The function of bursae sacs is to lubricate the pressure points so you can move without pain. Bursitis, an inflammation in these sacs, creates pain which, in effect, reverses their ability to function as intended. Bursitis most commonly occurs in the joints of the shoulders, hips, or elbows, but it can also affect the knees, heels, or that part of the big toes adjoining the foot. You can often ease the pain by self-treating, but if the pain lasts more than ten days, if it is disabling or sharp, if swelling, redness, or a rash is present, or if you have a fever which could indicate an infection, seek medical attention.

Symptoms

The more serious cases of bursitis exhibit a sharp, aching, or burning sensation. Generally, the pain worsens with any movement or pressure on the affected area. There can be a dull ache, or a feeling of stiffness in the joint, and you can experience swelling, heat, and/or redness.

Common Causes

The primary cause of bursitis is repetitive motion, or overuse of a joint, which may be occupational or sports-related. The function of the bursae is to protect your tendons from being damaged as they slide across your bones in movement. If you repeatedly move your body in the same way, correctly or not, the tendons in that area have to constantly be relubricated to continue their protective function, and, in time, this repetition can cause an inflammation of the affected bursae.

Other causes of bursitis can be:

- ❏ Arthritis;
- ❏ Calcium deposits;
- ❏ Gout;
- ❏ Infection;
- ❏ Trauma;
- ❏ Unknown.

Diagnosing the Problem

A doctor can determine if it is bursitis by seeing if there is a tenderness in the specific areas that are most susceptible to bursitis. Bursitis pain is usually confined to a particular area. X-rays do not show bursitis unless there is calcification present, but your doctor may order them to rule out other conditions.

Conventional Treatments

There are different approaches to treating this condition. One way is to encourage inaction, either by avoiding the motion causing the problem, or by resting and immobilizing the painful area. Other methods include physical therapy, surgery (rare), TENS units, trigger point therapy (a once-alternative treatment similar to acupressure and rolfing), or ultrasound. Drugs, or drug-related treatments, are also prescribed. They include:

- ❏ Bextra or Celebrex, for example, to relieve pain and inflammation;
- ❏ Corticosteroid injections into the bursa to relieve inflammation—an anesthetic may be included for pain relief;
- ❏ NSAIDs (nonsteroidal anti-inflammatory drugs) to relieve pain and inflammation.

Problems with Some Conventional Treatments

- ❏ The entire class of COX-2 inhibitors, including Bextra and Celebrex, may be linked to potentially damaging side effects to the heart.
- ❏ NSAIDs can cause internal bleeding, and even though bursitis has to do with inflammation, anti-inflammatory medications are not usually particularly helpful.

SELF-HELP ALTERNATIVE TREATMENTS

The following techniques can be done at home. Although they may not work as fast as drugs or surgery, natural alternatives help the body heal itself. All herbs, homeopathic remedies, packs, and supplements discussed here are available in health food stores and, increasingly, in large drug and grocery stores, as well as on the Internet.

Aromatherapy

Aromatherapy can relieve the pain of bursitis, particularly the essential oils of clove bud, marjoram, rosemary, and pine. Apply gently twice daily to the affected area. Do not use a vigorous massage over any swollen joint. (*See* AROMATHERAPY in PART 2 Treatment Section for additional information.)

Compresses, Packs, and Poultices

Soak a cloth or towel in cold water, warm herbal tea, or the appropriate aromatherapy oils (diluted). Apply the soaked cloth to the affected area, cover with a towel to retain the heat or the cold, and leave in place for twenty to thirty minutes. (*See* COMPRESSES, PACKS, and POULTICES in PART 2 Treatment Section for additional information.)

Diet

Even though bursitis is primarily a wear-and-tear condition, it is inflammatory in nature so certain dietary modifications may be helpful.

Good Foods

- Cilantro helps to clear heavy metals from the body.
- Dark green vegetables contain antioxidants that help scavenge and neutralize the free radicals causing the inflammation.
- Fish, particularly wild salmon, helps reduce inflammation.
- Garlic also reduces inflammation.

(*See* NUTRITIONAL THERAPY in PART 2 Treatment Section for additional information.)

Bad Foods

Gluten-containing foods are not good because they lead to inflammation in the tissues, thereby worsening the condition. You can remember which foods contain gluten by thinking B R O W—Barley, Rye, Oats, and Wheat.

Heat Therapy/Cold Therapy

Cold will help reduce swelling in the painful area of the bursitis and, once the swelling is reduced, heat will increase blood flow to the area. (*See* HEAT THERAPY/COLD THERAPY in PART 2 Treatment Section for additional information.)

Herbal Remedies

- Boswellia, per label, has anti-inflammatory properties and acts similarly to NSAIDs without the side effects of stomach irritation or ulceration.
- Cayenne ointment, applied topically, relieves pain.
- Turmeric helps protect your body from free radicals. Its active component is curcumin, a potent anti-inflammatory compound. Studies have shown that taking 400 mg of curcumin three times a day is as effective as taking the drug phenylbutazone, but without any side effects.
- White willow bark relieves inflammation and pain. Take 60–120 mg per day. Although its pain-relieving aspects are slower than aspirin, they last longer.

(*See* HERBAL REMEDIES in PART 2 Treatment Section for additional information.)

Homeopathic Remedies

You can self-treat with homeopathic remedies by selecting the one that most closely matches your symptoms. If you don't see improvement, try another, or a combination product. Follow the instructions on the label. If you do not have relief in a reasonable amount of time, consult a practitioner who specializes in homeopathic medicine.

- Arnica montana is useful when bursitis is caused by trauma and the area is sensitive to touch.
- Belladonna helps when the area is throbbing, inflammed, swollen, and sensitive to touch.
- Bryonia helps when pain worsens from motion, and heat aggravates the problem.
- Ferrum phosphoricum soothes pain, especially, in the right shoulder, and where the pain is relieved by cold applications.
- Kalmia latifolia relieves shoulder and hip pain that moves downward, and worsens at night and from motion.
- Rhus toxicodendron eases stiffness and pain that gets worse in cold damp weather, or while sleeping. It is also useful for those who find relief in hot applications or hot baths.
- Ruta graveolens is useful for bursitis that occurs from trauma, and for acute bursitis accompanied by swelling, stiffness, and severe pain.
- Sanguinaria helps shoulder pain (especially right shoulder pain) that extends down the arm when the shoulder is moved.
- Sulphur helps bursitis on the left side of the body that is accompanied by inflammation and burning pain.

(*See* HOMEOPATHY in PART 2 Treatment Section for additional information.)

Hydrotherapy

Use ice packs for twenty-minute periods as long as the area is inflamed. Then, after the inflammation has gone, when the joint no longer feels warm or appears red, use moist heat for twenty-minute periods. Cold damp weather can add to the discomfort of bursitis and hot applications or hot baths can bring relief, but always wait until the inflammation has gone before using heat. (*See* HYDROTHERAPY in PART 2 Treatment Section for additional information.)

Magnet Therapy

Magnet therapy relieves pain, accelerates healing, and reduces inflammation. Placing magnets on and around the painful bursa brings increased amounts of blood to the area which, in turn, brings oxygen and other healing substances to reduce the pain. (*See* MAGNET THERAPY in PART 2 Treatment Section for additional information.)

Meditation

Meditation helps reduce stress and increases production of your body's natural painkillers. (*See* MEDITATION in PART 2 Treatment Section for additional information.)

Supplements

Vitamin B_{12} or a combination of B_{12} and B_3 (niacin) injected intramuscularly have been shown to relieve bursitis symptoms and also decrease calcifications in the bursae that are chronically inflamed. Oral supplementation of these vitamins does not have the same effect. Consult a nutritionally oriented doctor for these injections. (*See* SUPPLEMENT THERAPY in PART 2 Treatment Section for additional information.)

ASSISTED ALTERNATIVE TREATMENTS

The following techniques may require specialized training or the aid of a healthcare professional.

Acupuncture and Acupressure

Acupuncture and acupressure create a smooth flow of vibratory energy throughout the body that can help alleviate the symptoms of bursitis. (*See* ACUPUNCTURE and ACUPRESSURE in PART 2 Treatment Section for additional information.)

Applied Kinesiology

Applied kinesiology is excellent for reducing pain rapidly, including the pain of bursitis. The AK practitioner tests your muscles to determine the origin of your problem and then decides on the best course of action, choosing from a wide variety of therapeutic methods at her or his disposal. (*See* APPLIED KINESIOLOGY in PART 2 Treatment Section for additional information.)

Bee Venom Therapy

Some components of bee venom are thought to stimulate the immune system. Other components are thought to modify the transmission of pain signals within the nervous system, and the therapy has proven consistently useful for painful conditions. (*See* BEE VENOM THERAPY in PART 2 Treatment Section for additional information.)

Compresses, Packs, and Poultices

Soak a cloth or towel in cold water, warm herbal tea, or the appropriate aromatherapy oils (diluted). Apply the soaked cloth to the affected area, cover with a towel to retain the heat or the cold, and leave in place for twenty to thirty minutes. (*See* COMPRESSES, PACKS, and POULTICES in PART 2 Treatment Section for additional information.)

Exercise

Exercise is important for the prevention of bursitis because, when you strengthen your muscles, it helps to protect the joint. But, if you already have the condition, you should not start an exercise program until the pain and inflammation have gone from the area, and when you do start, it should be carefully supervised to avoid further injury. (*See* EXERCISE, STRETCHING, and SPORTS in PART 2 Treatment Section for additional information).

Guided Imagery and Visualization Techniques

Guided imagery can help manage the pain of bursitis. To alleviate the burning sensation, visualize a temperature guage set on high and gradually turn down the heat. (*See* GUIDED IMAGERY and VISUALIZATION in PART 2 Treatment Section for additional information.)

Massage

Massage increases blood flow throughout your body so that all tissues are oxygenated and nourished and the cells are helped to get rid of lactic acid buildup which is a contributing cause of pain. (*See* MASSAGE in PART 2 Treatment Section for additional information.)

Osteopathic Manipulation

The goal of osteopathic manipulation is to increase range of motion, decrease muscle tension, and improve blood circulation, all of which can be helpful for bursitis. (*See* OSTEOPATHIC MANIPULATION in PART 2 Treatment Section for additional information.)

Physical Therapy

Physical therapy helps correct and improve your body's natural healing mechanisms. It increases the range of motion in the joints and is one of the recommended modalities for bursitis. (*See* PHYSICAL THERAPY in PART 2 Treatment Section for additional information.)

Reflexology

Reflexology massage therapy performed on the specific part of the foot and/or hand that corresponds with the bursitis area can be helpful. (*See* REFLEXOLOGY in PART 2 Treatment Section for additional information.)

Rolfing

Rolfing is very useful for treating impaired mobility and sports injuries, and has long-lasting effects in easing pain, including the pain of bursitis. (*See* ROLFING in PART 2 Treatment Section for additional information.)

PRACTICAL SUGGESTIONS

Elevating the affected area will help reduce swelling. In order to be effective, the joint must be higher than your heart.

(*See also* OSTEOARTHRITIS in PART 1 Conditions Section.)

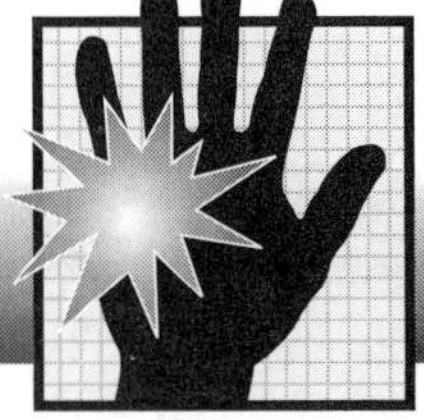

Carpal Tunnel Syndrome

Carpal tunnel syndrome is a painful affliction of the hand and wrist usually associated with repetitive stress injuries. Pain can be debilitating to the point where you cannot hold a pencil, brush your teeth, comb your hair, or hold a coffee cup.

Symptoms

The condition produces pain, burning, tingling, and weakness. The hands weaken and fall asleep, and, if left untreated, the nerves can eventually die, leading to atrophied muscles in the hand and fingers. The pain, described as burning or tingling, gets worse with motion and eases with rest.

Causes

Picture the wrist as a U-shaped cradle of bones, with the carpal ligament stretched across the open part of the U, forming the tunnel. Passing through this tunnel are the flexor tendons (they are attached to the fingers and enable the hand to close) and the median nerve in the wrist, which supplies nerve impulses to the mound at the base of the thumb and the next three fingers. The fifth, or pinky finger, is not affected because its nerve supply does not originate in the carpal tunnel. When the canal (the inside of the tunnel) becomes smaller, the nerve gets compressed, causing the problems in the hand. The most common cause of carpal tunnel syndrome is a flexion injury resulting from repeated wrist movements. Carpenters, computer operators, drummers, hairdressers, meat cutters, pianists, violinists, and people who knit and crochet are the most susceptible. Their repeated wrist movements cause irritation and swelling in the sheath of the flexor tendons, which can lead to fluid in the canal and cause pressure on the nerve. There are causes other than repetitive motion as well.

- ❏ Pregnancy can cause the canal to become smaller due to fluid retention, but this disappears after delivery in most cases.
- ❏ Rheumatoid arthritis causes the bones to thicken, leading to a narrowing of the canal.
- ❏ Tenosynovitis causes a chronic inflammation of the membranes around the tendon.
- ❏ Thyroid problems, diabetes, and injuries can lead to CTS, possibly because they can cause an increase of swelling in the tunnel, or interfere with circulation to the nerve.

Diagnosing the Problem

Carpal tunnel syndrome is suspected when pain is present in the thumb and next three fingers, but not in the pinky. It often occurs during the night, interrupting sleep. There are a number of tests for this condition.

- ❏ Electromyelegraphic studies test for hand-muscle strength, and they can detect abnormalities in the median nerve in the wrist.
- ❏ A nerve-conduction test determines the speed at which nerves carry a sensory message. If it is traveling slowly, that confirms a diagnosis of CTS.
- ❏ Phalen's test shows whether tingling occurs in at least one minute after arms and elbows are placed on the table in a flexed position while the wrists hang loosely over the edge.
- ❏ Tinel's sign is a test done to see if tingling in the fingers occurs when the doctor taps the skin over the median nerve in the wrist.
- ❏ X-rays can rule out arthritis and see if old fractures exist.

Conventional Treatments

The condition can be treated conservatively if diagnostic studies show no nerve injury is present. If there is no response to conservative treatment, surgery may have to be considered. The most frequently used treatments are:

- ❏ Anti-inflammatories;
- ❏ Cortisone injections;
- ❏ Ice;
- ❏ Night splint to keep the wrist straight while sleeping;
- ❏ Physical therapy;
- ❏ Reduction of repetitive hand motions;
- ❏ Surgery called carpal tunnel release opens the transverse carpal ligament, which releases pressure and allows more space in the tunnel for the median nerve;

  At one time, the surgical incision for CTT was made into the skin and muscle from the wrist through the entire length of the palm, and recovery took months. Fortunately, surgery is less complicated nowadays than it used to be. The newer procedure requires only a one-centimeter incision in the wrist. The ligament is cut with a special knife that resembles a seam ripper. Recovery is fast and patients can drive home.

Problems with Some Conventional Treatments

- ❑ Anti-inflammatories can cause gastrointestinal problems and bleeding.
- ❑ Casts and splints tend to weaken other areas of the wrist and hand.
- ❑ If your job requires repetitive hand motions, you may have to think about a career change.
- ❑ Surgery treats only the symptoms, but does not address the cause of carpal tunnel syndrome.

SELF-HELP ALTERNATIVE TREATMENTS

The following techniques can be done at home. Although they may not work as fast as drugs or surgery, natural alternatives help the body heal itself. They get at the root of the problem instead of just temporarily alleviating the symptoms. All herbs, homeopathic remedies, packs, and supplements discussed here are available in health food stores and, increasingly, in large drug and grocery stores, as well as on the Internet.

Compresses, Packs, and Poultices

Soak a cloth or towel in cold water, warm herbal tea, or the appropriate aromatherapy oils (diluted). Apply the soaked cloth to the affected area, cover with a towel to retain the heat or the cold, and leave in place for twenty to thirty minutes. (*See* COMPRESSES, PACKS, and POULTICES in PART 2 Treatment Section for additional information.)

Diet

Carpal tunnel syndrome is inflammatory in nature so certain dietary modifications may be helpful.

Good Foods

Eat foods that contain B-vitamins such as complex carbohydrates, fruits, nuts, seeds, vegetables, and whole grains. (*See* NUTRITIONAL THERAPY in PART 2 Treatment Section for additional information.)

Bad Foods

Alcohol, fast food, processed meats, saturated fats, simple sugars, and spicy foods can all trigger an inflammatory reaction in your body.

Exercise

If your job requires repetitive hand motions, do some warm-up exercises specifically for your hands. If you were a runner, you wouldn't do a marathon without warming up, would you?

- ❑ Squeeze a sponge ball for four or five minutes before starting work.
- ❑ Make a fist and bend your wrist down for five seconds. Repeat ten times.
- ❑ When you are finished exercising, shake your hands and wrists for a few seconds. Do this also at work periodically.

(*See* EXERCISE, STRETCHING, and SPORTS in PART 2 Treatment Section for additional information.)

Herbal Remedies

- ❑ Coltsfoot and comfrey, used externally in soaks or poultices, reduce fluid retention. (Note: Comfrey taken internally has the potential to cause liver damage and should be used only under supervision.)
- ❑ Hydrangea acts like cortisone.
- ❑ Watercress reduces fluid retention.
- ❑ Yucca is a precursor to cortisone. It enables your adrenal glands to produce and release their own cortisone into your system.

Take the above herbs as directed on label. They can also be used in teas and infusions. (*See* HERBAL REMEDIES in PART 2 Treatment Section for additional information.)

Homeopathic Remedies

You can self-treat with homeopathic remedies by selecting the one that most closely matches your symptoms. If you don't see improvement, try another, or a combination product. Follow the instructions on the label. If you do not have relief in a reasonable amount of time, consult a physician who specializes in homeopathic medicine.

- ❑ Arnica soothes inflammation. It is also available in cream and ointment form for external application.
- ❑ Calcarea phosphorica eases pain and stiffness.
- ❑ Causticum helps those who have had the condition for a long time.
- ❑ Hypericum eases nerve pain.
- ❑ Rhus toxicodendron is useful for stiffness and pain that eases with motion.
- ❑ Ruta graveolens helps ease stiffness and weakness.

Take the above remedies as indicated on label. Combination remedies sometimes work more effectively than single ones. (*See* HOMEOPATHY in PART 2 Treatment Section for additional information.)

Hydrotherapy

Use ice packs for twenty-minutes at a time as long as the area is inflamed. After the inflammation has gone, when the joint no longer feels warm or appears red, then use moist heat for twenty-minute periods. Always wait until the inflammation has gone before using heat. Running hot water over the painful spots while in the shower can alleviate the pain. (*See* HYDROTHERAPY in PART 2 Treatment Section for additional information.)

Supplements

- ❏ Bromelain acts as an anti-inflammatory. Take 500 mg twice daily on an empty stomach.
- ❏ Magnesium citrate, 500 mg three times daily, acts as a muscle antispasmodic.
- ❏ Vitamin B_6 aids the normal function of nerve cells and helps reduce swelling because it has a natural ability to eliminate water retention. Dr. Edward M. Wagner, ND, recommends 200 mg three times a day. He says it is more effective to use the pyrodoxal #5 phosphate form of B_6 which has a higher assimilation rate than plain pyrodoxine.
- ❏ Vitamin B_{12}, sublingual, helps prevent nerve damage. Take 500 mcg twice daily. Note: For balance when taking individual Bs, be sure to supplement with a B-complex once daily, or a multivitamin containing B-complex.
- ❏ Vitamin C (Ester-C), 1000 mg three times daily, is a general overall antioxidant.

(*See* SUPPLEMENT THERAPY in PART 2 Treatment Section for additional information.)

FAST-ACTING MINERAL SUPPLEMENT

SierraSil, dubbed "nature's ultimate mineral," is a recently formulated supplement blending more than sixty-five naturally occurring minerals in order to alleviate the pain, stiffness, and inflammation of arthritis and related conditions. One of its advocates is Ken Venturi, the former US Open golf champion, who had been forced into early retirement at the age of thirty-nine due to severe carpal tunnel syndrome. Since using SierraSil, Ken reports he has been able to successfully return to playing golf with no discomfort in his hands.

A double-blind, randomized, placebo-controlled study involving 120 patients, all age twenty or older, and all diagnosed with osteoarthritis of the knee, is currently evaluating the efficacy of SierraSil alone and SierraSil combined with vincaria, an extract of cat's claw. In both human and animal clinical tests, SierraSil has been found completely safe. It can be purchased in health food stores, or by calling 1-888-888-1464, or going to the website: *www.sierrasil.com.*

Additional Self-Help Treatments

For information on these therapies, refer to individual entries in PART 2 Treatment Section.

- ❏ Heat Therapy/Cold Therapy.
- ❏ Magnet Therapy.

ASSISTED ALTERNATIVE TREATMENTS

The following techniques may require specialized training or the aid of a healthcare professional.

Acupuncture and Acupressure

Acupuncture and acupressure create a smooth flow of vibratory energy throughout the body that can help alleviate the symptoms of carpal tunnel syndrome. (*See* ACUPUNCTURE and ACUPRESSURE in PART 2 Treatment Section for additional information.)

Applied Kinesiology

Applied Kinesiology is excellent for reducing pain rapidly. The AK practitioner tests your muscles to determine the origin of your problem and then decides on the best course of action, choosing from a wide variety of therapeutic methods at his or her disposal. (*See* APPLIED KINESIOLOGY in PART 2 Treatment Section for additional information.)

Chiropractic

By adjusting misaligned vertebrae (subluxations), the nervous system can function at its optimum level which enhances healing. (*See* CHIROPRACTIC in PART 2 Treatment Section for additional information.)

Reflexology

Reflexology helps your body heal itself by eliminating energy blockages, improving circulation, and relieving stress and tension. (*See* REFLEXOLOGY in PART 2 Treatment Section for additional information.)

Tai Chi, Qigong, and Yoga

These therapies help you relax and direct healing energy where it is needed in your hands and feet. (*See* TAI CHI, QIGONG, and YOGA in PART 2 Treatment Section for additional information.)

Additional Assisted Treatments

For information on these therapies, refer to individual entries in PART 2 Treatment Section.

- ❑ Guided Imagery and Visualizations.
- ❑ Massage.
- ❑ Osteopathic Manipulation.
- ❑ Physical Therapy.
- ❑ Rolfing.

PRACTICAL SUGGESTIONS

- ❑ Adjust your work area so you avoid using your wrist in a bent position. Just use your fingers to strike the keys.
- ❑ If you work at a computer, keep your palms up off the keyboard. You might want to investigate keyboards that have been ergonomically designed to help with CTS.
- ❑ Try changing the height of your desk or chair.
- ❑ Support your elbows on the armrest of your chair.

Problem for One Leads to Solution for Many

Julie got carpal tunnel syndrome in her left hand from the repetitive nature of the massages she gave and was forced to close her practice. It was one thing to be out of work, she said, but quite another when her problem almost caused her to drop her infant granddaughter—that's when she knew she needed to do something serious, so she experimented on herself until she came up with a therapy that worked. It involved finding and fixing the spasms in all the muscles that, in the case of CTS, interact with the median nerve which originates in the neck, goes across the front of the shoulder, down the inside of the arm, through the carpal tunnel, and into the hands.

Julie, who refers to herself as a deep-tissue muscular therapist, and who co-authors books and works with an MD, has since helped hundreds of people, including Earl. Paralyzed with a stroke on his left side, Earl relied on his good right side for all movements, and the constant pressure of putting the weight of his right hand onto his cane (without which he was completely chairbound) caused his right wrist to develop very painful CTS. One treatment by Julie gave him immediate relief and taught him how to self-treat daily to maintain his pain-free status. Monique was another success story. A carriage driver in New York's Central Park, she had CTS and ulna entrapment in both hands, which made her wrists hurt and her hands numb, thereby threatening her ability to continue with the livelihood she enjoyed. Monique found her way to Julie, but treatment for her took a little longer. There was one visit to teach her what to do, then one month of self-treating daily to get rid of the pain and reverse the whole situation. All three of these people now go about their lives pain-free, as do the many others who have been helped at Julie's center.

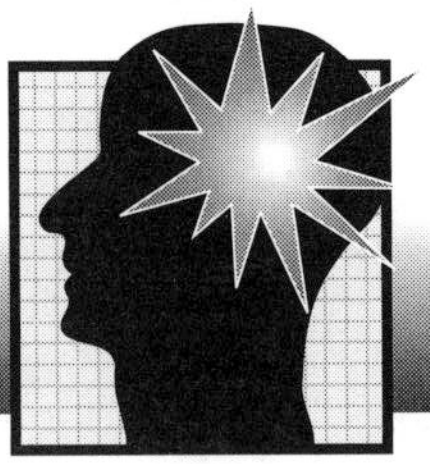

Cluster Headaches

All headaches, including cluster headaches, are symptoms of underlying conditions, not diseases in themselves, and all are almost universal. Each year, more than forty million Americans seek treatment for relief of their headache pain. If you have a headache accompanied by breathing problems, fever, or a stiff neck, or if it occurs after a head injury or respiratory infection, you should seek medical help immediately because it could be a symptom of a life-threatening condition. Medical help should also be sought if you have headaches that: occur daily; do not respond to simple pain relievers; become progressively worse; are caused by exertion from coughing, sneezing or exercise; or are accompanied by numbness, loss of consciousness, or hallucinations.

Symptoms

Cluster headache pain is usually in the area of one eye. It can be severe and has been described as vise-like. These headaches usually begin with an agonizing sensation of pain that is often described as burning or piercing. Some say it feels like a hot poker is stuck in the eye. The pain occurs in groups or clusters, most frequently in the spring and fall. It may be there every day for weeks or months, then disappear for several months, but for an approximate 20 percent, it's an everyday occurrence that doesn't recede, and makes them scream or pound their heads against a wall.

The Silent Epidemic

According to the director of the Jefferson Headache Center in Philadelphia, PA, Dr. Stephen Silberstein, rebound headaches are becoming a silent epidemic, and as many as half the chronic daily headache patients he sees developed their problem from overuse of headache medications. Referring to one patient who came to him in desperate pain from headaches that had shriveled her life down to a near-hermetic existence, he said the probable cause of her pain was her headache medicine. It had interfered with her body's own natural pain-control system, thereby causing her headaches to come back as soon as the medicine's effects wore off. Subsequent withdrawal from the medications did, in fact, help her return to a more normal life.

People with cluster headaches often have accompanying nasal congestion, a runny nose, or a flushed face, and the eye on the side where the pain is located may tear and droop. The attacks generally last about forty-five minutes until the pain subsides, only to return again in several hours. Cluster headaches affect about one million Americans, 90 percent of whom are men, with the onset usually between the ages of twenty and forty-five.

Common Causes

Cluster headaches may result from overactive nerve endings inside the dilated blood vessels. There are many more factors which can trigger a headache. Some of the most common are:

- ❑ Air pollution;
- ❑ Alcohol consumption;
- ❑ Bruxism (grinding of teeth);
- ❑ Change in altitude;
- ❑ Clenching the jaw;
- ❑ Constipation;
- ❑ Dehydration;
- ❑ Eye problems, or improper eyeglass prescriptions;
- ❑ Glare from fluorescent lights;
- ❑ Hormonal changes;
- ❑ Imbalance in brain chemicals and nerve pathways;
- ❑ Insomnia or too much sleep;
- ❑ Low barometric pressure;
- ❑ Low levels of fresh air, as found in airplane cabins or poorly ventilated buildings;
- ❑ Low serotonin levels;
- ❑ Narrowing of the blood vessels going into the brain, muscles, and tissues of the neck and scalp;
- ❑ Overexposure to sun;
- ❑ Side effects of prescribed medications, including hormone replacement therapy, nitroglycerin (taken for angina), and some asthma drugs;
- ❑ Smoking and second-hand tobacco smoke;
- ❑ Stress;
- ❑ Tension;
- ❑ TMJ misalignment;

- ❑ Video display terminals and television screens.

Diagnosing the Problem

Before any treatment can begin, a proper diagnosis is essential in order to rule out the possibility of brain tumors, intracranial pressure changes, or meningeal inflammation, an inflammation of the membranes surrounding the brain and spinal cord. Once a potentially serious condition has been ruled out, a cluster headache can be determined by the symptoms described above.

Conventional Treatments

Some medications prevent the onset of headaches, others relieve them after they've begun. These are the most frequently used medications.

- ❑ Analgesics (painkillers). These reduce or relieve pain without addressing its cause.
- ❑ Antidepressants. They help soothe the tension contributing to headaches.
- ❑ Anti-inflammatory drugs. They reduce the inflammation that contributes to the pain.
- ❑ Beta blockers and calcium channel blockers. They stabilize blood vessels.
- ❑ Cafergot (ergotamine). This works as abortive treatment to prevent the full onset of cluster headaches.
- ❑ Histamine infusions. They are thought by some professionals to stop the pain of cluster headaches. Others prescribe antihistamines for them.
- ❑ Imitrex (Sumatriptan). This intensifies the activity of serotonin receptors in the brain and can relieve a cluster headache that has already become severe.
- ❑ Oxygen. Breathing in pure oxygen helps the blood get rid of toxic material that arteries are producing, and this helps them constrict and dilate in a normal fashion which helps ward off cluster headaches. (*See also* OXYGEN THERAPIES in PART 2 Treatment Section.)

Problems with Some Conventional Treatments

- ❑ At first, caffeine constricts blood vessels, easing pain, but when it wears off, rebound swelling occurs, and that can ultimately worsen the pain.
- ❑ Overuse of analgesics can be counterproductive by causing the blood vessels to become less sensitive to the medication. When this happens, higher doses are needed, setting up a vicious cycle.
- ❑ Over-the-counter analgesics (painkillers), even used as infrequently as five times a week, can turn periodic headaches into chronic rebound headaches.
- ❑ Long-term use of nonsteroidal anti-inflammatory drugs (NSAIDs) may cause kidney, liver, or stomach problems.
- ❑ Histamine infusions have to be administered in a hospital and can require a twelve-day stay.
- ❑ Methysergide may lead to fibroid growth in the kidneys. It can also cause permanent scar tissue around the heart and lungs. Anyone using this drug must be closely supervised.
- ❑ Vasoconstrictors constrict all other arteries in the body. If, for example, a heart problem is present, vasoconstrictors could ultimately make things worse.

SELF-HELP ALTERNATIVE TREATMENTS

The following techniques for alleviating cluster headaches can be done at home. Although they may not work as fast as drugs or surgery, natural alternatives help the body heal itself. All herbs, homeopathic remedies, packs, and supplements discussed here are available in health food stores and, increasingly, in large drug and grocery stores, as well as on the Internet.

Aromatherapy

Aromatherapy is useful for headaches, particularly the essential oils of basil, cajeput, eucalyptus, lavender, niaouli, peppermint, and rosemary. They are available in health food stores and stores specializing in aromatherapy products listed in the yellow pages. (*See* AROMATHERAPY in PART 2 Treatment Section for additional information.)

Compresses, Packs, and Poultices

Alternate hot and cold compresses. Use heat for three minutes and cold for one minute and keep switching for about fifteen minutes. Castor oil packs have also been recommended for cluster headaches. Soak a piece of white flannel in warm castor oil, wring it out and place it over the area of the cluster headache. Cover with plastic and apply a heating pad. Do this twice a day for an hour each time.(*See* COMPRESSES, PACKS, and POULTICES, HEAT THERAPY/COLD THERAPY, and HYDROTHERAPY in PART 2 Treatment Section for additional information.)

Diet

Knowing which foods to eat and which to avoid can help ameliorate or even ward off cluster headaches.

Good Foods

- ❑ Caffeinated beverages taken in small amounts raise serotonin levels and help constrict dilated blood vessels, but sometimes, when caffeine wears off, a rebound effect occurs, causing swelling of the blood vessels. Do not overdo the caffeine. If a small amount helps, more will not necessarily be better.

(*See* NUTRITIONAL THERAPY in PART 2 Treatment Section for additional information.)

Bad Foods

The following list of substances can bring on, or worsen, a headache.

- ❑ Aged cheese.
- ❑ Alcohol.
- ❑ Aspartame—an artificial sweetener.
- ❑ Avocados.
- ❑ Bananas.
- ❑ Chicken livers.
- ❑ Chocolate.
- ❑ Cured meats.
- ❑ Fermented foods, such as sour cream and yogurt.
- ❑ Herring.
- ❑ Hot dogs.
- ❑ Monosodium glutamate (MSG).
- ❑ Nuts.
- ❑ Onions.
- ❑ Red wine.
- ❑ Salami.
- ❑ Vinegar.
- ❑ Wheat.

Other Substances to Avoid

Aftershave lotion, molds, perfume, and tobacco can all bring on headaches.

Herbal Remedies

- ❑ Burdock root helps purify the blood.
- ❑ Cayenne aids circulation.
- ❑ Feverfew makes your body less responsive to the chemicals that cause spasms in the muscles surrounding your brain.
- ❑ Goldenseal has anti-inflammatory properties.
- ❑ Lobelia is a relaxant.
- ❑ Mint helps relieve nausea.
- ❑ Peppermint helps oxygenate the bloodstream.
- ❑ White willow bark has an effect similar to aspirin.

Take according to label instructions. (*See* HERBAL REMEDIES in PART 2 Treatment Section for additional information.)

Homeopathic Remedies

You can self-treat with homeopathic remedies by selecting the one that most closely matches your symptoms. If you don't see improvement, try another, or a combination product. Follow the instructions on the label. If you do not have relief in a reasonable amount of time, consult a physician who specializes in homeopathic medicine.

- ❑ Belladonna relieves headaches that start at the back of the head or upper neck.
- ❑ Bryonia helps relieve splitting headaches that settle over one eye.
- ❑ Cimicifuga relieves headaches with throbbing pain that worsens with motion.
- ❑ Ignatia helps headaches caused by emotional upsets or grief.
- ❑ Spigelia relieves left-sided throbbing headaches accompanied by pain above or through the eyeball.

Instructions for use are usually printed on the label. (*See* HOMEOPATHY in PART 2 Treatment Section for additional information.)

Magnet Therapy

Magnet therapy can help relieve head pain. Placing magnets on the area of the head that is in pain brings increased amounts of blood to the area which, in turn brings oxygen and other healing substances to ease the pain. (*See* MAGNET THERAPY in PART 2 Treatment Section for additional information.)

Meditation

Meditation helps reduce stress, which contributes to head pain. (*See* MEDITATION in PART 2 Treatment Section for additional information.)

Supplements

- ❑ Calcium. Take 1500 mg daily to help transmission of nerve impulses.

- ❑ Fish Oil. Take 1 gram per pound of body weight. Fish oil modifies prostaglandins, hormone-like substances made by the body that may cause headaches.
- ❑ 5-HTP. This amino acid helps raise serotonin levels, and people with headaches often have low serotonin levels. Take per instructions on label.
- ❑ Magnesium. 400 mg three times daily helps relieve pain.
- ❑ Potassium. 100 mg daily aids in proper sodium and potassium balance, necessary to avoid fluid retention, which may put pressure on the brain.
- ❑ SAMe (S-adenosyl-L-methionine) is a mood stabilizer and helps regenerate nerves. Take per instructions on label.
- ❑ Vitamin B-complex. 50 mg taken twice daily relieves stress.
- ❑ Vitamin E. 400 IU taken twice a day aids circulation.

(*See* SUPPLEMENT THERAPY in PART 2 Treatment Section for additional information.)

ASSISTED ALTERNATIVE TREATMENTS

The following techniques may require specialized training or the aid of a healthcare professional.

Acupuncture and Acupressure

Acupuncture and acupressure create a smooth flow of vibratory energy throughout the body. Practitioners aim to move the energy away from the head. For self-treatment, knead the area between your thumb and index finger. (*See* ACUPUNCTURE and ACUPRESSURE in PART 2 Treatment Section for additional information.)

Applied Kinesiology

Applied Kinesiology can help reduce headache pain. The AK practitioner tests your muscles to determine the origin of your problem and then decides on the best course of action, choosing from a wide variety of therapeutic methods at her or his disposal. (*See* APPLIED KINESIOLOGY in PART 2 Treatment Section for additional information.)

Biofeedback

Biofeedback works by reducing stress and the physical responses, such as a headache, associated with it. (*See* BIOFEEDBACK in PART 2 Treatment Section for additional information.)

Chiropractic

Poor vertebral alignment, often the result of wearing high heels or having flat feet, may reduce blood flow to the brain, which can cause headaches. Chiropractic manipulation can help correct this situation. (*See* CHIROPRACTIC in PART 2 Treatment Section for additional information.)

Craniosacral Therapy

Cluster headaches caused by pressure of cranial fluid can be eased by gently manipulating the cranial bones. (*See* CRANIOSACRAL THERAPY in PART 2 Treatment Section for additional information.)

Cupping

Cupping can ease cluster headaches that are caused by a lack of oxygen in the cells. It helps promote energy flow and reduces swelling and pain. (*See* CUPPING in PART 2 Treatment Section for additional information.)

Exercise

Aerobic activity, which needs to be supervised at first to avoid further damage, reduces stress and increases the production of endorphins. This helps to raise the pain threshold. (*See* EXERCISE, STRETCHING, and SPORTS in PART 2 Treatment Section for additional information.)

Guided Imagery and Visualization Techniques

Guided imagery can help manage the pain of cluster headaches. Since most cluster headaches are described as vise-like, or as a feeling of tightness, picture a tool that can loosen the vise. (*See* GUIDED IMAGERY and VISUALIZATION in PART 2 Treatment Section for additional information.)

Hypnosis

Hypnosis helps you relax, and relaxation alleviates stress, which contributes to headache pain. (*See* HYPNOSIS in PART 2 Treatment Section for additional information.)

Massage

A massage can help your body relax, thereby reducing head pain caused by stress. There are many kinds of massage therapies available and you can ask your practitioner to suggest the appropriate one for your cluster headache. Many conventional doctors are now extolling the benefits of massage. (*See* MASSAGE in PART 2 Treatment Section for additional information.)

Osteopathic Manipulation

Osteopathic manipulation can help decrease muscle tension, which is a contributing factor to many types of headaches. (*See* OSTEOPATHIC MANIPULATION in PART 2 Treatment Section for additional information.)

Oxygen Therapy

Oxygen therapy, also listed in conventional therapies in this entry (which underscores its dual role as a therapy), is a useful adjunct for treating cluster headaches. (*See* OXYGEN THERAPIES in PART 2 Treatment Section for additional information.)

Physical Therapy

Physical therapy helps correct and improve your body's natural healing mechanisms and can help prevent the return of symptoms. (*See* PHYSICAL THERAPY in PART 2 Treatment Section for additional information.)

Reflexology

Reflexology massage therapy performed on the specific part of the foot and/or hand that corresponds with the head can be helpful. (*See* REFLEXOLOGY in PART 2 Treatment Section for additional information.)

Tai Chi, Qigong, and Yoga

These therapies induce a profoundly relaxed state and help bring healing energy to the body. Relaxation techniques and concentrating on your breathing can relieve tension. One technique is to take six deep breaths, counting to four as you inhale and as you exhale. (*See* TAI CHI, QIGONG, and YOGA in PART 2 Treatment Section for additional information.)

PASS THE OXYGEN

On the morning show, *Good Morning America*, Dr. Nancy Snyderman told millions of listeners that pure oxygen is the most popular treatment for stopping headaches, and that it is safer than other treatments, which can have powerful side effects. One guest who had frequent cluster headaches told her that he keeps oxygen tanks in his house and his car, sometimes stopping by the side of the road to take a hit so he can keep working.

PRACTICAL SUGGESTIONS

- ❏ Capsaicin ointment rubbed on your nose can relieve cluster headaches.
- ❏ Stay hydrated. Drink eight to ten glasses of water a day, and if your indoor air is dry, use a humidifier.
- ❏ Improve the quality of your indoor air. A negative ion generator or HEPA filter will remove unhealthy particles. If you live in an unpolluted area, open your windows at least fifteen minutes a day. Houseplants also filter indoor pollution from the air.
- ❏ Use incandescent bulbs rather than fluorescent light tubes. The flickering in the latter may not be noticeable, but it can be enough to bring on a headache.

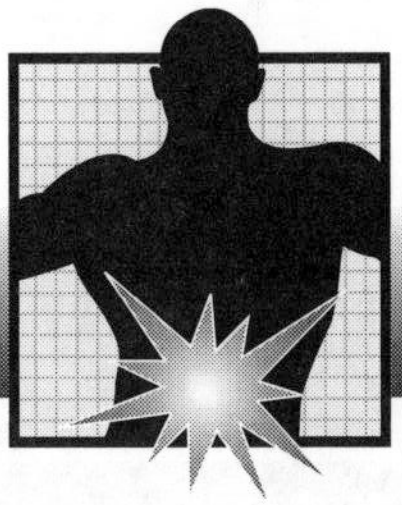

Crohn's Disease (Inflammatory Bowel Disease)

Inflammatory bowel diseases (IBD) are disorders in which the bowel becomes inflamed, resulting in cramps and diarrhea. The IBD known as Crohn's disease is named for Burrill Crohn, MD, a physician who wrote a paper in 1932 describing the condition. It is a chronic inflammation of the intestinal wall that usually occurs in the ileum (the lowest part of the small intestine) and in the large intestine. Sometimes referred to as ileitis when it is in the small intestine, it affects all layers of the intestinal wall. It is occasionally seen in other parts of the digestive tract, which extends from the mouth to the anus, and can also occur in the skin around the anus. Normal areas may be present between the affected places. Crohn's can occur in both sexes equally, and the condition can first appear anywhere between the relatively early age of fourteen and thirty years of age. It is most prevalent among Jewish people, is least seen among blacks and Asians, and tends to run in families. During flare-ups, inflammation may also occur elsewhere in the body, particularly in the joints, mouth, skin, and whites of the eyes.

Symptoms

Attacks of Crohn's disease come on quickly and can include:

- ❑ Abdominal cramps;
- ❑ Diarrhea;
- ❑ Fever;
- ❑ Pain and tenderness, especially in the right lower abdomen (the condition may be misdiagnosed as appendicitis due to pain occurring in the same area);
- ❑ Recurring intestinal obstructions;
- ❑ Weight loss due to loss of appetite.

Note: Children with Crohn's disease may not exhibit abdominal symptoms. If they have anemia, a persistent fever, joint inflammation, or slow growth patterns, Crohn's disease should be suspected.

Common Causes

It is not known why symptoms of Crohn's come and go, or what initiates new episodes. Although no definitive cause has yet been isolated, possibilities include diet, a poorly functioning immune system, or an infection.

Diagnosing the Problem

A physician may suspect Crohn's disease in anyone who complains of abdominal cramps and diarrhea accompanied by eye, joint, and skin inflammation. Blood tests do not specifically identify the condition, but may show anemia, a high white-cell count, and low albumin levels, which are indicative of inflammation. There are several diagnostic tests that can be performed. A barium enema study of the large intestine can show the characteristic appearance of Crohn's disease. And, a colonoscopy with a biopsy can be performed. Here, a flexible tube is passed through the large intestine and pieces of tissue are removed by a pathologist for tests to show whether or not Crohn's is present.

Conventional Treatments

- ❑ Azathioprine and mercaptopurine modify the action of the immune system, heal fistulas, and decrease the need for corticosteroids.
- ❑ Codeine relieves cramps and diarrhea.
- ❑ Corticosteroids reduce fever and diarrhea and relieve pain and tenderness.
- ❑ Deodorized opium tincture controls diarrhea.
- ❑ Diphenoxylate relieves cramps and diarrhea.
- ❑ Loperamide also relieves cramps and diarrhea.
- ❑ Metronidazole (a broad-spectrum antibiotic) relieves symptoms, especially those that lead to abscesses and fistulas.
- ❑ Methyl cellulose helps make stools firmer.
- ❑ Psyllium preparations help make stools firmer.
- ❑ Sulfasalazine suppresses mild inflammation,
- ❑ Surgery can be performed, in extreme cases, to remove diseased sections of the intestine.

Problems with Some Conventional Treatments

- ❑ Azathioprine and mercaptopurine take three to six months to be effective and can lead to allergic reactions, pancreatitis (inflammation of the pancreas), and a low white blood-cell count.
- ❑ Corticosteroids have side effects, such as fluid retention, a puffy face, bone loss, eye problems (glaucoma

and cataracts), elevated blood pressure, and a lowered resistance to infections. Corticosteroids given to children for prolonged periods of time can suppress their growth.

- ❑ Metronidazole can cause nerve damage that results in pins-and-needles sensations in the extremities. Discontinuing the drug relieves its side effects, but once discontinued, a relapse of the Crohn's disease usually occurs.
- ❑ Psyllium should not be taken within thirty to forty-five minutes of taking supplements as it can interfere with their absorption.
- ❑ Sulfasalazine is not effective for severe flare-ups. Some who take this drug may be allergic to it and can experience difficulty breathing, or hives, rashes, and swelling of the tissues in the area around the eyes.
- ❑ Surgery relieves symptoms temporarily, but does not cure Crohn's disease. About half the people who undergo surgery need a second operation because the area where the intestine was rejoined tends to become inflamed again.

SELF-HELP ALTERNATIVE TREATMENTS

Many medications for bowel problems have undesirable side effects so you may want to try the following alternative techniques, which can be done at home, to promote wellness. All herbs, homeopathic remedies, packs, and supplements discussed here are available in health food stores and, increasingly, in large drug and grocery stores, as well as on the Internet.

Aromatherapy

Aromatherapy is particularly useful for relieving symptoms related to the digestive system. To relieve constipation, black pepper, cardamom, cinnamon leaf, citronella, ginger, and peppermint oils have a stimulating effect. Mix two or three drops of these oils with a carrier oil, such as sweet almond oil, and use to massage the abdomen in a clockwise direction. You can also add up to ten drops of these oils to your bath water, or soak a piece of flannel in hot water containing four or five drops of oil and apply it as a compress.

For control of diarrhea, chamomile, cinnamon, clove, geranium, ginger, lavender, nutmeg, tea tree oils, and thyme are beneficial. Use as above.

Do not ingest essential oils or use them full strength as they are very powerful compounds. They are available in health food stores and stores specializing in aromatherapy products which you can find in the yellow pages. (*See* AROMATHERAPY in PART 2 Treatment Section for additional information.)

Castor Oil Packs

Dip a piece of white flannel into some warm castor oil. Wring it out and place it over the affected area of the intestines. Cover with plastic and apply a heating pad for one hour. Do this twice daily. (*See* COMPRESSES, PACKS, and POULTICES in PART 2 Treatment Section for additional information.) (*See also* AROMATHERAPY in this entry.)

Diet

If you have any kind of bowel problem, you may have food intolerances. These are not true allergies caused by an immune system response, but are metabolic in nature and can best be evaluated by an elimination diet whereby suspected foods are avoided and then gradually reintroduced. This should be monitored by a qualified nutritionist.

Good Foods

According to the Crohn's and Colitis Foundation, eating to help the gut heal itself is a new concept in IBD treatment, and fish, especially white fish, and flaxseed oils can help fight the inflammation. To alleviate the painful symptoms of Crohn's, it is important to drink lots of pure water and vegetable juices, and eat fresh fruit. Also, be sure to eat fresh vegetables that are non-acidic, such as broccoli, Brussels sprouts, cabbage, carrots, celery, kale, spinach, and turnips. (*See* NUTRITIONAL THERAPY in PART 2 Treatment Section for additional information.)

Bad Foods

The following foods may exacerbate your condition.

- ❑ Chocolate.
- ❑ Dairy products.
- ❑ Meat and other animal products.
- ❑ Processed foods.
- ❑ Spicy foods.
- ❑ Wheat.

Other Substances to Avoid

Anyone who has a bowel disorder has a problem with alcohol, caffeine, carbonated beverages, and tobacco because they are irritating to the gastrointestinal tract. Additionally, all artificial sweeteners, especially aspartame, minnitol, and sorbitol, can cause diarrhea.

Herbal Remedies

- ❑ Echinacea has anti-inflammatory properties and stimulates the immune system.
- ❑ Garlic is a natural antibiotic and is useful for intestinal problems.
- ❑ Ginger relieves most digestive problems.
- ❑ Goldenseal helps cleanse mucous membranes and has anti-inflammatory and antibacterial properties.
- ❑ Pau d'arco aids healing.
- ❑ Rose hips help heal infections.
- ❑ Yerba maté helps relieve constipation and stimulates the body's natural cortisone production.

Take the above herbs as directed on label. They can also be used in teas and infusions. (*See* HERBAL REMEDIES in PART 2 Treatment Section for additional information.)

Homeopathic Remedies

You can self-treat with homeopathic remedies by selecting the one that most closely matches your symptoms. If you don't see improvement, try another, or a combination product. Follow the instructions on the label. If you do not have relief in a reasonable amount of time, consult a physician who specializes in homeopathic medicine.

The following homeopathic remedies are useful for Crohn's disease.

- ❑ Argentum nitricum eases bloating, flatulence, and diarrhea that occurs after drinking water.
- ❑ Bismuth relieves diarrhea.
- ❑ Bryonia relieves constipation.
- ❑ Carbo veg controls diarrhea alternating with constipation.
- ❑ Chamomilla relieves diarrhea.
- ❑ Colocynthis eases abdominal pain and cramping that eases by bending over or applying pressure.
- ❑ Dulcamara helps control diarrhea containing mucous.
- ❑ Hydrastis relieves constipation.
- ❑ Iris ver also relieves constipation.
- ❑ Kali sulph relieves diarrhea containing mucous.
- ❑ Lycopodium helps control bloating, constipation, gas, heartburn, and pain.
- ❑ Mag phos is an antispasmodic.
- ❑ Nat mur aids digestion.
- ❑ Nux vomica helps relieve gas, cramps, and muscular soreness in the abdomen.
- ❑ Podophyllum helps control diarrhea that alternates with constipation and is accompanied by weakness.
- ❑ Sulphur is useful for anyone with morning diarrhea and excessive gas.

Combination remedies sometimes work more effectively than single ones. (*See* HOMEOPATHY in PART 2 Treatment Section for additional information.)

Meditation

Meditation can help if the bowel problem is stress-related. (*See* MEDITATION in PART 2 Treatment Section for additional information.)

Supplements

The following help your body function better and make it more resistant to Crohn's disease.

- ❑ Acidophilus, per label, aids digestion.
- ❑ Aloe vera juice, 4 ounces three times daily, helps soften stools.
- ❑ Garlic capsules, per label, aid healing and help reduce free-radical formation.
- ❑ A high-quality multivitamin and mineral complex helps to avoid nutritional deficiencies.
- ❑ Protein supplements, per label, aid intestinal healing.

(*See* SUPPLEMENT THERAPY in PART 2 Treatment Section for additional information.

ASSISTED ALTERNATIVE TREATMENTS

The following techniques may require specialized training or the aid of a healthcare professional.

Acupuncture and Acupressure

Acupuncture involves the insertion of extremely thin solid needles into specific points of your body to stimulate its own healing mechanism and improve blood flow to the affected areas. It also reduces inflammation, relieves pain, improves mobility, and there are rarely any risks or side effects. (*See* ACUPUNCTURE and ACUPRESSURE in PART 2 Treatment Section for additional information.)

Applied Kinesiology

Applied kinesiology is a non-invasive, non-toxic method

that can correct imbalances in the body. It is excellent for reducing pain rapidly, including the pain of Crohn's disease. (*See* APPLIED KINESIOLOGY in PART 2 Treatment Section for additional information.)

Biofeedback

Biofeedback is useful for reducing stress in anyone with painful bowel problems. (*See* BIOFEEDBACK in PART 2 Treatment Section for additional information.)

Chiropractic

Chiropractic theory is based on the assumption that a properly aligned spine is essential for good health, and that any misalignment of the vertebrae in the spine causes pressure on the spinal nerves, leading to pain. The chiropractor makes spinal adjustments to move misaligned vertebrae to more normal positions which helps the nervous system to function properly. (*See* CHIROPRACTIC in PART 2 Treatment Section for additional information.)

Craniosacral Therapy

Craniosacral therapy is a form of energy healing that can help balance your system. It has been shown to be effective for soothing bowel problems. (*See* CRANIOSACRAL THERAPY in PART 2 Treatment Section for additional information.)

Cupping

Cupping helps to promote energy flow and reduce pain. (*See* CUPPING in PART 2 Treatment Section for additional information.)

Exercise and Stretching

Stretching exercises can help to improve digestion, but they must be carefully supervised to avoid further damage to the affected area. (*See* EXERCISE, STRETCHING, and SPORTS in PART 2 Treatment Section for additional information.)

Guided Imagery

Guided imagery helps relieve stress and manage pain. Visualizing your bowel area as relaxed can be useful to help relieve the stress associated with inflammatory bowel disease. (*See* GUIDED IMAGERY and VISUALIZATION in PART 2 Treatment Section for additional information.)

Hypnosis

Hypnosis is useful for reducing stress in those with Crohn's disease. (*See* HYPNOSIS in PART 2 Treatment Section for additional information.)

Massage

A massage helps bring blood to the affected area to relieve the pain. There are many kinds of massage therapies available and you can ask your practitioner to suggest the appropriate one for your problem. (*See* MASSAGE in PART 2 Treatment Section for additional information.) (*See also* AROMATHERAPY in this entry.)

Oxygen Therapy

Oxygen therapy helps enhance your body's ability to heal itself. Crohn's disease responds well to hyperbaric oxygen therapy (HBOT) and ultraviolet irradiation of blood (UVIB). (*See* OXYGEN THERAPIES in PART 2 Treatment Section for additional information.)

Reflexology

Reflexology massage therapy can be performed on the part of the foot or hand corresponding to the bowel area that is in pain due to Crohn's disease. (*See* REFLEXOLOGY in PART 2 Treatment Section for additional information.)

Tai Chi, Qigong, and Yoga

These therapies help your body to enter a relaxed state and also increase production of endorphins, which are natural painkillers. (*See* TAI CHI, QIGONG, and YOGA in PART 2 Treatment Section for additional information.)

PRACTICAL SUGGESTIONS

Do not wear tight clothing around your waist.

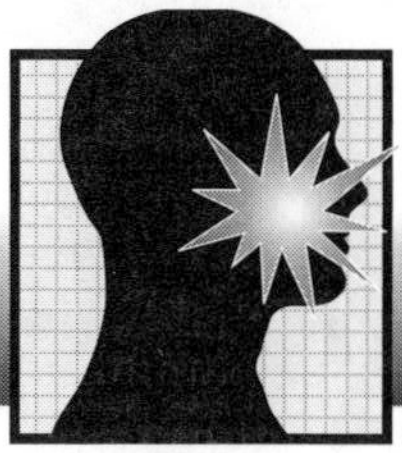

Dental Pain

Dental pain is often more bothersome at night when you are trying to sleep because more blood goes to your head when you lie down, and that causes pressure.

Symptoms

The primary symptoms of dental problems are: loose teeth; sensitivity to heat, cold, or sweets; small holes or brown spots on a tooth. If you have a fever, if your gums appear red or swollen, or if your face is swollen, you may have a serious infection and should seek medical attention promptly. And, even more critical, if the pain is accompanied by sweating or chest discomfort below your breast bone, or if it travels to your arm, get to an emergency room promptly because these symptoms could indicate a heart attack.

Common Causes

- ❑ Cracked teeth.
- ❑ Decayed teeth.
- ❑ Dental abscesses or infections.
- ❑ Gum infections.
- ❑ Lost fillings.

Diagnosing the Problem

Diagnosis is based on history and symptoms.

Conventional Treatments

The routine treatments for dental problems include antibiotics, extractions, fillings, and root canals.

Problems with Some Conventional Treatments

- ❑ Antibiotics have side effects, including gastrointestinal disturbances and yeast infections. Overuse of antibiotics leads to antibiotic-resistant strains of germs.
- ❑ If a tooth is extracted, after the area heals, it should be replaced in order to prevent malocclusion, which could lead to TMJ.
- ❑ When you have a cavity filled, insist that material other than a mercury alloy (amalgam) be used, since mercury has been shown to have toxic effects on the system.
- ❑ Root canals are painful and expensive and do not always prevent a future extraction.

SELF-HELP ALTERNATIVE TREATMENTS

The following techniques can all be done at home. Although they may not work as fast as drugs or surgery, natural alternatives help the body heal itself. They get at the root of the problem instead of just temporarily alleviating the symptoms. All herbs, homeopathic remedies, packs, and supplements discussed here are available in health food stores and, increasingly, in large drug and grocery stores, as well as on the Internet.

Aromatherapy

Aromatherapy, particularly the essential oils of cinnamon, fennel, peppermint, sage, spearmint, and thyme, are antibacterial and help to stimulate blood flow to the gums. They are available in health food stores and stores specializing in aromatherapy products which you can find in the yellow pages. (*See* AROMATHERAPY in PART 2 Treatment Section for additional information.)

Castor Oil Packs

Dip a piece of white flannel into some warm castor oil. Wring it out and place it over the affected mouth area. Cover with plastic and apply a heating pad for one hour. Do this twice daily. (*See* COMPRESSES, PACKS, and POULTICES in PART 2 Treatment Section for additional information.)

Diet

Dental pain is inflammatory in nature so certain dietary modifications may be helpful.

Good Foods

The following dietary modifications can be useful for maintaining good dental hygiene.

- ❑ Eat calcium-rich foods, such as cheese, low fat milk, and yogurt.
- ❑ Cheeses, such as cheddar consumed at the end of a meal, can help prevent dental decay.
- ❑ Fresh fruits and vegetables are high in vitamins and minerals. The act of chewing these foods rich in phytonutrients (plant nutrients) promotes healthy gums

by stimulating saliva flow, and the saliva helps to wash away food particles that can get lodged in the teeth and cause decay.

(*See* NUTRITIONAL THERAPY in PART 2 Treatment Section for additional information.)

Bad Foods

Avoid these foods because they can lead to cavities and exacerbate your pain.

- ❑ Candy and all other refined simple sugars. If you must have something sweet, eat chocolate rather than hard candy. It does not remain in contact with your teeth as long, and it contains tannins and cocoa which counteract its sugar content. Additionally, dark chocolate contains beneficial antioxidants. Look for an organic variety at a health food store.
- ❑ Dried fruits are high in sugar and cling to the teeth.
- ❑ Sodas.
- ❑ Spicy food.
- ❑ Sticky food because it can lodge between the teeth and lead to more sensitivity and pain.

Heat Therapy/Cold Therapy

Applying cold in the form of a cloth soaked in ice water, or rubbing the painful area of the mouth with an ice cube will help reduce swelling. Heat will increase blood flow to the area and aid healing after the swelling is gone. (*See* HEAT THERAPY/COLD THERAPY in PART 2 Treatment Section for additional information.)

Herbal Poultice

Chamomile used as a poultice reduces pain and swelling. (*See* COMPRESSES, PACKS, and POULTICES in PART 2 Treatment Section for additional information.)

Herbal Remedies

The following herbs help your body heal itself when you have gum or tooth problems.

- ❑ Aloe vera gel, applied topically, soothes inflamed gums.
- ❑ Anise is an anti-inflammatory.
- ❑ Bloodroot inhibits bacteria.
- ❑ Chamomile tea used as a mouthwash soothes inflamed gums.
- ❑ Clove oil, applied topically, helps stop toothache pain.
- ❑ Echinacea strengthens your immune system and aids healing. Take internally and use the diluted tincture as a mouthwash.
- ❑ Evening primrose oil, applied topically, relieves inflamed gums.
- ❑ Eucalyptus oil, applied topically, relieves inflamed gums.
- ❑ Hops (tincture), applied topically, helps stop toothache pain.
- ❑ Garlic is a natural antibiotic.
- ❑ Ginseng aids circulation and helps repair gum tissue.
- ❑ Goldenseal is an anti-inflammatory and antibacterial. Take internally and/or use as a mouthwash.
- ❑ Horsetail used as a mouthwash relieves gum infections.
- ❑ Kelp helps promote healthy gums.
- ❑ Myrrh is an anti-inflammatory.
- ❑ Peppermint oil put on a small piece of cotton, then placed in a cavity, helps ease a toothache.
- ❑ Plantain is an anti-inflammatory.
- ❑ Sage reduces gum inflammation (use as a mouthwash).
- ❑ Tea tree oil, applied topically, relieves sore gums. It can also be diluted and used as a mouthwash.
- ❑ Usnea has antibiotic properties.
- ❑ Wintergreen oil has antiseptic properties. It can be applied directly to a sore tooth, or rubbed on inflamed gums.

Take the above herbs as directed on label. They can also be used in teas and infusions. (*See* HERBAL REMEDIES in PART 2 Treatment Section for additional information.)

Homeopathic Remedies

You can self-treat with homeopathic remedies by selecting the one that most closely matches your symptoms. If you don't see improvement, try another, or a combination product. Follow the instructions on the label. If you do not have relief in a reasonable amount of time, consult a physician who specializes in homeopathic medicine.

- ❑ Arnica relieves toothache that gets worse at night.
- ❑ Arsenicum album relieves tooth pain that is worse at night.
- ❑ Belladonna relieves toothaches and abscesses.
- ❑ Bismuthum eases toothaches that are relieved with cold water, and soothes swollen gums.

- ❏ Calcarea carbonica eases pulsating pain and pain caused by hot or cold foods or liquids.
- ❏ Hepar sulphuris reduces swelling and treats infection.
- ❏ Hypericum treats nerve injuries and is useful to control pain following dental surgery.
- ❏ Kali phos treats nerve pain.
- ❏ Magnesium carbonica eases toothache pain.
- ❏ Plantago major relieves tooth pain caused by touch and sensitive to cold beverages.
- ❏ Silicea aids gums that are sensitive to cold and treats abscesses.

Combination remedies sometimes work more effectively than single ones. (*See* HOMEOPATHY in PART 2 Treatment Section for additional information.)

Magnet Therapy

Magnet therapy relieves pain, accelerates healing, and reduces inflammation. (*See* MAGNET THERAPY in PART 2 Treatment Section for additional information.)

Meditation

Meditation helps alleviate stress, which contributes to pain. (*See* MEDITATION in PART 2 Treatment Section for additional information.)

Supplements

- ❏ Bromelain, 500 mg twice daily between meals, acts as an anti-inflammatory.
- ❏ Calcium, 1500–2000 mg, is necessary for strong bones and teeth and also helps prevent muscle cramps. For better absorption, take calcium in divided doses throughout the day and at bedtime (since most calcium is lost at night).
- ❏ Garlic, 2 capsules three times daily, is a natural antibiotic and immune-system stimulator.
- ❏ Propolis, per label, has antiviral and antibacterial properties.
- ❏ Vitamin B_6 has anti-inflammatory properties. Take 200 mg three times a day.
- ❏ Vitamin C, 3000–5000 mg daily, aids tissue repair. Take to bowel tolerance (if diarrhea occurs, reduce the dosage until normal bowel function returns). It is preferable to take Ester-C because more of the vitamin is absorbed in this form.

ASSISTED ALTERNATIVE TREATMENTS

The following techniques may require specialized training or the aid of a healthcare professional.

Acupuncture and Acupressure

Acupuncture involves the insertion of extremely thin solid needles into specific points of your body to stimulate its own healing mechanism and improve blood flow to the affected mouth areas. It also reduces inflammation, relieves pain, improves mobility, and there are rarely any risks or side effects. (*See* ACUPUNCTURE and ACUPRESSURE in PART 2 Treatment Section for additional information.)

Applied Kinesiology

Applied Kinesiology is excellent for reducing pain rapidly. The AK practitioner tests your muscles to determine the origin of your dental problem and then decides on the best course of action, choosing from a wide variety of therapeutic methods at his or her disposal. (*See* APPLIED KINESIOLOGY in PART 2 Treatment Section for additional information.)

Chiropractic

Chiropractic theory is based on the assumption that a properly aligned spine is essential for good health, and that any misalignment of the vertebrae in the spine causes pressure on the spinal nerves, leading to pain. The chiropractor makes spinal adjustments to move misaligned vertebrae to more normal positions, which helps the nervous system to function properly, and can help relieve dental pain. (*See* CHIROPRACTIC in PART 2 Treatment Section for additional information.)

Craniosacral Therapy

A trained craniosacral practitioner can feel areas in the mouth where healthy tissue function is restricted, usually due to physical or emotional trauma. The theory is that physical injuries and emotional traumas are stored or frozen in the body until they are released by gentle craniosacral treatment. (*See* CRANIOSACRAL THERAPY in PART 2 Treatment Section for additional information.)

Guided Imagery and Visualization Techniques

These help to relieve stress and minimize pain in the mouth area. The technique of changing your pain into an object can be helpful for treating dental pain. (*See* GUIDED

IMAGERY and VISUALIZATION in PART 2 Treatment Section for additional information.)

Osteopathic Manipulation

Osteopathic manipulation can correct faulty structure and function and rebalance your body's system, enabling it to function better, and easing the dental pain. (*See* OSTEOPATHIC MANIPULATION in PART 2 Treatment Section for additional information.)

Reflexology

Reflexology massage therapy can be performed on the part of the hand or foot corresponding to the mouth area that is in pain. (*See* REFLEXOLOGY in PART 2 Treatment Section for additional information.)

Rolfing

Rolfing is helpful for conditions caused by compressed nerves. (*See* ROLFING in PART 2 Treatment Section for additional information.)

PRACTICAL SUGGESTIONS

- ❑ See your dentist on a regular basis, usually every six months, and it might be a good idea to have a checkup before a vacation, especially if you are going to an area where dental care might not be available.
- ❑ In your medical kit, carry temporary filling material. If you lose a filling or a cap, or break a tooth and you don't have filling material, you can use candle wax.
- ❑ Do not drink anything that is extremely hot or cold.
- ❑ Hold an ice pack on the area of the mouth that is in pain.
- ❑ Hold warm salt water in your mouth at the site of the pain.

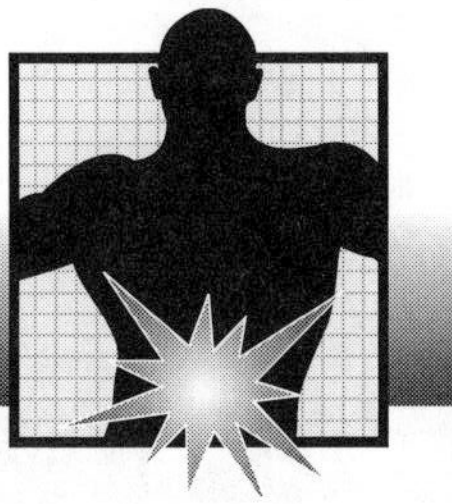

Diverticulitis

Diverticulitis is an inflammation of the diverticula, small sac-like herniations of the colon's lining. Approximately 20 to 50 percent of Americans over fifty have small hernias in the bowel wall, and this condition, known as diverticulosis, becomes diverticulitis when the hernias are inflamed. Most diverticular disease is benign, but a proper diagnosis is important to rule out bowel cancer or inflammatory bowel disease. It is important to treat the condition because, untreated, it can lead to abscesses, fistulas, or a rupture of the diverticula into the peritoneal cavity, which could lead to peritonitis if feces were to leak into this cavity from the colon.

Symptoms

Symptoms can include:

- Constipation;
- Cramping;
- Diarrhea;
- Nausea;
- Lower left-sided abdominal pain.

Causes

Constipation is a primary cause of diverticulitis. When the stool is hard and dry, and you have to strain, the increased bowel pressure causes weak spots in the intestinal lining to bulge and form small sacs called diverticula. Then bits of undigested food and waste tend to collect in these sacs, causing inflammation and infection. Consuming processed foods, and lack of fiber in the diet are other causes.

Diagnosing the Problem

An accurate diagnosis is important to rule out colon cancer. A barium enema x-ray study and a sigmoidoscopy are effective diagnostic tools. During a barium enema procedure, a barium solution, which will show up on an x-ray, is given through the anus and the exam is done in a darkened room by a radiologist using a fluoroscope. During a sigmoidoscopy, an illuminated tubular surgical instrument is inserted into the anus for examination of the sigmoid colon.

Conventional Treatments

- Antibiotics help fight infection.
- Antispasmodic drugs, such as belladonna and lomotil, can relieve spasms.
- Drugs, such as GasX, can relieve colonic pressure.
- Psyllium is a good source of fiber, and helps promote regular bowel movements.
- Surgery can remove the affected portion of the bowel.

Problems with Some Conventional Treatments

- Psyllium should not be taken within thirty to forty-five minutes of taking supplements as it can interfere with their absorption.
- Surgery does not address the underlying condition and can cause scar tissue and adhesions to form.

SELF-HELP ALTERNATIVE TREATMENTS

Many medications for bowel problems have undesirable side effects so you may want to try the following alternative techniques, which can be done at home, to promote wellness. All herbs, homeopathic remedies, packs, and supplements discussed here are available in health food stores and, increasingly, in large drug and grocery stores, as well as on the Internet.

Aromatherapy

Aromatherapy is particularly useful for relieving symptoms related to the digestive system. To relieve constipation, black pepper, cardamom, cinnamon leaf, citronella, ginger, and peppermint oils have a stimulating effect. Mix two or three drops of these oils with a carrier oil, such as sweet almond oil, and use to massage the abdomen in a clockwise direction. You can also add up to ten drops of these oils to your bath water, or soak a piece of flannel in hot water containing four or five drops of oil and apply it as a compress.

For control of diarrhea, chamomile, cinnamon, clove, geranium, ginger, lavender, nutmeg, tea tree oils, and thyme are beneficial. Use as above.

Do not ingest essential oils or use them at full strength, as they are very powerful compounds. They are available in health food stores and stores specializing in aromatherapy products which you can find in the yellow pages. (*See* AROMATHERAPY in PART 2 Treatment Section for additional information.)

Castor Oil Packs

Dip a piece of white flannel into some warm castor oil. Wring it out and place it over the affected area. Cover with plastic and apply a heating pad for one hour. Do this twice daily. (*See* COMPRESSES, PACKS, and POULTICES in PART 2 Treatment Section for additional information.) (*See also* AROMATHERAPY in this entry.)

Diet

If you have any kind of bowel problem, you may have food intolerances. These are not true allergies caused by an immune system response, but are metabolic in nature and can best be evaluated by an elimination diet whereby suspected foods are avoided and then gradually reintroduced. This should be monitored by a qualified nutritionist.

Good Foods

A whole-food, high-fiber diet can prevent and relieve diverticulitis. It is easier to prevent the condition than treat it. Foods high in fiber include barley, beans, brown rice, fruit, guar gum, oat bran, peas, psyllium, and vegetables, which can all help to absorb water as they pass through the colon and lead to bulkier stools that are more easily passed. Cabbage and carrot juices are nutritious and also have a cleansing effect.

(*See* NUTRITIONAL THERAPY in PART 2 Treatment Section for additional information.)

Bad Foods

The following foods may exacerbate your condition.

- ❏ Berries that contain small seeds, such as raspberries and blackberries.
- ❏ Dairy products.
- ❏ Fried foods.
- ❏ Grains.
- ❏ Nuts.
- ❏ Processed foods.
- ❏ Red meat.
- ❏ Seeds.
- ❏ Spicy and sugary type foods.

Other Substances to Avoid

Anyone with a bowel disorder has a problem with alcohol, caffeine, carbonated beverages, and tobacco because they are irritating to the gastrointestinal tract. Additionally, all artificial sweeteners, especially aspartame, minnitol, and sorbitol, can cause diarrhea.

(*See* NUTRITIONAL THERAPY in PART 2 Treatment Section for additional information.)

Herbal Remedies

The following are beneficial for diverticulitis.

- ❏ Alfalfa, per label, is a good source of vitamin K (a deficiency of vitamin K has been linked to intestinal disorders).
- ❏ Cramp bark is an antispasmodic that helps alleviate pain.
- ❏ Garlic is a natural antibiotic and is useful for intestinal problems.
- ❏ Ginger relieves most digestive problems.
- ❏ Peppermint is an antispasmodic, has anti-inflammatory properties, and relieves gas pains.
- ❏ Wild yam is an antispasmodic and has anti-inflammatory properties.
- ❏ Valerian relieves gas pains.

Take the above herbs as directed on label. They can also be used in teas and infusions. (*See* HERBAL REMEDIES in PART 2 Treatment Section for additional information.)

Homeopathic Remedies

You can self-treat with homeopathic remedies by selecting the one that most closely matches your symptoms. If you don't see improvement, try another, or a combination product. Follow the instructions on the label. If you do not have relief in a reasonable amount of time, consult a physician who specializes in homeopathic medicine.

The following homeopathic remedies are useful for *all* painful bowel problems, including diverticulitis.

- ❏ Argentum nitricum eases bloating, flatulence, and diarrhea that occurs after drinking water.
- ❏ Bismuth relieves diarrhea.
- ❏ Bryonia relieves constipation.
- ❏ Carbo veg controls diarrhea alternating with constipation.
- ❏ Chamomilla relieves diarrhea.
- ❏ Colocynthis eases abdominal pain and cramping that eases by bending over or applying pressure.
- ❏ Dulcamara helps control diarrhea containing mucus.
- ❏ Hydrastis relieves constipation.
- ❏ Iris ver also relieves constipation.
- ❏ Kali sulph relieves diarrhea containing mucus.

- ❑ Lycopodium helps control bloating, constipation, gas, heartburn, and pain.
- ❑ Mag phos is an antispasmodic.
- ❑ Nat mur aids digestion.
- ❑ Nux vomica helps relieve gas, cramps, and muscular soreness in the abdomen.
- ❑ Podophyllum helps control diarrhea that alternates with constipation and is accompanied by weakness.
- ❑ Sulphur is useful for anyone with morning diarrhea and excessive gas.

Combination remedies sometimes work more effectively than single ones. (*See* HOMEOPATHY in PART 2 Treatment Section for additional information.)

Meditation

Meditation can help if your diverticulitis is causing you stress. (*See* MEDITATION in PART 2 Treatment Section for additional information.)

Supplements

The following help your body function better and make it more resistant to diverticulitis.

- ❑ Acidophilus, per label, helps maintain normal intestinal flora. It is also very important to use when taking antibiotics.
- ❑ Charcoal, take four tablets or capsules with eight ounces of water to help absorb trapped gas. Take at least one hour before or after taking medication or vitamins.
- ❑ Proteolytic enzymes, per label, aid in protein digestion and reduce inflammation.
- ❑ Vitamin B-complex, 100 mg three times daily.

(*See* SUPPLEMENT THERAPY in PART 2 Treatment Section for additional information.)

ASSISTED ALTERNATIVE TREATMENTS

The following techniques may require specialized training or the aid of a healthcare professional.

Acupuncture and Acupressure

Acupuncture involves the insertion of extremely thin solid needles into specific points of your body to stimulate its own healing mechanism and improve blood flow to the affected areas. It also reduces inflammation, relieves pain, improves mobility, and there are rarely any risks or side effects. (*See* ACUPUNCTURE and ACUPRESSURE in PART 2 Treatment Section for additional information.)

Applied Kinesiology

Applied kinesiology is a non-invasive, non-toxic method that can correct imbalances in the body. It is excellent for reducing pain rapidly, including the pain caused by diverticulitis. (*See* APPLIED KINESIOLOGY in PART 2 Treatment Section for additional information.)

Biofeedback

Biofeedback is useful for reducing stress in anyone with painful bowel problems. (*See* BIOFEEDBACK in PART 2 Treatment Section for additional information.)

Chiropractic

Chiropractic theory is based on the assumption that a properly aligned spine is essential for good health, and that any misalignment of the vertebrae in the spine causes pressure on the spinal nerves, leading to pain. The chiropractor makes spinal adjustments to move misaligned vertebrae to more normal positions, which helps the nervous system to function properly. (*See* CHIROPRACTIC in PART 2 Treatment Section for additional information.)

Craniosacral Therapy

Craniosacral therapy is a form of energy healing that can help balance your system. It has been shown to be effective for soothing bowel problems. (*See* CRANIOSACRAL THERAPY in PART 2 Treatment Section for additional information.)

Cupping

Cupping helps to promote energy flow and reduce pain. (*See* CUPPING in PART 2 Treatment Section for additional information.)

Exercise and Stretching

Stretching exercises help improve digestion and relieve constipation, which is a leading cause of diverticulitis. To avoid further damage, the exercises must be carefully supervised at the beginning. (*See* EXERCISE, STRETCHING, and SPORTS in PART 2 Treatment Section for additional information.)

Guided Imagery

Guided imagery helps relieve stress and manage pain.

Visualizing your bowel area as soft and relaxed can be useful to help relieve the stress associated with diverticular pain. (*See* GUIDED IMAGERY and VISUALIZATION in PART 2 Treatment Section for additional information.)

Hypnosis

Hypnosis is useful for reducing stress in those with diverticulitis. (*See* HYPNOSIS in PART 2 Treatment Section for additional information.)

Massage

A massage helps bring blood to the affected area to relieve the pain. There are many kinds of massage therapies available and you can ask your practitioner to suggest the appropriate one for diverticulitis. (*See* MASSAGE in PART 2 Treatment Section for additional information.) (*See also* AROMATHERAPY in this entry.)

Reflexology

Reflexology massage therapy can be performed on the part of the foot or hand corresponding to the bowel area that is in pain. (*See* REFLEXOLOGY in PART 2 Treatment Section for additional information.)

Tai Chi, Qigong, and Yoga

These therapies help your body to enter a relaxed state and also increase production of endorphins, which are natural painkillers. (*See* TAI CHI, QIGONG, and YOGA in PART 2 Treatment Section for additional information.)

PRACTICAL SUGGESTIONS

Do not wear tight clothing around your waist.

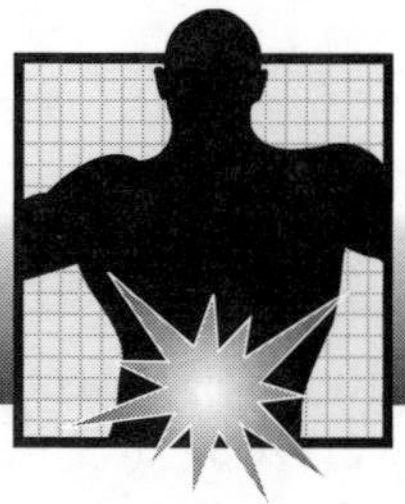

Endometriosis

Endometriosis is a chronic disorder in women that results when pieces of tissue from the lining of the uterus, the endometrium, spread and grow outside the uterine wall and throughout the pelvic area, particularly around the ovaries and fallopian tubes. Then, when estrogen is released during the normal menstrual cycle, this misplaced tissue responds to it and grows and spreads further. As endometrial cells break away, they can migrate to other parts of the body, including the bladder, bowel, kidneys, lungs, and nasal passages, where they also respond to the hormones regulating the menstrual cycle, and bleed monthly. Endometriosis eventually builds up destructive scar tissue which can be a major, often unrecognized, cause of infertility. It affects 4 to 12 million American women who are usually diagnosed with it in their thirties or forties, but it has also been known to occur in teenagers.

Symptoms

The most common symptoms are:

- ❑ Chronic crampy lower abdominal pain, and dull back pain throughout the month;
- ❑ Excruciating pain before and during menstruation;
- ❑ Heavy bleeding;
- ❑ Infertility;
- ❑ Painful bowel movements during menstruation;
- ❑ Painful sexual intercourse;
- ❑ Painful urination;
- ❑ Rectal bleeding during periods.

Common Causes

- ❑ A deficient intake of essential fatty acids.
- ❑ A diet lacking sufficient grains, nuts, and seeds.
- ❑ Environmental toxins, such as the pesticide dioxin, which adversely affect your hormones and may be a leading reason for the prevalence of endometriosis.
- ❑ Genetic predisposition. There is a 7 to 10 percent increase in your chances of developing endometriosis if your mother or sister has the condition.
- ❑ Excessive estrogen in your system.
- ❑ An immune-system deficiency that can prevent the body's natural defenses from destroying the transplanted endometrial cells.
- ❑ A high-fat diet containing too many animal fats and dairy products.
- ❑ A magnesium deficiency.
- ❑ Retrograde menstruation. This theory for the cause of endometriosis holds that, instead of flowing downward and out through the vagina, some menstrual blood and tissue move back up through the fallopian tubes and spill into the pelvic cavity. Although it gets absorbed in most cases, some of this retrograde flow can become implanted outside the uterus where it continues to grow, become inflamed, and form scar tissue.

Diagnosing the Problem

An accurate diagnosis is crucial before beginning treatment. The history and symptoms of the problem must be carefully evaluated in order to determine that the cause of the pain is, in fact, endometriosis because a misdiagnosis could lead to inappropriate or useless treatment. After that, two studies, ultrasound and laparoscopy, can be performed, and both can diagnose and treat endometriosis. In performing a laparascopy, a thin tube with a light on it (a fiber-optic instrument) is inserted into the abdomen through a small incision below the navel to look into the pelvic cavity and determine the precise nature of the condition. Once an accurate diagnosis is made, appropriate treatment can be instituted.

Conventional Treatments

- ❑ Birth control pills to stop ovulation.
- ❑ Cauterizing or laser treatment at the time of the laparoscopy.
- ❑ Complete hysterectomy (removal of the uterus and ovaries).
- ❑ Danazol, a synthetic male hormone that stops ovulation which causes the endometrial tissue to shrivel.
- ❑ Lupron, which blocks the production of reproductive hormones.
- ❑ Nafarelin (Synarel), a nasal spray that helps shrink endometrial lesions.
- ❑ Nonsteroidal anti-inflammatory agents (NSAIDs).
- ❑ Pregnancy. Interrupting menstruation for nine months helps shrink misplaced endometrial tissue. Some women get permanent relief following a pregnancy.

Problems with Some Conventional Treatments

- ❑ Birth control pills can cause abdominal bloating, sore breasts, ankle swelling, and deep vein thrombosis.
- ❑ Complete hysterectomy results in early menopause, and about a third of the women still have pain afterwards. Additionally, this procedure is not an option for anyone wishing to have children.
- ❑ Danazol has side effects, including acne, growth of facial hair, voice changes, a decrease in breast size, and weight gain.
- ❑ Endometriosis can recur after treatment with hormones is stopped, usually after four to six months. About 50 percent of the women taking them have a recurrence of endometriosis within five years.
- ❑ Lupron can cause hot flashes, vaginal dryness, and other menopausal symptoms.
- ❑ Nafarelin can induce hot flashes, vaginal dryness, headaches, and nasal irritation.
- ❑ NSAIDs can cause gastrointestinal bleeding.
- ❑ Pregnancy results in children, who can be a joy (or not).
- ❑ Surgical treatment of any kind can create more scar tissue that will worsen the pain.
- ❑ Younger women have an increased risk of developing osteoporosis.

SELF-HELP ALTERNATIVE TREATMENTS

The following techniques can be done at home. Although they may not work as fast as drugs or surgery, natural alternatives help the body heal itself. All herbs, homeopathic remedies, packs, and supplements discussed here are available in health food stores and, increasingly, in large drug and grocery stores, as well as on the Internet.

Aromatherapy

Aromatherapy, particularly the essential oils of bergamot, chamomile, clary sage, fennel, geranium, grapefruit, jasmine, lavender, melissa, neroli, nutmeg, palmarosa, parsley seed, rose, vetiver, and ylang ylang all help regulate hormonal balance. They also relieve spasms and help heal tissues. You can either put a few drops into a hot bath and soak, or add a few drops to vegetable oil and massage into the affected area. Do not ingest essential oils or use them full strength, as they are very powerful compounds. They are available in health food stores and stores specializing in aromatherapy products, which you can find in the yellow pages. (*See* AROMATHERAPY in PART 2 Treatment Section for additional information.)

Castor Oil Packs

Dip a piece of white flannel into some warm castor oil. Wring it out and place it over your uterine area. Cover with plastic and apply a heating pad for one hour. Do this twice daily. (*See* COMPRESSES, PACKS, and POULTICES in PART 2 Treatment Section for additional information.)

Diet

What you eat can play a role in endometriosis so certain dietary modifications can be helpful. There may be a relationship between yeast infections and endometriosis so a yeast-free diet could be helpful.

Good Foods

- ❑ Acidophilus-containing foods, such as yogurt.
- ❑ Beans (all kinds) and bean sprouts contain beneficial phytoestrogens (plant estrogens) that bind to the cell's estrogen receptor sites and prevent the harmful types of estrogen from binding to the receptors.
- ❑ Foods with a high-fiber content.
- ❑ Iron-containing foods, such as dark green leafy vegetables and their juices, are beneficial because the heavy menstrual bleeding experienced by some women with endometriosis can lead to an iron deficiency.
- ❑ Peanuts contain many of the helpful substances found in beans and soy- beans.
- ❑ Soybeans and soy-containing foods, such as tofu, contain large amounts of the plant estrogens genistein and daidzein, which bind to the cell's estrogen-receptor sites and keep harmful types of estrogen from binding to these sites.

(*See* NUTRITIONAL THERAPY in PART 2 Treatment Section for additional information.)

Bad Foods

It's a good idea to avoid the following foods as they can worsen your symptoms.

- ❑ Dairy products, eggs, and meat from non-organic sources because most animals are raised on hormones which can affect your system.
- ❑ Dried fruits, fermented foods, overripe fruits, and sugars all cause yeast proliferation.
- ❑ Estrogen-producing foods, such as alfalfa, carrots, endive, legumes, liver, oatmeal, wheat germ, and yams (except for wild Mexican yams).
- ❑ Fatty foods because hormones store in fatty tissue.

Other Substances to Avoid

- ❑ Dioxin Exposure. Use only unbleached tampons and sanitary napkins.
- ❑ Do not use an IUD for contraception because it increases menstrual flow.
- ❑ PABA produces estrogen, so be sure your multivitamin does not contain it. And do not use sunscreens containing PABA because it can be absorbed through the skin.

Heat Therapy/Cold Therapy

Some women find that ice, in the form of frozen gel packs, frozen peas, or a frozen wet cloth in a plastic bag wrapped in a second cloth, relieves their pain better than heat. It reduces tissue swelling. Others prefer to apply heat to the lower abdomen, using a hot water bottle or a heating pad. The heat helps to relieve cramps, as can a hot bath. See what works for you. You might want to try alternating heat and cold. (*See* HEAT THERAPY/COLD THERAPY, and HYDROTHERAPY in PART 2 Treatment Section for additional information.)

Herbal Remedies

- ❑ Blessed thistle aids in menstrual disorders.
- ❑ Dandelion root eases cramps and helps rid the body of excess fluid.
- ❑ False unicorn helps uterine disorders.
- ❑ Red clover enhances liver function.
- ❑ Red raspberry contains nutrients to strengthen the uterine wall.
- ❑ Sarsaparilla helps regulate hormones.

Take the above herbs as directed on label. They can also be used in teas and infusions. (*See* HERBAL REMEDIES in PART 2 Treatment Section for additional information.)

Homeopathic Remedies

You can self-treat with homeopathic remedies by selecting the one that most closely matches your symptoms. If you don't see improvement, try another, or a combination product. Follow the instructions on the label. If you do not have relief in a reasonable amount of time, consult a physician who specializes in homeopathic medicine.

- ❑ Calcarea relieves dull achy lower back pain that occurs during menstrual periods.
- ❑ Lachesis relieves lower abdominal pain that that occurs premenstrually.

(*See* HOMEOPATHY in PART 2 Treatment Section for additional information.)

Meditation

Meditation helps reduce stress, which contributes to endometriosis. (*See* MEDITATION in PART 2 Treatment Section for additional information.)

Supplements

- ❑ Bioflavanoids, per label, strengthen capillaries and aid healing. They also work synergistically with Vitamin C.
- ❑ Evening primrose oil, per label, relieves pain and inflammation.
- ❑ Fish oil, per label, is an anti-inflammatory.
- ❑ Lipotropic factor, 2000 mg with meals. Dr. Edward M. Wagner, ND, recommends taking this supplement in divided doses twice daily. It contains choline, inositol, and methionine, and the combination helps the liver break down the active forms of estrogen (estradiol and estrone) into inactive estrogen (estriol). That way, Dr. Wagner says, the cells are not overly activated to boost endometrial growth.
- ❑ Oxynutrients, as directed on label. Dr. Wagner also recommends this high antioxidant supplement containing coenzyme Q_{10}, germanium, DMG, inosine, gamma oryzanol, and L-carnitine. Additionally, it contains ascorbal palmitate, a fat-soluble form of vitamin C that activates the antioxidant property of this vitamin in fatty tissue.
- ❑ Vitamin B_5, 100 mg three times daily, aids hormone balance.
- ❑ Vitamin B_6, 50 mg three times daily, helps rid your system of excess fluids. Note: For balance, when taking individual Bs, be sure to supplement with a B-complex once daily, or a multivitamin containing Bs.
- ❑ Vitamin E helps balance hormones. Start with 400 IU daily and work up gradually to 1000 IU.

(*See* SUPPLEMENT THERAPY in PART 2 Treatment Section for additional information.)

ASSISTED ALTERNATIVE TREATMENTS

The following techniques may requite specialized training or the aid of a healthcare professional.

Acupuncture and Acupressure

Acupuncture involves the insertion of extremely thin solid needles into specific points of your body to stimulate its own healing mechanism and improve blood flow to the uterine area. It also reduces inflammation and relieves pain, and there are rarely any risks or side effects. (*See* ACUPUNCTURE and ACUPRESSURE in PART 2 Treatment Section for additional information.)

Applied Kinesiology

Applied Kinesiology is excellent for reducing pain rapidly. The AK practitioner tests your muscles to determine the origin of your problem and then decides on the best course of action, choosing from a wide variety of therapeutic methods at his or her disposal. (*See* APPLIED KINESIOLOGY in PART 2 Treatment Section for additional information.)

Bee Venom Therapy

Some components of bee venom are thought to stimulate the immune system. Other components are thought to modify the transmission of pain signals within the nervous system, and the therapy has proven consistently useful for the pain of endometriosis. (*See* BEE VENOM THERAPY in PART 2 Treatment Section for additional information.)

Chiropractic

Chiropractic theory is based on the assumption that a properly aligned spine is essential for good health, and that any misalignment of the vertebrae in the spine causes pressure on the spinal nerves, leading to pain. The chiropractor makes spinal adjustments to move misaligned vertebrae to more normal positions, which helps the nervous system to function properly. In pelvic disorders, a chiropractor can determine if the pelvic bones are out of alignment and if the muscles attached to them are able to properly relax. (*See* CHIROPRACTIC in PART 2 Treatment Section for additional information.)

Craniosacral Therapy

Craniosacral therapy is a form of energy healing that can help balance your system. It has been shown to be effective for alleviating endometriosis. (*See* CRANIOSACRAL THERAPY in PART 2 Treatment Section for additional information.)

Exercise and Stretching

Regular exercise started in your early twenties can lower your risk of developing endometriosis, because it lowers estrogen levels. It also increases the ratio of muscle to fat which helps reduce estrogen levels. Regular aerobic exercise, which must be carefully supervised at the beginning to avoid further damage, aids circulation, helps oxygenate the blood, and relaxes the uterus. (*See* EXERCISE, STRETCHING, and SPORTS in PART 2 Treatment Section for additional information.)

Guided Imagery and Visualization Techniques

Guided imagery can help manage endometriosis. To relieve any sensation of chronic heaviness, change the pain into a light object that you can easily handle. (*See* GUIDED IMAGERY and VISUALIZATION in PART 2 Treatment Section for additional information.)

Massage

A massage helps bring blood to the uterine area and relieves the pain. There are many kinds of massage therapies available and you can ask your practitioner to suggest the appropriate one for your endometriosis. (*See* MASSAGE in PART 2 Treatment Section for additional information.)

Osteopathic Manipulation

The goal of osteopathic manipulation in the treatment of endometriosis is to reduce uterine congestion, relieve pain, and improve blood circulation. (*See* OSTEOPATHIC MANIPULATION in PART 2 Treatment Section for additional information.)

Reflexology

Reflexology massage therapy can be performed on the part of the foot or hand corresponding to the uterine area that is in pain. (*See* REFLEXOLOGY in PART 2 Treatment Section for additional information.)

Tai Chi, Qigong, and Yoga

These therapies induce a profoundly relaxed state and help bring healing energy to the body. (*See* TAI CHI, QIGONG, and YOGA in PART 2 Treatment Section for additional information.)

PRACTICAL SUGGESTIONS

- ❏ Orgasms cause uterine contractions, which can be helpful in flushing out retrograde tissue.
- ❏ Progesterone cream, available in health food stores, helps relieve the effects of excess estrogen. Use according to instructions on label.
- ❏ Seek a practitioner who specializes in treating endometriosis. Not all ob/gyns have enough experience.
- ❏ Using tampons instead of sanitary napkins helps absorb the retrograde menstrual tissue that can migrate to the area surrounding the fallopian tubes and ovaries.

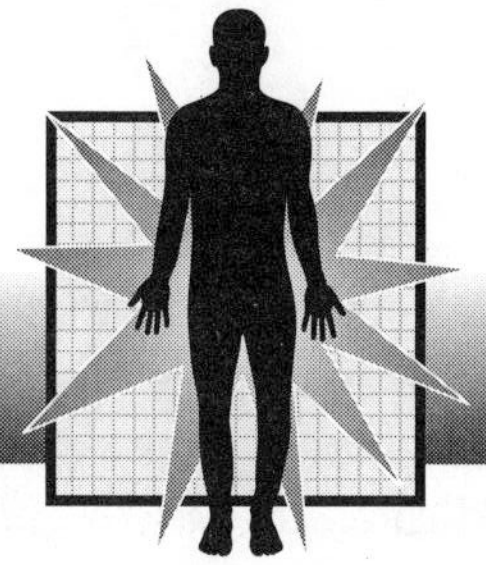

Fibromyalgia

Fibromyalgia is a chronic pain disease of unknown origin. When people with this disorder seek help, they are often shunted from one specialist after another, only to be eventually informed it is all in their heads or they are suffering from depression. Although dismissively told that psychological distress is the cause of their pain, fibromyalgia is not a psychiatric illness. The opposite is, in fact, most probably the case—that their distressed psychological state is the *result* of attempting, unsuccessfully, to cope with the pain, not the cause of it.

Prior to 1990, fibromyalgia was not even recognized by mainstream medicine as a medical musculoskeletal disorder. Even now, on average the person has had the condition for about five years on average before being accurately diagnosed with it, and has often undergone extensive testing and unnecessary surgery. It is a progressive illness that, in its early stages, appears for only a few days at a time, and, as with many conditions involving pain, it is usually worse in the morning, easing up somewhat in the early afternoon. It is estimated that up to 10 million people in the United States have the disease, which is known to strike four times as many women as men, usually those between the ages of twenty and forty-five.

Symptoms

Fibromyalgia is characterized by terrible pain in the muscles, ligaments, tendons, and fascial connective tissue. The pain has been described as as burning, stabbing, or throbbing, and is accompanied by extreme fatigue, very likely caused by disrupted sleep patterns—besides having difficulty falling asleep, people with the condition also have a problem staying asleep. Although x-rays do not show any evidence of damage to the joints, severe joint pain is often present and may or may not be accompanied by swelling, redness, and heat. Some people with fibromyalgia say they feel like they have rigor mortis, or they are turning into marble.

Fibromyalgia's many symptoms mimic those of other conditions, which is one reason why it is so hard to pin down. These also include achy, flu-like symptoms (some complain that every day they feel they are coming down with a terrible case of the flu); frequent urination, accompanied by burning and a pungent odor; vulvar pain; and dyspareunia (painful intercourse). For women, the symptoms are usually worse premenstrually. Hair loss may occur, nails can become brittle, and the skin often becomes super sensitive to touch. People complain of blurred vision; dry eyes; headaches; heart palpitations; mottled skin; nasal congestion; post-nasal drip; a feeling of numbness or tingling in the arms, legs, hands, and feet; a heightened sensitivity to lights, odors, and sounds; a metallic taste; and sugar cravings. Fingernails may peel and dental tartar may accumulate on the teeth and break off. Those affected may also experience anxiety, digestive disturbances, irritable bowel syndrome, a lack of energy, a lowered threshold of pain, and weight gain.

The pain is usually most severe in the low back and hips, the neck, or the shoulders, and is generally accompanied by muscle twitching, with increased sensitivity to heat or cold, and any changes in the weather. The pain does not go away while resting and it may even worsen when not moving.

Common Causes

The causes of fibromyalgia are unclear, but the condition may be triggered by such factors as infection, stress, or surgery. Symptoms may begin following some emotional or physical trauma, and may appear following an accident that did not result in a physical injury. The cause may be an internal acid condition, low serotonin levels, or a phosphate accumulation. Serotonin regulates sleep patterns and low levels of it can cause pain, sleep disturbances, and changes in how the central nervous system processes pain. There may be an infectious origin because symptoms often appear following a flu-like illness. Another theory for its cause involves leaky gut syndrome. If the lining of the gut is not intact, large food particles can get into the circulatory system, triggering the immune system to recognize them as invaders. Then antibodies form and latch onto joint tissue, leading to inflammation, which causes pain. From then on, every time that particular food is consumed, the inflammatory action occurs.

Diagnosing the Problem

It wasn't until 1990 that fibromyalgia was accepted as a diagnosis, and it took until 1993 for it to be incorporated into the International Statistical Classification of Diseases and Related Health Problems by the World Health Organization.

There are no definitive blood tests or diagnostic x-ray

tests. Doctors should suspect fibromyalgia when there is more diffuse pain than that seen with rheumatoid arthritis, which results only in localized joint swelling.

The condition is difficult to diagnose because there are no diagnostic tests other than a process called mapping, which is finding tender points in eighteen precise locations in muscles, or areas where muscles join tendons, that have been present for at least three months. There can be sensitivity to moderate finger pressure in at least eleven of these eighteen specific points located primarily in the back of the head and neck, on the lower back and hips, between the shoulder blades, the upper shoulders, the upper chest, the inside of the knees, and the elbows.

Conventional Treatments

- ❑ Amitriptyline helps induce sleep.
- ❑ Cyclobenzaprine eases muscle spasms.
- ❑ Doxepin is good to treat depression.
- ❑ Elavil helps increase serotonin levels.
- ❑ Probenecid helps reverse symptoms.
- ❑ Sulfinpyrazone also helps reverse symptoms.
- ❑ Over-the-counter pain-relievers, such as Advil, Aleve, or Tylenol.

Problems with Some Conventional Treatments

- ❑ Some people are allergic to sulfanomides (probenecid).
- ❑ Sulfinpyrazone can cause hyperacidity.
- ❑ Amitriptyline, Dyclobenzaprine, Doxepan, and Elavil can react adversely with other medications. Another annoying side effect is dry mouth, which can lead to dental problems.
- ❑ Advil and Aleve, when taken for long periods, can lead to internal bleeding and gastric disturbances.

Effective Conventional Treatment for Fibromyalgia

R. Paul St. Armand, MD, Assistant Clinical Professor, Endocrinology at Harbor/UCLA Medicine, has had some remarkable results treating his patients with guaifenesin, a component of many cough and cold preparations that has almost no side effects, with the possible exception of a runny nose. Guaifenesin, used to liquefy mucous, increases the excretion of phosphate, and phosphate accumulation is believed by some to be a prime cause of fibromyalgia. The suggested dosage is 300 milligrams twice a day for one week. If symptoms worsen, that is the correct dosage. If they do *not* worsen, the dosage is increased to 600 mg. This may sound backward, but when symptoms worsen, it indicates that the condition has begun to reverse itself. Two months at the proper dosage will reverse one year of accumulated metabolic debris, so the longer the condition has been present, the more time you need for relief.

Unfortunately, guaifenesin will not work in the presence of salicylates, which are naturally occuring chemicals in many plants that protect them against harmful bacteria and fungi. Any form of salicylate, even the small amounts in cosmetics or other topical preparations, will block the beneficial effects of guaifenesin. Salicylates are present in many natural and synthetic preparations, including aspirin and similar products for pain relief, and in other over-the-counter items, such as alka seltzer and urised, an OTC preparation for urinary tract infections.

Herbal medications, such as blue-green algae, echinacea, ginko biloba, ginseng, nonni juice, St. John's Wort, and saw palmetto also contain salicylates, as does mint. Additionally, they are present in many vitamin supplements, especially those containing alfalfa, bioflavanoids, parsley, and vitamins E or C derived from rose hips. It is important to be diligent in reading labels on all shampoos and cosmetics to be sure they don't contain saliclyate components, such as aloe, cucumber, lavender, almond or grape seed oils, or camphor or castor oils. It is also very important, while gardening, to wear protective gloves so the plant juices do not adhere to your skin.

Dr. St. Armand says he will assume guaifenesin is not working if his patients do not completely remove salicylates from their environment.

Relief on the Internet

Before Victoria found Dr. St. Armand's website and learned about his methods of treating fibromyalgia, the quality of her life from the debilitating disease had gone downhill to the point that she was forced to stop working and had to be hospitalized regularly when the symptoms, including pain, completely overwhelmed her. The guaifenesin and accompanying protocol that Dr. St. Armand recommended to Victoria easily cleared up these symptoms and allowed her to go on with her life, the only side effect being a runny nose that she was happy to trade for the fibromyalgia nightmare she had just been through.

SELF-HELP ALTERNATIVE TREATMENTS

Although fibromyalgia tends to stubbornly resist most forms of treatment, there are alternative measures to alleviate your worst symptoms, and the following techniques can be done at home. All herbs, homeopathic remedies, and supplements discussed here are available in health food stores and, increasingly, in large drug and grocery stores, as well as on the Internet.

Aerobic Exercises

Biking, jogging, swimming, and walking raise body levels of endorphins, your body's natural pain relievers, and these and similar aerobic exercises also increase your levels of serotonin. (*See* EXERCISE, STRETCHING, and SPORTS in PART 2 Treatment Section for additional information.)

Aromatherapy

Aromatherapy can help relieve the pain of fibromyalgia, particularly the essential oils of chamomile, ginger, lavaender, marjoram, rosemary, and yarrow. (*See* AROMATHERAPY in PART 2 Treatment Section for additional information.)

Diet

A proper, balanced diet can be a positive therapeutic factor for this condition.

Good Foods

The following foods should be added to your diet because they all contain magnesium, which has a calming effect and helps relax the muscles. It also aids in removing toxins from the body.

- ❑ Brown rice.
- ❑ Buckwheat.
- ❑ Chickpeas.
- ❑ Green vegetables.
- ❑ Kidney beans.
- ❑ Lentils.
- ❑ Millet.
- ❑ Nuts.
- ❑ Seeds.

(*See* NUTRITIONAL THERAPY in PART 2 Treatment Section for additional information).

Bad Foods

If you are using guaifenesin, you must diligently avoid all foods containing salycilates. (*See* above.)

Other Substances to Avoid

As with bad foods previously mentioned, when using guaifenesin all products containing salycilates are to be avoided.

Heat Therapy/Cold Therapy

Heat will increase blood flow to the painful area and cold will help reduce swelling. (*See* HEAT THERAPY/COLD THERAPY in PART 2 Treatment Section for additional information.)

Herbal Remedies

- ❑ Deglycyrrhizinated licorice, two grams three times a day, helps reduce fatigue.
- ❑ Devil's claw, per label, reduces inflammation and aids in removing toxins from the body.
- ❑ Hypericum (St. John's Wort), per label, increases serotonin levels.

(*See* HERBAL REMEDIES in PART 2 Treatment Section for additional information.)

Homeopathic Remedies

- ❑ Arnica is beneficial when body areas feel bruised and sore after exertion, injury, or overuse of muscles.
- ❑ Bryonia helps those whose pain is worse following motion.
- ❑ Calcarea carbonica eases muscle soreness and weakness that worsen with exertion and cold.
- ❑ Causticum eases soreness, weakness and muscle stiffness that worsen from exposure to cold and overuse.
- ❑ Cimicifuga helps relieve soreness and stiffness accompanied by headaches, shooting pains, and tightness in the neck.
- ❑ Kalmia latifolia is for severe muscular pain accompanied by stiffness and numbness that worsens at night.
- ❑ Ranunculus bulbosus is beneficial for muscle stiffness accompanied by stabbing pains in the back and neck.
- ❑ Rhus toxicodendron aids those who have stiffness and pain upon waking in the morning and after resting.
- ❑ Ruta graveolena soothes muscle stiffness accompanied by lameness and weakness.

Take the above remedies as indicated on label. Combination remedies sometimes work more effectively than single ones. (*See* HOMEOPATHY in PART 2 Treatment Section for additional information.)

Hydrotherapy

Warm baths and hot tubs help relax your body and relieve pain. (*See* HYDROTHERAPY in PART 2 Treatment Section for additional information).

Magnets

Magnet therapy relieves pain, accelerates healing, and reduces inflammation. Magnets on and around painful areas can bring blood to the area which, in turn, brings oxygen and other healing substances to reduce the pain. Hold the magnets in place with a velcro strip, or tape them on. (*See* MAGNET THERAPY in PART 2 Treatment Section for additional information.)

Meditation

Meditation helps reduce stress and increases production of your body's natural painkillers. (*See* MEDITATION in PART 2 Treatment Section for additional information.)

Supplements

- ❑ Coenzyme Q_{10} speeds up metabolism and increases serotonin levels. According to Dr. Edward M. Wagner, ND, a 400-mg daily intake should be the minimum for fibromyalgia, and you could go as high as 1000 mg because the digestive disturbances associated with the condition can lead to problems of assimilation.
- ❑ Magnesium taken at bedtime aids in relaxation and helps reduce joint sensitivity. Start by taking 150 mg once a day and gradually increase to 150 mg three times daily.
- ❑ It takes about two months to see an improvement, but magnesium malate—150 mg magnesium mixed with 600 mg malic acid extract from apples, pears, or certain other fruits, has been shown to bring relief.
- ❑ Malic acid is a natural muscle relaxant. Take 1200–2400 mg per day.
- ❑ Melatonin helps regulate sleep patterns. The usual dose is 3 mg at bedtime. Use caution with this supplement as prolonged use can interfere with the body's own internal clock.
- ❑ Vitamin E. 100–300 IU per day.

(*See* SUPPLEMENT THERAPY in PART 2 Treatment Section for additional information.)

ASSISTED ALTERNATIVE TREATMENTS

The following techniques may require specialized training or the aid of a healthcare professional.

Acupuncture and Acupressure

Acupuncture and acupressure create a smooth flow of vibratory energy throughout the body that can help alleviate the symptoms of fibromyalgia. (*See* ACUPUNCTURE and ACUPRESSURE in PART 2 Treatment Section for additional information.)

Bee Venom Therapy

Some components of bee venom are thought to stimulate the immune system. Other components are thought to modify the transmission of pain signals within the nervous system, and the therapy has proven consistently useful for the pain of fibromyalgia. (*See* BEE VENOM THERAPY in PART 2 Treatment Section for additional information.)

Biofeedback

Electrodes taped to the skin transmit impulses to a computer screen so you can actually see when you tense and relax your muscles. (*See* BIOFEEDBACK in PART 2 Treatment Section for additional information.)

Guided Imagery and Visualization Techniques

Guided imagery can help manage the pain of fibromyalgia. Since so many different symptoms are associated with fibromyalgia, it is most helpful to focus on them individually and mentally bring in the appropriate tools to deal with them. (*See* GUIDED IMAGERY and VISUALIZATION in PART 2 Treatment Section for additional information.)

Osteopathic Manipulation

The goal of osteopathic manipulation is to increase range of motion, decrease muscle tension, and improve blood circulation, all of which can relieve the pain of fibromyalgia. (*See* OSTEOPATHIC MANIPULATION in PART 2 Treatment Section for additional information.)

Oxygen Therapy

Oxygen therapy, particularly HBOT, is a useful adjunct for treating those with fibromyalgia. (*See* OXYGEN THERAPIES in PART 2 Treatment Section for additional information.)

Physical Therapy

Physical therapy helps correct and improve your body's natural healing mechanism. It increases the range of motion in the joints. (*See* PHYSICAL THERAPY in PART 2 Treatment Section for additional information.)

Reflexology

Reflexology massage therapy performed on the specific part of the foot and/or hand that corresponds with the affected area can be helpful. (*See* REFLEXOLOGY in PART 2 Treatment Section for additional information.)

Rolfing

Rolfing is very useful for treating impaired mobility and sports injuries and has long-lasting effects in easing pain. (*See* ROLFING in PART 2 Treatment Section for additional information.)

Tai Chi, Qigong, and Yoga

These therapies induce a profoundly relaxed state and help bring healing energy to the body. (*See* QIGONG, TAI CHI, and YOGA in PART 2 Treatment Section for additional information.)

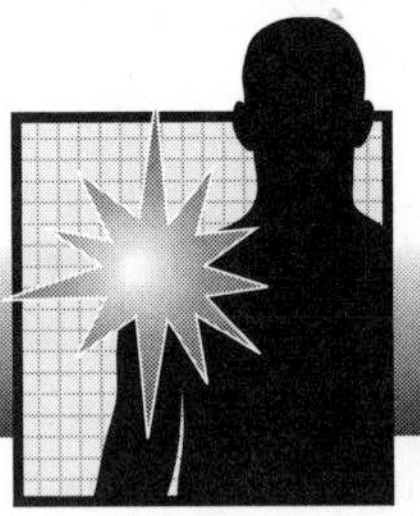

Frozen Shoulder

Of all the joints in your body, your shoulder is among the most complex and has one of the widest ranges of motion when it is working properly. When frozen shoulder (adhesive capsulitis) develops, however, the flexible tissue surrounding the shoulder joint that allows it to move smoothly thickens and stiffens, making movement painful and difficult.

Symptoms

Frozen shoulder can hit awake or asleep. It has been described as coming on like a white-hot poker (one person referred to it as a 12 on a pain scale of 1–10), completely immobilizing the shoulder and requiring a manual readjustment of it with the hand on the other side.

Common Causes

Frozen shoulder can occur following an injury, especially if the shoulder has had to be immobilized while it is healing; the resulting scar tissue (adhesions) can shrink the shoulder capsule, freezing the shoulder. It can also occur following activities that overuse the shoulder, such as sports, heavy construction labor, or other work-related activities. And, for some as-yet-unknown reason, it is five times more likely to happen in people with diabetes.

Diagnosing the Problem

A clinical diagnosis can be made by rotating the shoulder and noting the stiffness and painful movement.

Conventional Treatments

- ❏ Painkillers.
- ❏ Surgery.

Problems with Some Conventional Treatment

- ❏ Painkillers can have harmful side effects.
- ❏ Surgery often leads to complications and is to be avoided wherever possible.

SELF-HELP ALTERNATIVE TREATMENTS

Fortunately, there are a number of self-help treatments that can be utilized for frozen shoulder. As with all conditions in this book, anyone with frozen shoulder can benefit from proper nutrition, herbs, homeopathic remedies, and supplements. If these treatments, which can be done at home, are started early, the prognosis is good, and more aggressive, invasive methods, surgery included, can often be avoided. Herbs, homeopathic remedies, packs, and supplements are available in health food stores and, increasingly, in large drug and grocery stores, as well as on the Internet. (*See* HERBAL REMEDIES, HOMEOPATHY, and NUTRITIONAL THERAPY in PART 2 Treatment Section for additional information.)

Baths

Soaking in a hot bath, or taking a whirlpool bath can relax the muscles. (*See* HEAT THERAPY/COLD THERAPY and HYDROTHERAPY in PART 2 Treatment Section for additional information.)

Ice Packs

Some find that ice packs relieve the pain of frozen shoulder as much as anything. (*See* COMPRESSES, PACKS, and POULTICES in PART 2 Treatment Section for additional information.)

Supplements

MSM (methylsulfonylmethane), a natural sulfur compound available in capsule, tablet, or powder form, is said to be helpful for frozen shoulder. (*See* SUPPLEMENT THERAPY in PART 2 Treatment Section for additional information.)

ASSISTED ALTERNATIVE TREATMENTS

The following techniques may require specialized training or the aid of a healthcare professional.

Acupuncture and Acupressure

Acupuncture involves the insertion of extremely thin solid needles into specific points of your body to stimulate its own healing mechanism and improve blood flow to the affected shoulder. It also reduces inflammation, relieves pain, improves mobility, and there are rarely any risks or side effects. (*See* ACUPUNCTURE and ACUPRESSURE in PART 2 Treatment Section for additional information.)

Deep Tissue Massage

Kinesiologists trained in rolfing, or rolfers themselves, can use deep tissue massage, applying deep pressure to certain muscle trigger points, and these therapies can be followed up with supervised stretching and exercises. (*See* APPLIED KINESIOLOGY and ROLFING in PART 2 Treatment Section for additional information.)

Physical Therapy

Physical therapy, also a conventional treatment, helps correct and improve your body's natural healing mechanisms. It increases the range of motion in the joints. With frozen shoulder, physical therapy to gently stretch the tissues, followed by a supervised exercise and stretching program, is also recommended. (*See* EXERCISE, STRETCHING, and SPORTS and PHYSICAL THERAPY in PART 2 Treatment Section for additional information.)

Shoulder Manipulations

More severe cases may respond to having a chiropractor or an osteopath do shoulder manipulations of the muscle and skeletal structure to break up the adhesions and unfreeze the shoulder. (*See* CHIROPRACTIC and OSTEOPATHIC MANIPULATION in PART 2 Treatment Section for additional information.)

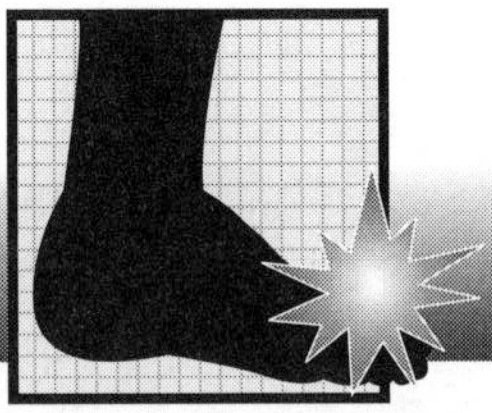

Gout

Gout is an arthritis condition that produces acute joint pain. Unlike rheumatoid or osteoarthritis, which in many instances are chronic, gout pain is of a more sporadic nature. It usually occurs in the early morning, eases up during the day, comes back severely at night, and generally lasts about one week. This condition occurs in men 90 to 95 percent of the time, and those over forty are the most vulnerable. Gout has been referred to as the rich man's disease, or the disease of kings, because it most often strikes those who overindulge in food and drink.

Symptoms

The primary symptom of gout is sudden severe joint pain in the big toe, but wrists, ankles, or knees can also be affected. The afflicted joint often becomes red (sometimes dark red), shiny and swollen because the skin is stretched. There can be cutting, lightning-like pains that radiate through the joints and fever may also be present. Some people describe the pain as radiating and freezing. During this time, any pressure put on the inflamed joint is so excruciating that some people take to bed for the entire duration of an attack, leaving the affected area uncovered as they cannot bear even the weight of a sheet covering the area. Gout attacks usually strike without warning, but sometimes you can tell when an attack is imminent.

Cause

An overabundance of uric acid is the cause of gout. Uric acid, a component of urine, is an organic substance resulting from the breakdown of purines (*See* definition below). Uric acid is dissolved in the blood, passes through the kidneys and is normally eliminated daily through the skin and the urinary tract. When uric acid is *not* eliminated normally, as with those who are experiencing a gout attack, and there is too much uric acid in the blood, causing above-normal concentrations of it in your tissues, the uric acid crystallizes in the joint spaces, which then become swollen, inflamed, and very painful. And small wonder! Look at a microscopic enlargement of uric acid crystals and you'll see they have *razor-sharp spikes*. Interestingly, it has been found that high uric acid levels are often present in overachievers and very intelligent people, not much of a consolation, however, if you happen to be one of these highly intelligent people in the midst of an acute attack of gout.

Causes of Uric-Acid Buildup

- ❑ Alcohol abuse is why people, mostly men, develop the uric-acid buildup that leads to gout.
- ❑ Foods containing purines are another reason for the buildup of uric acid. Purines are those elements of human tissue that break down to form uric acid, leading to the onslaught of the gout condition. (Purines are components of nucleoproteins that are associated with the building process of cells that is necessary for optimum health.) In some people's systems, the uric acid is synthesized too quickly and when those with this problem ingest products that are high in purines, the normal breakdown of nucleoproteins in their bodies leads instead to the formation of uric-acid crystals and salts, which can, in turn, lead to gout. To avoid this, these individuals should stay away from foods high in purines.
- ❑ Overeating and being overweight. Besides the usual problems created by the additional weight placing

Gout and Alcohol

A study in *The Lancet* reports that, for the first time ever, there is documented evidence of the long-held belief that alcohol and gout, a painful inflammatory type of arthritis, are related. As reported in *The New York Times,* the Harvard-affiliated authors of the study say that "alcohol intake strongly increases the risk of developing gout," but the risk level depends on the type of alcohol consumed. Drinking twelve ounces of beer or more was found to increase the gout risk two and a half times, they said, and two shots of hard liquor increased it approximately one and a half times. For some reason though, drinking two or more four-ounce glasses of wine a day did *not* increase it. Although this study was the first to document the alcohol/gout link and determine which kinds of alcohol were most likely to trigger the condition, more research will be needed to determine whether as-yet-unidentified, non-alcoholic elements of beer and spirits promote gout, as they suspect, and what, if any, substance in wine protects against gout.

more stress on the joints, these factors may also increase the body's production of uric acid.

- ❑ Rapid weight loss is another primary reason for uric-acid buildup. If you are overweight, it's important to lose weight slowly. A too-rapid weight loss may increase the concentration of uric acid in your body and cause your uric acid to rise too fast to levels that are too high, which can lead to a gout condition if you are one of those susceptible to it.
- ❑ Taking diuretics. Diuretics, which help you lose water, decrease the amount of uric acid excreted in the urine, allowing for a possible buildup in the system. People with high blood pressure often take diuretics.

Diagnosing the Problem

Gout is generally diagnosed by its obvious symptoms. Or, if the diagnosis is uncertain, a doctor can insert a needle into the affected joint, withdraw some of the fluid and examine it under a microscope to see if uric-acid crystals are present.

Conventional Treatments

Some medications prevent the attack while others treat it after it has happened. In general there are two types of drugs offered, over-the-counter and by prescription. The following are the most frequently used drugs.

- ❑ Allopurinol. This prescription drug decreases the amount of uric acid in the body.
- ❑ Colchine. Instead of lowering the amount of uric acid in the body, this prescription drug acts to inhibit the white blood cell response and works to prevent an attack by decreasing the amount of harmful chemicals the body produces in response to the crystals formed in the joints.
- ❑ NSAIDs. Over-the-counter non-steroidal anti-inflammatory drugs include aspirin, ibuprofen, and naproxen. They reduce inflammation and function as painkillers for temporary relief. Prescription NSAIDs include higher strengths of ibuprofen and naproxen, and there are new prescription NSAIDs coming onto the market regularly.
- ❑ Prescription painkillers. In addition to prescribed NSAIDs, stronger medications, including narcotics, such as codeine and morphine, are available by prescription from a doctor.
- ❑ Probenecid. This drug helps to eliminate uric acid from the body.

Problems with Some Conventional Treatments

- ❑ Allopurinol causes inflammation of blood vessels, liver and kidney problems, and skin eruptions.
- ❑ Colchine can cause abdominal pain, abnormal bleeding, bruising, fever, hair loss, nausea, vomiting, and weakness, and may make your hands and feet feel numb.
- ❑ Drugs that lower uric acid levels may weaken your kidneys.
- ❑ NSAIDs, over-the-counter and by prescription, may cause internal bleeding.
- ❑ Painkillers can be habit-forming, even addictive. They can lead to secondary problems, such as constipation, or drowsiness, which makes it unsafe to drive or operate machinery. Further, painkillers only mask symptoms rather than address the underlying cause of the problem which, in the case of gout, is uric acid buildup.

SELF-HELP ALTERNATIVE TREATMENTS

The following techniques can be done at home. Although a gout attack is usually acute and sudden, if you know you are susceptible and are given enough warning, you can ward one off, or at least reduce its severity, by resting, diligently following the dietary advice here, drinking lots of pure water, and avoiding alcohol. If you do this, it may keep you from having to pop pills with harmful side effects. All herbs, homeopathic remedies, packs, and supplements discussed here are available in health food stores and, increasingly, in large drug and grocery stores, as well as on the Internet.

Begin with Rest and Relaxation

During an acute attack of gout, it is of primary importance to rest and elevate the affected joint. This natural treatment is also recommended by practitioners of conventional medicine.

Aromatherapy

Aromatherapy is useful for gout, particularly the essential oils of carrot seed, chamomile, lavender, and yarrow. They are available in health food stores and stores specializing in aromatherapy products, listed in the yellow pages. (*See* AROMATHERAPY in PART 2 Treatment Section for additional information.)

Castor Oil Packs

Soak a piece of white flannel in warm castor oil, wring it out, and place over the inflamed joint. Cover with plastic and apply a heating pad. Do this twice a day for an hour each time.(*See* COMPRESSES, PACKS, and POULTICES in PART 2 Treatment Section for additional information.)

Diet

Diet is extremely important in any attack of gout and can either help alleviate the condition or exacerbate it, primarily because of the presence or absence of purines in the diet. Eating a diet low in purines is important because purines are present in nucleoproteins and, as previously mentioned, it is the breakdown of these nucleoproteins that leads to the formation of uric acid crystals and salts in the joints of certain individuals and, in turn, causes the painful gout condition.

There are two types of low purine foods. High-fiber foods are one type. Not only are they low in purines, but they have the additional benefit of helping to neutralize or eliminate purines. Eggs and dairy products are the other type. While they do not necessarily neutralize or eliminate purines, they are good for you simply because they are nourishing and are low in purines.

A high-fiber diet, consisting mainly of fruits and vegetables, plus nuts, seeds, and whole grains, is helpful because it works to eliminate uric acid by absorbing bile acids formed in the liver. This is important for people who are susceptible to gout because these bile acids act as a precursor to the buildup of uric acid, the root cause of the painful gout condition.

Good Foods

The following foods all have beneficial therapeutic powers because they can help stop the aggressive buildup of uric acid crystals. Fruits and vegetables and their juices are particularly beneficial because of their high potassium content (potassium helps to neutralize uric acid).

- ❑ Blueberries and strawberries contain substances that keep uric acid crystals from forming.
- ❑ Celery juice acts as a natural diuretic and, unlike the prescribed versions, does not decrease the amount of uric acid excreted in the urine. Juicing is preferable to pulverizing or blending because it removes indigestible fiber so more nutrients are available to your body in much larger quantities (an eight-ounce glass contains the juice from an entire bunch of celery). Although fiber is important, says Dr. Edward M. Wagner, ND, it should not be consumed in a pulverized state because fiber must be chewed thoroughly and mixed with saliva in order to break it down properly in your digestive system.
- ❑ Cherries. This fruit stops uric acid crystals from forming and causing the gout condition. During an attack, start eating fifteen to twenty-five cherries a day. Then, as the attack subsides, you can cut back to six to eight a day to prevent future attacks. Red or black, sweet, sour, or frozen cherries are all equally effective. You can also drink unsweetened cherry juice, which has the beneficial side effect of preventing tooth decay, and there is a cherry juice herbal concentrate that is very effective. It is available in health food stores and some specialty markets. You should drink one glassful a day.
- ❑ Fish, except those listed below as *bad foods*, is a good source of potassium, and potassium-rich foods protect your body against gout. Additionally, almost all types of fish, but particularly halibut, mackerel, salmon and tuna, are good because they aid in the production of omega-3 essential fatty acids which help regulate cellular metabolism and help keep your body on an even keel.
- ❑ Grapes are high in alkalines, which lessen the acidity of uric acid and aid in its elimination from the body.
- ❑ Parsley acts as a natural diuretic which, like celery, does not decrease the amount of uric acid excreted in the urine.
- ❑ Pears relieve inflammation of the kidneys.
- ❑ Pineapples contain bromelain, a natural anti-inflammatory.
- ❑ Vegetables (preferably raw) and their juices, such as beets, carrots, corn, leafy greens, legumes, potatoes, and yams, are all rich in potassium and fiber.
- ❑ Water is good because it dilutes the concentration of urine in the body. Drink eight to ten glasses a day and make sure it is pure water.

(*See* NUTRITIONAL THERAPY in PART 2 Treatment Section for additional information.)

Bad Foods

The following list of foods that contain purines may trigger an attack of gout, or may prolong the duration of one. By avoiding these foods in your diet, you can cut down on the amount and severity of gout attacks.

- ❑ Anchovies.
- ❑ Asparagus.

- ❑ Cauliflower.
- ❑ Herring.
- ❑ Mushrooms.
- ❑ Oatmeal.
- ❑ Organ meats, such as kidneys, liver, and sweetbreads.
- ❑ Peas.
- ❑ Poultry.
- ❑ Red meat, and meat-based broth and gravies.
- ❑ Sardines.
- ❑ Shrimp.
- ❑ Spinach.
- ❑ Sugar.
- ❑ White refined flour.

Other Substances to Avoid

- ❑ Alcohol, especially beer. Alcohol increases uric acid production.
- ❑ Aspirin. When you have pain, the first thing you usually reach for is the aspirin bottle, but if you have gout, it will make your pain worse because aspirin causes the retention of uric acid.
- ❑ Caffeine. This impairs kidney function, and good kidney functioning is needed to get uric acid out of the your system.

Heat Therapy/Cold Therapy

When a gout attack begins, ice and coldwater treatments are useful for controlling pain, swelling, and inflammation. Apply a crushed ice compress to the affected joint, or plunge it into cold water for ten minutes every half-hour. This therapy is most effective when used immediately after symptoms appear. (*See* COMPRESSES, PACKS, and POULTICES, HEAT THERAPY/COLD THERAPY, and HYDROTHERAPY in PART 2 Treatment Section for additional information.)

Herbal Remedies

- ❑ Black cohash moderates blood acidity.
- ❑ Burdock relieves gout symptoms.
- ❑ Devil's claw cleanses the body of toxic impurities.
- ❑ Guggulu, an ayurvedic herb, is very effective for arthritis conditions and is recommended for gout.
- ❑ Hydrangea is an anti-inflammatory.
- ❑ Juniper reduces inflammation.
- ❑ Nettle contains alkaloids, which neutralize uric acid.
- ❑ Psyllium leaves soothe the pain of gout.
- ❑ Saffron neutralizes uric acid buildup.

Take the above herbs as directed on label. They can also be used in teas and infusions. (*See* HERBAL REMEDIES in PART 2 Treatment Section for additional information.)

Homeopathic Remedies

You can self-treat with homeopathic remedies by selecting the one that most closely matches your symptoms. If you don't see improvement, try another or a combination product. Follow the instructions on the label. If you do not have relief in a reasonable amount of time, consult a physician who specializes in homeopathic medicine.

- ❑ Aconite 30c is good to use at the start of an attack when the joint is red, shiny, and very painful.
- ❑ Belladonna 6c is useful for typical gout symptoms when joints are swollen, red and shiny and when there are cutting, lightning-like pains that radiate through them.
- ❑ Colchinum 6c is beneficial when the pain is worse in the evenings and the afflicted parts are swollen and dark red.
- ❑ Urtica 30c is for acute attacks.

Take the above remedies as indicated on label. Combination remedies sometimes work more effectively than single ones. (*See* HOMEOPATHY in PART 2 Treatment Section for additional information.)

Hydrotherapy

Make a paste of half a cup of activated charcoal powder and water in a bowl. Stir in enough hot water to cover your foot and mix throroughly, then soak your foot in this for half an hour to an hour. (*See* HYDROTHERAPY in PART 2 Treatment Section for further information.)

Supplements

- ❑ Bromelain. 500 mg twice daily. This enzyme acts as an anti-inflammatory.
- ❑ Charcoal. Take $^1/_2$ to 1 teaspoon of activated charcoal four times daily. Charcoal can help reduce uric acid levels in the blood. Be aware that the use of charcoal can turn your stools black so don't be alarmed if this happens. You can also use charcoal for a foot bath. (*See* HYDROTHERAPY above in this entry.)

- ❏ DL-phenylalanine (DLPA). Take 500 mg four times daily on an empty stomach. This amino acid decreases pain.
- ❏ Fish oil. Take two 1000 mg capsules three times daily. Acts as an anti-inflammatory.
- ❏ Folic Acid. Take two 800 mcg tablets three times daily. Aids in nucleoprotein metabolism.
- ❏ L-Glutamine. Take 500 mg four times daily on an empty stomach. This amino acid acts as an antacid and, as such, helps to neutralize uric acid.
- ❏ L-Glutathione. Take 100 mg twice daily on an empty stomach. This amino acid increases cleansing of uric acid in the kidneys.
- ❏ L-Glycine. Take 500 mg four times daily between meals. Like L-Glutamine, this amino acid acts as an antacid.
- ❏ L-Methionine. Take 250 mg twice daily on an empty stomach. This amino acid detoxifies purines.
- ❏ Magnesium citrate. Take 400 mg three times daily. This mineral acts as an anti-spasmodic that relieves pain.
- ❏ Vitamin B_5 (Pantothene). Take 300 mg three times daily. This vitamin acts as an anti-inflammatory.
- ❏ Vitamin C, preferably Ester-C. Take at least 3000–5000 mg. You can take more, to bowel tolerance (when diarrhea occurs). If this happens, reduce the dosage until normal bowel function returns. Vitamin C reduces the levels of uric acid.

(*See* SUPPLEMENT THERAPY in PART 2 Treatment Section for additional information.)

ASSISTED ALTERNATIVE TREATMENTS

The following techniques may require specialized training or the aid of a healthcare professional.

Acupuncture and Acupressure

Acupuncture and acupressure reduce inflammation, relieve pain, and improve mobility. Acupuncture involves the insertion of extremely thin solid needles into specific points of your body to stimulate its own healing mechanism, improve blood flow to the affected areas, and create a smooth flow of vibratory energy throughout the body that can alleviate the pain of gout. There are rarely any risks or side effects. (*See* ACUPUNCTURE and ACUPRESSURE in PART 2 Treatment Section for additional information.)

Guided Imagery

Guided imagery can relieve stress and manage your pain. This pain-guage technique could help. Try visualizing your pain as a ten on a scale of one to ten, and then lower the reading on the guage. (*See* GUIDED IMAGERY and VISUALIZATION in PART 2 Treatment Section for additional information.)

Reflexology

Reflexology massage therapy can be performed on the unaffected foot or on the hands. (*See* REFLEXOLOGY in PART 2 Treatment Section for additional information.)

Tai Chi, Qigong, and Yoga

By helping you achieve a profoundly relaxed state, these therapies are useful for relieving your pain and boosting your general health. (*See* TAI CHI, QIGONG, and YOGA in PART 2 Treatment Section for additional information.)

(*See also* OSTEOARTHRITIS in PART 1 Conditions Section.)

Irritable Bowel Syndrome (IBS)

Irritable bowel syndrome (IBS), sometimes called spastic colon or mucous colitis, is a condition of abnormally increased movement of the small and large intestines, leading to pain and a change of bowel patterns, and causing excessive mucus and toxins to form in the bowels. IBS occurs most frequently in women, usually beginning between twenty to thirty-years-old. Up to 20 percent of the American population has symptoms of IBS, but very few people seek treatment. It is not a life-threatening condition, but it is a frequent health-related reason for missing work. And, although it is unrelated to other problems of the digestive system, such as the inflammatory bowel diseases (Crohn's or ulcerative colitis), and does not cause inflammation, it is possible to have both irritable bowel syndrome and an inflammatory bowel disease at the same time.

Symptoms

- Abdominal pain after eating that is relieved by a bowel movement.
- Abdominal pain, bloating, distention, and tenderness.
- Diarrhea that alternates with constipation.
- Flatulence.
- Loss of appetite.
- Mucus in the stools.
- Nausea.
- Vomiting.

Causes

The exact causes are not known, but some possibilities include dietary fats, food allergies, and stress.

Diagnosing the Problem

Diagnosis is made from the person's history. A screening for colon cancer and inflammatory bowel disease should also be performed.

Conventional Treatments

- Antidepressants can help block pain.
- Antispasmodics, such as belladonna and lomotil, can relieve pain.
- Lotronex can control diarrhea.
- Psyllium is a good source of fiber, and helps promote regular bowel movements.
- Zelnorm relieves bloating, constipation, and pain.

Problems with Some Conventional Treatments

- Antidepressants and antispasmodics have side effects, such as dry mouth, visual blurriness, and dizziness.
- Lotronex can cause such serious problems as constipation and inflammation of the large bowel. It was removed from the market in November, 2000 after causing several deaths, but in June, 2002 the FDA allowed the drug to return to the market. If this drug is recommended to you, be sure to get a second opinion from a gastroenterologist who is more qualified to make a differential diagnosis between IBS and other conditions with similar symptoms and knows who *not* to treat with Lotronex.

  Note: Although the FDA hasn't blocked its use for men, at this time the drug has only been approved for treating women.
- Psyllium can cause bloating and flatulence and should not be taken within thirty to forty-five minutes of taking supplements as it can interfere with their absorption.
- Zelnorm is approved for short-term use only. It can lead to diarrhea, which usually stops after the first week. Its safety and effectiveness in men has not been evaluated at this time.

SELF-HELP ALTERNATIVE TREATMENTS

Many medications for bowel problems have undesirable side effects so you may want to try the following self-help alternative techniques, which can be done at home, to promote wellness. All herbs, homeopathic remedies, packs, and supplements discussed here are available in health food stores and, increasingly, in large drug and grocery stores, as well as on the Internet.

Aromatherapy

Aromatherapy is particularly useful for relieving symptoms related to the digestive system. To relieve constipation, black pepper, cardamom, cinnamon leaf, citronella, ginger, and peppermint oils have a stimulating effect. Mix two or three drops of these oils with a carrier oil, such as sweet almond oil, and use to massage the abdomen in a clockwise direction. You can also add up to ten drops of these oils to your bath water, or soak a piece of flannel in hot water containing four or five drops of oil and apply it as a compress.

For control of diarrhea, chamomile, cinnamon, clove, geranium, ginger, lavender, nutmeg, tea tree oils, and thyme are beneficial. Use as above.

Do not ingest essential oils or use them full strength as they are very powerful compounds. They are available in health food stores and stores specializing in aromatherapy products which you can find in the yellow pages. (*See* AROMATHERAPY in PART 2 Treatment Section for additional information.)

Castor Oil Packs

Dip a piece of white flannel into some warm castor oil. Wring it out and place it over the affected abdominal area. Cover with plastic and apply a heating pad for one hour. Do this twice daily. (*See* COMPRESSES, PACKS, and POULTICES in PART 2 Treatment Section for additional information.) (*See also* AROMATHERAPY above.)

Diet

If you have any kind of bowel problem, you may have food intolerances. These are not true allergies caused by an immune system response, but are metabolic in nature and can best be evaluated by an elimination diet whereby suspected foods are avoided and then gradually reintroduced. This should be monitored by a qualified nutritionist.

Good Foods

IBS is best treated by reducing irritation to the digestive system, so certain dietary modifications may be helpful. Try to eat foods containing fiber from a source other than wheat because wheat may cause food sensitivities. Good sources of fiber are barley, beans, brown rice, fruit, guar gum, oat bran, peas, psyllium, and vegetables.

Note: Although psyllium is a good source of fiber, it can cause bloating so it is probably better to get fiber from whole foods. (*See* NUTRITIONAL THERAPY in PART 2 Treatment Section for additional information.)

Bad Foods

The following foods may exacerbate your condition.

- ❏ Animal fats.
- ❏ Citrus fruits.
- ❏ Corn.
- ❏ Dairy products (for those who are lactose intolerant).
- ❏ Eggs.
- ❏ Fried foods.
- ❏ Nuts.
- ❏ Pastries.
- ❏ Peanuts.
- ❏ Processed foods.
- ❏ Seeds.
- ❏ Spicy foods.
- ❏ Sugars (not easily digested, and intestinal microbes feed on them and further injure the intestinal walls).
- ❏ Wheat.

Other Substances to Avoid

Anyone who has a bowel disorder has a problem with alcohol, caffeine, carbonated beverages, and tobacco because they are irritating to the gastrointestinal tract. Additionally, all artificial sweeteners, especially aspartame, minnitol, and sorbitol, can cause diarrhea.

Herbal Remedies

- ❏ Artichoke leaf extract has anti-inflammatory properties.
- ❏ Balm has an antispasmodic effect on the intestines,
- ❏ Cat's claw has healing properties for the digestive tract.
- ❏ Chamomile has an antispasmodic effect on the intestines and can help relieve alternating bouts of constipation and diarrhea.
- ❏ Charcoal tablets, per label, relieve gas and bloating. Note: For occasional use only, as charcoal also absorbs nutrients.
- ❏ Ginger is known to relieve most digestive problems.
- ❏ Peppermint oil, enteric-coated to avoid its being absorbed into the upper digestive tract. (When a product is enteric-coated, that means it is specially prepared so it breaks down in the intestines, not the stomach, and only intestinal enzymes can digest it.) Peppermint helps relieve gas, bloating, and cramps, soothes irritation, and relaxes the muscles in the bowel.
- ❏ Rosemary has an antispasmodic effect on the intestines.
- ❏ Valerian also has an antispasmodic effect on the intestines.

Take the above herbs as directed on label. They can also be used in teas and infusions. (*See* HERBAL REMEDIES in PART 2 Treatment Section for additional information.)

Homeopathic Remedies

You can self-treat with homeopathic remedies by selecting the one that most closely matches your symptoms. If you don't see improvement, try another, or a combination product. Follow the instructions on the label. If you do not have relief in a reasonable amount of time, consult a physician who specializes in homeopathic medicine.

The following homeopathic remedies are useful for *all* painful bowel problems, including irritable bowel syndrome.

- ❑ Argentum nitricum eases bloating, flatulence, and diarrhea that occurs after drinking water.
- ❑ Bismuth relieves diarrhea.
- ❑ Bryonia relieves constipation.
- ❑ Carbo veg controls diarrhea alternating with constipation, a frequent symptom of irritable bowel syndrome.
- ❑ Chamomilla relieves diarrhea.
- ❑ Colocynthis eases abdominal pain and cramping that eases by bending over or applying pressure.
- ❑ Dulcamara helps control diarrhea containing mucous.
- ❑ Hydrastis relieves constipation.
- ❑ Iris ver also relieves constipation.
- ❑ Kali sulph relieves diarrhea containing mucous.
- ❑ Lycopodium helps control bloating, constipation, gas, heartburn, and pain.
- ❑ Mag phos is an antispasmodic.
- ❑ Nat mur aids digestion.
- ❑ Nux vomica helps relieve gas, cramps, and muscular soreness in the abdomen.
- ❑ Podophyllum helps control diarrhea that alternates with constipation and is accompanied by weakness.
- ❑ Sulphur is useful for anyone with morning diarrhea and excessive gas.

Combination remedies sometimes work more effectively than single ones. (*See* HOMEOPATHY in PART 2 Treatment Section for additional information.)

Meditation

Meditation can help with the stress that can cause irritable bowel syndrome. (*See* MEDITATION in PART 2 Treatment Section for additional information.)

Supplements

The following help your body function better and make it more resistant to irritable bowel syndrome (IBS).

- ❑ Acidophilus, per label, replenishes friendly bacteria.
- ❑ Evening primrose oil, per label, supplies essential fatty acids.
- ❑ 5-HTP helps raise serotonin levels naturally. Serotonin is a neurotransmitter helpful for reducing pain and anxiety and regulating sleep patterns. Start by taking 30–50 mg at bedtime. The dose can be increased to 100 mg three times a day on an empty stomach over a three to four week period.
- ❑ Garlic capsules, per label, help destroy toxins in the colon.
- ❑ Grapefruit seed extract, per label, helps relieve constipation and flatulence.
- ❑ A high-potency multivitamin and mineral complex is important for replacing nutrients that have not been absorbed. Note: Check label to see if recommended amounts of vitamin A, the Bs, and zinc are present. Do not overdose.
- ❑ Lactase enzymes, per label, should be taken before consuming dairy products.
- ❑ Proteolytic enzymes, per label, aid in protein digestion and reduce inflammation.
- ❑ Vitamin A aids tissue repair. Take 25,000 IU daily.
- ❑ Zinc promotes healing. Take 30 mg daily.

(*See* SUPPLEMENT THERAPY in PART 2 Treatment Section for additional information.)

ASSISTED ALTERNATIVE TREATMENTS

The following techniques may require specialized training or the aid of a healthcare professional.

Acupuncture and Acupressure

Acupuncture involves the insertion of extremely thin solid needles into specific points of your body to stimulate its own healing mechanism and improve blood flow to the affected areas. It also reduces inflammation, relieves pain, improves mobility, and there are rarely any risks or side effects. (*See* ACUPUNCTURE and ACUPRESSURE in PART 2 Treatment Section for additional information.)

Applied Kinesiology

Applied kinesiology is a non-invasive, non-toxic method that can correct imbalances in the body. It is excellent for reducing pain rapidly, including the abdominal pain often experienced by those with irritable bowel syndrome. (*See*

APPLIED KINESIOLOGY in PART 2 Treatment Section for additional information.)

Biofeedback

Biofeedback is useful for reducing stress in anyone with irritable bowel syndrome. (*See* BIOFEEDBACK in PART 2 Treatment Section for additional information.)

Chiropractic

Chiropractic theory is based on the assumption that a properly aligned spine is essential for good health, and that any misalignment of the vertebrae in the spine causes pressure on the spinal nerves, leading to pain. The chiropractor makes spinal adjustments to move misaligned vertebrae to more normal positions which helps the nervous system to function properly. (*See* CHIROPRACTIC in PART 2 Treatment Section for additional information.)

Craniosacral Therapy

Craniosacral therapy is a form of energy healing that can help balance your system. It has been shown to be effective for soothing irritable bowel problems. (*See* CRANIOSACRAL THERAPY in PART 2 Treatment Section for additional information.)

Cupping

Cupping helps to promote energy flow and reduce pain. (*See* CUPPING in PART 2 Treatment Section for additional information.)

Exercise and Stretching

Stretching exercises help improve digestion. To avoid further damage to the affected area, they must be carefully supervised in the beginning. (*See* EXERCISE, STRETCHING, and SPORTS in PART 2 Treatment Section for additional information.)

Guided Imagery

Guided Imagery helps relieve stress and manage pain. Visualizing your abdominal area as soft and relaxed can be useful to help relieve the stress associated with irritable bowel pain. (*See* GUIDED IMAGERY and VISUALIZATION in PART 2 Treatment Section for additional information.)

Hypnosis

Hypnosis is useful for reducing stress in those with irritable bowel syndrome. (*See* HYPNOSIS in PART 2 Treatment Section for additional information.)

Massage

A massage helps bring blood to the affected area to relieve the pain. There are many kinds of massage therapies available and you can ask your practitioner to suggest the appropriate one to relieve the pain associated with irritable bowel syndrome. (*See* MASSAGE in PART 2 Treatment Section for additional information.) (*See also* AROMATHERAPY in this entry.)

Reflexology

Reflexology massage therapy can be performed on the part of the foot or hand corresponding to the abdominal area that is in pain. (*See* REFLEXOLOGY in PART 2 Treatment Section for additional information.)

Tai Chi, Qigong, and Yoga

These therapies help your body to enter a relaxed state and also increase production of endorphins, which are natural painkillers. (*See* TAI CHI, QIGONG, and YOGA in PART 2 Treatment Section for additional information.)

PRACTICAL SUGGESTIONS

❑ Do not wear tight clothing around your waist.

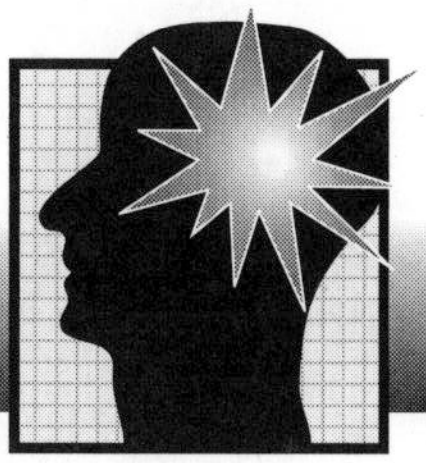

Migraine Headaches

Headaches are symptoms of underlying conditions, not diseases in themselves, and are almost universal. Each year, more than 40 million Americans seek treatment for relief of their headache pain. (For more information on the overall problem of headaches, see inset, THE SILENT EPIDEMIC, on page 34.) If you have a headache accompanied by breathing problems, fever, or a stiff neck, or if it occurs after a head injury or respiratory infection, you should seek medical help immediately because it could be a symptom of a life-threatening condition. Medical help should also be sought if you have headaches that: occur daily; do not respond to simple pain relievers; become progressively worse; are caused by exertion from coughing, sneezing or exercise; or are accompanied by numbness, loss of consciousness, or hallucinations.

Symptoms

Migraine headaches are very painful and most often begin on one side of the head, near an eye; they sometimes worsen with exposure to light. The pain is described as a severe throbbing sensation, often accompanied by nausea, vomiting, and visual changes. Prior to the onset of pain, people with migraines frequently have visual disturbances—they see flashing or jagged lights. Women account for about 70 percent of those with migraines and the onset is typically under the age of forty. Migraine headaches can occur anywhere from several times a week to several times a year. They usually last from four to eight hours, but can sometimes last for days. Often a family history is present.

Common Causes

Migraines occur when blood vessels contract and then expand. They may be triggered by allergies or sensitivities to specific foods, such as aged cheese, chocolate, nuts, shellfish, and red wine.

There are many more factors that can trigger a headache. Some of the most common are:

- Air pollution;
- Alcohol consumption;
- Bruxism (grinding of teeth);
- Change in altitude;
- Clenching the jaw;
- Constipation;
- Dehydration;
- Eye problems, or improper eyeglass prescriptions;
- Glare from fluorescent lights;
- Hormonal changes;
- Imbalance in brain chemicals and nerve pathways;
- Insomnia or too much sleep;
- Low barometric pressure;
- Low levels of fresh air, as found in airplane cabins or poorly ventilated buildings;
- Low serotonin levels;
- Narrowing of the blood vessels going into the brain, muscles, and tissues of the neck and scalp;
- Overexposure to sun;
- Side effects of prescribed medications, including hormone replacement therapy, nitroglycerin (taken for angina), and some asthma drugs;
- Smoking and second-hand tobacco smoke;
- Stress;
- Tension;
- TMJ misalignment;
- Video display terminals and television screens.

Diagnosing the Problem

Diagnosis is made by evaluating the person's history. A proper diagnosis is essential to rule out the possibility of brain tumors, intracranial pressure changes, or meningeal inflammation—an inflammation of the membranes surrounding the brain and spinal cord. Once these potentially serious conditions have been ruled out, the type of headache can be determined by its symptoms, which are described above.

Conventional Treatments

Some medications prevent the onset of headaches, others relieve them after they've begun. The following are the most frequently used medications.

- ❑ Analgesics (painkillers). These reduce or relieve pain without addressing its cause.
- ❑ Antidepressants. They help soothe the tension contributing to headaches.
- ❑ Anti-inflammatory drugs. They reduce the inflammation that contributes to the pain.
- ❑ Antiseizure medications. They can reduce the frequency of migraine headaches when taken daily. (No one knows exactly how they work, but they have been found effective.)
- ❑ Beta blockers and calcium channel blockers. They stabilize blood vessels.
- ❑ Cafergot (ergotamine). This works as an abortive treatment for migraine headaches. Abortive treatments help keep a mild headache from becoming worse.
- ❑ Caffeine. It constricts blood vessels, reducing swelling, and this is helpful in migraines.
- ❑ DHE intranasal spray. This relatively new drug gets absorbed more quickly.
- ❑ Imitrex (Sumatriptan). This intensifies the activity of serotonin receptors in the brain and can relieve a headache that has already become severe.
- ❑ Methysergide, a vasoconstrictor, helps to prevent migraine headaches because it is involved in constricting the blood vessels.
- ❑ Midrin and Norgesic Forte. Both are abortive treatments.
- ❑ Oxygen Therapy.
- ❑ Stadol. Inhaled through the nose, this spray helps relieve chronic tension headaches.

Problems with Some Conventional Treatments

- ❑ At first, caffeine constricts blood vessels, easing some types of headache pain, including migraines, but when it wears off, rebound swelling occurs, and that can ultimately worsen the pain.
- ❑ Overuse of analgesics can be counterproductive by causing the blood vessels to become less sensitive to the medication. When this happens, higher doses are needed, setting up a vicious cycle.
- ❑ In connection with this, over-the-counter analgesics (painkillers), even used as infrequently as five times a week, can turn periodic headaches into chronic rebound headaches.
- ❑ Long-term use of nonsteroidal anti-inflammatory drugs (NSAIDs) may cause kidney, liver, or stomach problems.
- ❑ Methysergide may lead to fibroid growth in the kidneys. It can also cause permanent scar tissue around the heart and lungs. Anyone using this drug must be closely supervised.
- ❑ Stadol is potentially addictive and subject to abuse.
- ❑ Vasoconstrictors constrict all other arteries in the body. If, for example, a heart problem is present, vasoconstrictors could ultimately make things worse.

Botox as Painkiller?

Botulinum toxin (botox) may be a poison, but it is also an organic product derived from a common bacterium that is taking its place alongside other natural poisons with medicinal uses. Researchers all over the world are now testing it, often successfully, for a wide variety of treatments, including migraine headaches and back pain, with one researcher even comparing it to penicillin for its versatility.

SELF-HELP ALTERNATIVE TREATMENTS

The following techniques for alleviating migraine headaches can be done at home. Although they may not work as fast as drugs or surgery, natural alternatives help the body heal itself. All herbs, homeopathic remedies, packs, and supplements discussed here are available in health food stores and, increasingly, in large drug and grocery stores, as well as on the Internet.

Aromatherapy

Aromatherapy is useful for headaches, particularly the essential oils of basil, cajeput, eucalyptus, lavender, niaouli, peppermint, and rosemary. They are available in health food stores and stores specializing in aromatherapy products listed in the yellow pages. (*See* AROMATHERAPY in PART 2 Treatment Section for additional information.)

Compresses, Packs, and Poultices

Alternate hot and cold compresses. Use heat for three minutes and cold for one minute and keep switching for about fifteen minutes. Castor oil packs have also been recommended for headaches. Soak a piece of white flannel in warm castor oil, wring it out and place it over the headache area. Cover with plastic and apply a heating pad. Do this twice a day for an hour each time.(*See* COMPRESSES, PACKS, and POULTICES, HEAT THERAPY/COLD THERAPY, and HYDROTHERAPY in PART 2 Treatment Section for additional information.)

Diet

Knowing which foods to eat and which to avoid can help ameliorate or even ward off headaches.

Good Foods

- ❑ Caffeinated beverages taken in small amounts raise serotonin levels and help constrict dilated blood vessels, but sometimes, when caffeine wears off, a rebound effect occurs, causing swelling of the blood vessels. Do not overdo the caffeine. If a small amount helps, more will not necessarily be better.
- ❑ Raw fruits, vegetables, and juices, especially carrot and celery juices, help relieve migraine headaches by keeping the system more alkaline. (According to Dr. Edward M. Wagner, ND, migraines are basically an acid condition.)

(*See* NUTRITIONAL THERAPY in PART 2 Treatment Section for additional information.)

Bad Foods

The following substances can bring on, or worsen, a headache.

- ❑ Aged cheese.
- ❑ Alcohol.
- ❑ Aspartame—an artificial sweetener.
- ❑ Avocados.
- ❑ Bananas.
- ❑ Chicken livers.
- ❑ Chocolate.
- ❑ Cured meats.
- ❑ Fermented foods, such as sour cream and yogurt.
- ❑ Herring.
- ❑ Hot dogs.
- ❑ Monosodium glutamate (MSG).
- ❑ Nuts.
- ❑ Onions.
- ❑ Red wine.
- ❑ Salami.
- ❑ Vinegar.
- ❑ Wheat.

Other Substances to Avoid

Aftershave lotion, molds, perfume, and tobacco can all bring on headaches.

Herbal Remedies

- ❑ Burdock root helps purify the blood.
- ❑ Cayenne aids circulation.
- ❑ Feverfew makes your body less responsive to the chemicals that cause spasms in the muscles surrounding your brain.
- ❑ Various forms of ginger teas and capsules help alleviate nausea accompanying migraines.
- ❑ Ginkgo biloba reduces the formation of platelet-activating factor which may contribute to migraines.
- ❑ Goldenseal has anti-inflammatory properties.
- ❑ Lobelia is a relaxant.
- ❑ Mint helps relieve nausea.
- ❑ Peppermint helps oxygenate the bloodstream.
- ❑ White willow bark has an effect similar to aspirin.

Take according to label instructions. (*See* HERBAL REMEDIES in PART 2 Treatment Section for additional information.)

Homeopathic Remedies

You can self-treat with homeopathic remedies by selecting the one that most closely matches your symptoms. If you don't see improvement, try another, or a combination product. Follow the instructions on the label. If you do not have relief in a reasonable amount of time, consult a physician who specializes in homeopathic medicine.

- ❑ Belladonna relieves headaches that start at the back of the head or upper neck.
- ❑ Bryonia helps relieve splitting headaches that settle over one eye.

- ❑ Cimicifuga relieves headaches with throbbing pain that worsens with motion.
- ❑ Cyclamen helps migraines that start with visual effects, such as flickering in the eyes or dim vision.
- ❑ Ignatia helps headaches caused by emotional upsets or grief.
- ❑ Iris versicolor relieves intense migraines accompanied by blurred vision.
- ❑ Kali bichromicum is useful for migraines that start with light sensitivity.
- ❑ Lachesis relieves left-sided migraines.
- ❑ Natrum muriaticum relieves migraines that usually occur on the right side and worsen from emotional upsets.
- ❑ Sanguinaria relieves right-sided migraines accompanied by tension in the neck and shoulder that extends to the forehead, with extreme pain in the eye.
- ❑ Sepia relieves left-sided migraines accompanied by dizziness and nausea.
- ❑ Silica relieves migraines that occur after mental exertion and that worsen with exposure to cold.
- ❑ Spigelia relieves left-sided throbbing headaches accompanied by pain above or through the eyeball.

Instructions for use are usually printed on the label. (*See* HOMEOPATHY in PART 2 Treatment Section for additional information.)

Magnet Therapy

Magnet therapy can help relieve head pain. Placing magnets on the area of the head that is in pain brings increased amounts of blood to the area which, in turn brings oxygen and other healing substances to ease the pain. (*See* MAGNET THERAPY in PART 2 Treatment Section for additional information.)

Meditation

Meditation helps reduce stress, which contributes to head pain. (*See* MEDITATION in PART 2 Treatment Section for additional information.)

Supplements

- ❑ Calcium. Take 1500 mg daily to help transmission of nerve impulses.
- ❑ Fish Oil. Take 1 gram per pound of body weight. Fish oil modifies prostaglandins, hormone-like substances made by the body that may cause headaches.
- ❑ 5-HTP. This amino acid helps raise serotonin levels, and people with migraines often have low serotonin levels. Take per instructions on label.
- ❑ Magnesium. 400 mg three times daily helps relieve pain. Women with pre-menstrual migraines might benefit from a single 400-mg dose.
- ❑ Potassium. 100 mg daily aids in proper sodium and potassium balance, necessary to avoid fluid retention, which may put pressure on the brain.
- ❑ SAMe (S-adenosyl-L-methionine) is a mood stabilizer and helps regenerate nerves. Take per instructions on label.
- ❑ Vitamin B-complex. 50 mg taken twice daily relieves stress.
- ❑ Vitamin E. 400 IU taken twice a day aids circulation.

(*See* SUPPLEMENT THERAPY in PART 2 Treatment Section for additional information.)

ASSISTED ALTERNATIVE TREATMENTS

The following techniques may require specialized training or the aid of a healthcare professional.

Acupuncture and Acupressure

Acupuncture and acupressure create a smooth flow of vibratory energy throughout the body. Practitioners aim to move the energy away from the head. For self-treatment with acupressure, knead the area between your thumb and index finger. (*See* ACUPUNCTURE and ACUPRESSURE in PART 2 Treatment Section for additional information.)

Applied Kinesiology

Applied Kinesiology can help reduce migraine pain. The AK practitioner tests your muscles to determine the origin of your problem and then decides on the best course of action, choosing from a wide variety of therapeutic methods at her or his disposal. (*See* APPLIED KINESIOLOGY in PART 2 Treatment Section for additional information.)

Bee Venom Therapy

Some components of bee venom are thought to stimulate the immune system. Other components are thought to modify the transmission of pain signals within the nervous system, and the therapy has proven consistently useful for painful conditions. (*See* BEE VENOM THERAPY in PART 2 Treatment Section for additional information.)

Biofeedback

Biofeedback works by reducing stress and the physical responses, such as a headache, associated with it. (*See* BIOFEEDBACK in PART 2 Treatment Section for additional information.)

Chiropractic

Poor vertebral alignment, often the result of wearing high heels or having flat feet, may reduce blood flow to the brain, which can cause headaches. Chiropractic manipulation can help correct this situation. (*See* CHIROPRACTIC in PART 2 Treatment Section for additional information.)

Craniosacral Therapy

Headaches caused by pressure of cranial fluid can be eased by gently manipulating the cranial bones. (*See* CRANIOSACRAL THERAPY in PART 2 Treatment Section for additional information.)

Cupping

Cupping can ease headaches that are caused by a lack of oxygen in the cells. It helps promote energy flow and reduces swelling and pain. (*See* CUPPING in PART 2 Treatment Section for additional information.)

Exercise

Aerobic activity reduces stress and increases the production of endorphins, which helps to raise the pain threshold. In the beginning, these should be carefully supervised to avoid damage. (*See* EXERCISE, STRETCHING, and SPORTS in PART 2 Treatment Section for additional information.)

Guided Imagery and Visualization Techniques

Guided imagery can help manage headache pain. Since most headaches are described as vise-like, or as a feeling of tightness, picture a tool that can loosen the vise. (*See* GUIDED IMAGERY and VISUALIZATION in PART 2 Treatment Section for additional information.)

Hypnosis

Hypnosis helps you relax and relaxation alleviates stress, which contributes to headache pain. (*See* HYPNOSIS in PART 2 Treatment Section for additional information.)

Massage

A massage can help your body relax, thereby reducing head pain caused by stress. There are many kinds of massage therapies available and you can ask your practitioner to suggest the appropriate one for your migraine problem. Many conventional doctors are now extolling the benefits of massage. (*See* MASSAGE in PART 2 Treatment Section for additional information.)

Osteopathic Manipulation

Osteopathic manipulation can help decrease muscle tension, which is a contributing factor to many types of headaches. (*See* OSTEOPATHIC MANIPULATION in PART 2 Treatment Section for additional information.)

Oxygen Therapy

Oxygen therapy, also listed in conventional therapies in this entry (which underscores its dual role as a therapy), is a useful adjunct for treating headaches, especially migraines. (*See* OXYGEN THERAPIES in PART 2 Treatment Section for additional information.)

Physical Therapy

Physical therapy helps correct and improve your body's natural healing mechanisms and can help to prevent the return of symptoms. (*See* PHYSICAL THERAPY in PART 2 Treatment Section for additional information.)

Reflexology

Reflexology massage therapy performed on the specific

PASS THE OXYGEN

Millions of listeners to *Good Morning America* heard Dr. Nancy Snyderman extol the benefits of oxygen therapy for headaches. Pure oxygen is the most popular treatment for stopping headaches, she said, because it is highly effective and it is safer than other treatments, which can have powerful side effects.

part of the foot and/or hand that corresponds with the head can be helpful. (*See* REFLEXOLOGY in PART 2 Treatment Section for additional information.)

Tai Chi, Qigong, and Yoga

These therapies induce a profoundly relaxed state and help bring healing energy to the body. Relaxation techniques and concentrating on your breathing can relieve tension. One technique is to take six deep even breaths, counting to four as you inhale and as you exhale. (*See* TAI CHI, QIGONG, and YOGA in PART 2 Treatment Section for additional information.)

PRACTICAL SUGGESTIONS

- ❑ Stay hydrated. Drink eight to ten glasses of water a day; if your indoor air is dry, use a humidifier.
- ❑ Improve the quality of your indoor air. A negative ion generator or HEPA filter will remove unhealthy particles. If you live in an unpolluted area, open your windows at least fifteen minutes a day. Houseplants also filter indoor pollution from the air.
- ❑ Use incandescent bulbs. The flickering in fluorescent light tubes may not be noticeable, but it can be enough to bring on a headache.

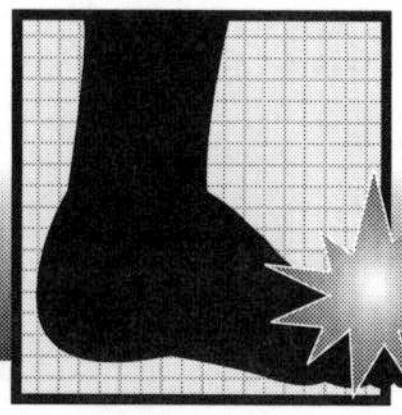

Neuroma (Foot Ailment)

Although there are many types of neuromas, the one we are concerned with in this book is Morton's neuroma, a benign, painful, swollen growth of nerve tissue, usually occurring between the base of the third and fourth toes, although it can occur between any two toes. The neuroma, which may be soft or hard and can vary in size, usually occurs on one foot only and affects more women than men.

There are several other kinds of neuromas, which include acoustic neuroma, a benign tumor of the acoustic nerve (the eighth cranial nerve) leading from the brain to the inner ear that can cause dizziness and lead to hearing loss. If the tumor grows very large, it can press on the trigeminal nerves (*see* TRIGEMINAL NEURALGIA in PART 1 Conditions Section). Cystic neuroma, also called false neuroma, is a tumor of the nerve tissue that has become sac-like (cystic). Ganglionar neuroma occurs in the stomach area, usually in children. Multiple neuroma, also known as endocrine neoplasias (type IIB), or neuromatosis, is numerous benign tumors of nerve cells and fibers in the mucous membrane. Myelinic neuroma, also known as medullated neuroma or fascicular neuroma is a tumor made of covered nerve fibers. Traumatic neuroma occurs after severe injury to a nerve.

Symptoms

In the early stages, there may only be a mild ache around the toe (usually the fourth), accompanied by a burning or tingling sensation, along with numbness, in the ball of your foot. You might feel like you have gravel or pebbles in your shoe under the ball of your foot. As the condition progresses, the pain can move from the tumor to the ends of the affected nerve, and a constant burning sensation can spread to the tips of the toes. The pain can be aggravated by improper footwear and also by walking, running, or going up and down stairs. Symptoms can usually be relieved by taking off your shoes and massaging your foot, but if any pain occurs while you are resting, it is possible that the neuroma is worsening.

Common Causes

Several factors can contribute to the development of a neuroma, primarily anything that causes constriction or irritation of the nerve. The most common factors are:

- ❑ Bunions, because they don't allow the foot to move properly;
- ❑ High heels;
- ❑ Inflammatory conditions, such as arthritis;
- ❑ Tight shoes;
- ❑ Trauma from recreational or occupational activities.

Diagnosing the Problem

It is easier to cure a neuroma when it is diagnosed early because the nerve becomes thicker and more painful over time if not treated. Diagnosis is based on a history of symptoms. If you have shooting, stabbing, or radiating pain while walking that is relieved by removing your shoes and massaging the area, the doctor will suspect a neuroma, especially if a moveable mass is present, and pressing on it, or moving it, replicates the pain. A clicking sensation may also be present. X-rays can rule out other causes, but they do not actually show a neuroma. An MRI will show it, as will an ultrasound, which is increasingly used to help determine the exact location of the neuroma.

Conventional Treatments

The goal of treatment is to relieve the symptoms, and it may be surgical or non-surgical. Treatments include the following:

- ❑ Anti-inflammatories;
- ❑ Cortisone injections mixed with a local anesthetic help relieve pain and swelling of the nerve;
- ❑ Icing your foot helps reduce swelling near the nerve (*See* HYDROTHERAPY in PART 2 Treatment Section for additional information);
- ❑ Orthotics and other shoe inserts, such as arch supports and metatarsal pads to help reposition body weight and prevent nerve irritation;
- ❑ Pads, and wider, more supportive, shoes to help decrease abnormal pressure on the neuroma;
- ❑ Surgical removal of the neuroma (neurectomy).

Problems with Some Conventional Treatments

- ❑ Anti-inflammatories can cause gastrointestinal problems.
- ❑ Cortisone injections should be given only by an experienced orthopedic surgeon or podiatrist who has made a correct diagnosis. If an infection has been mis-

taken for an injury, cortisone can make the infection worse. In inexperienced hands, a cortisone injection can introduce an infection through the skin. Cortisone should never be injected directly into a nerve or tendon because of the possibility of a rupture. In addition, overuse of cortisone causes bone death. Even short-term use can weaken tendons and cause further damage to the nerves. You should never have more than three cortisone injections a year in any one area.

- No surgical procedure is completely risk-free. Following a neurectomy, there can be recurrence of bleeding, infection, pain, or a painful scar. A small percentage of those who have had surgery experience a regrowth of the nerve and have worse pain than they did before the surgery. There is a permanent numbness between the toes where the nerve was removed, but most of those who have had the surgery say it is preferable to the pain.

SELF-HELP ALTERNATIVE TREATMENTS

The following techniques can be done at home. Although they may not work as fast as drugs or surgery, natural alternatives help the body heal itself. All herbs, homeopathic remedies, packs, and supplements discussed here are available in health food stores and, increasingly, in large drug and grocery stores, as well as on the Internet.

Aromatherapy

Aromatherapy, particularly the essential oils of cinnamon leaf, clove, eucalyptus, lavender, pine, rosemary, tea tree, and thyme, stimulate the immune system. (*See* AROMATHERAPY in PART 2 Treatment Section for additional information.)

Compresses, Packs, and Poultices

A poultice consisting of a combination of comfrey, pau d'arco, ragwort, and wood sage helps relieve pain and inflammation. (*See* COMPRESSES, PACKS, and POULTICES in PART 2 Treatment Section for additional information.)

Diet

What you eat may play a role in the development of tumors, so certain dietary modifications can be helpful.

Good Foods

A strict macrobiotic regime can be helpful, but it is difficult for many people to follow. Try to eat as many macrobiotic foods, such as brown rice, cabbage and other cruciferous vegetables, as possible, avoiding bananas, potatoes, tomatoes, and meats. In general, eat lots of fruits and vegetables and drink their juices. The darker colored fruits and vegetables have higher amounts of antioxidants, which help stimulate your immune system. Maitake, reishi, and shiitake mushrooms also stimulate the immune system.

(*See* NUTRITIONAL THERAPY in PART 2 Treatment Section for additional information.)

Bad Foods

Eliminating, or greatly reducing animal protein helps to starve tumors.

Other Substances to Avoid

Chemicals found in aerosol products, cleaning products, paints, and pesticides all promote the formation of free radicals in your body. Free radicals play havoc with your immune system. And, of course, don't smoke, and avoid second-hand smoke.

Herbal Remedies

- Chapparal has anti-tumor properties and is a painkiller.
- Burdock root stimulates the immune system.
- Dandelion cleanses the blood and liver.
- Pau d'arco is one of the strongest immune-system stimulants.
- Red clover reduces inflammation and helps purify the blood.

Take the above herbs as directed on label. They can also be used in teas and infusions. (*See* HERBAL REMEDIES in PART 2 Treatment Section for additional information.)

Homeopathic Remedies

You can self-treat with homeopathic remedies by selecting the one that most closely matches your symptoms. If you don't see improvement, try another, or a combination product. Follow the instructions on the label. If you do not have relief in a reasonable amount of time, consult a physician who specializes in homeopathic medicine. Helpful remedies are listed below.

- Arnica is useful following surgery.
- Berberis vulgaris is recommended for stabbing pain that occurs between the metatarsal bones when standing, or if you have pain on the ball of your foot when walking.
- Causticum is useful for numbness that alternates with pain.
- Cuprum helps relieve severe cramping.
- Hypericum eases biting or stitching pain between the ball of the foot and the toes.

- ❑ Ledum eases stabbing pain in the third toe that is relieved by cold applications.
- ❑ Rhus toxicodendron is useful for pain and cramping that is worse with initial motion and eases with continued activity.
- ❑ Ruta graveolens is helpful with pain in the ball of the foot that shoots into the toes, is aggravated by cold, damp weather, worsens with excessive activity, and eases after light activity.

Combination remedies sometimes work more effectively than single ones. (*See* HOMEOPATHY in PART 2 Treatment Section for additional information.)

Hydrotherapy

Use ice packs for twenty-minute periods as long as the area is inflamed. Then, after the inflammation has gone, when the area no longer feels warm or appears red, use moist heat for twenty-minute periods. Always wait until the inflammation has gone before using heat. (*See* HYDROTHERAPY in PART 2 Treatment Section for additional information).

Supplements

- ❑ Bromelain, 500 mg twice daily, acts as an anti-inflammatory.
- ❑ Coenzyme Q_{10}, 30 mg daily, aids immune function and helps oxygenate cells.
- ❑ Cynara (from artichokes), dosage per label, helps detoxify the liver and promote immune function.
- ❑ Garlic capsules, per label, may help reduce tumor size.
- ❑ Milk thistle (silymarin), per label, detoxifies the liver, prevents free-radical damage, and promotes immune function.
- ❑ Selenium is a powerful antioxidant. (Note: selenium and vitamin E act synergistically, which means one enhances the effect of the other so it is helpful to take them together.) Take 100 mcg. daily.
- ❑ Vitamin A (beta-carotene), 25,000 IU daily, is an antioxidant and aids tissue repair.
- ❑ Vitamin B-complex, per label, is useful to maintain healthy nerve function.
- ❑ Vitamin C, 3000–10,000 mg daily in divided doses, helps promote immune function.
- ❑ Vitamin E, 400–800 IU, is an antioxidant and also helps repair tissue.

(*See* SUPPLEMENT THERAPY in PART 2 Treatment Section for additional information.)

Additional Self-Help Treatment

- ❑ Heat Therapy/Cold Therapy.

For information on this therapy, refer to individual entry in PART 2 Treatment Section.

ASSISTED ALTERNATIVE TREATMENTS

The following techniques may require specialized training or the aid of a healthcare professional.

Acupuncture and Acupressure

Acupuncture involves the insertion of extremely thin solid needles into specific points of your body to stimulate its own healing mechanism and improve blood flow to the affected neuroma in the foot. It also reduces inflammation, relieves pain, and improves mobility, and there are rarely any risks or side effects. (*See* ACUPUNCTURE and ACUPRESSURE in PART 2 Treatment Section for additional information.)

Reflexology

Reflexology can help your body heal itself naturally by eliminating energy blockages. The unaffected foot can be treated. (*See* REFLEXOLOGY in PART 2 Treatment Section for additional information.

Rolfing

Rolfing helps place your body in balance with gravity by releasing stress patterns that keep it out of alignment. It can have long-lasting effects in easing pain. (*See* ROLFING in PART 2 Treatment Section for additional information.)

Additional Assisted Treatments

- ❑ Guided Imagery.
- ❑ Osteopathic Manipulation.

For information on these therapies, refer to individual entries in PART 2 Treatment Section.

PRACTICAL SUGGESTIONS

- ❑ Be sure your shoes are wide enough not to constrict your toes.
- ❑ A metatarsal pad (available in the footcare section of most drug stores) can help relieve pressure by spreading the bones in the foot.

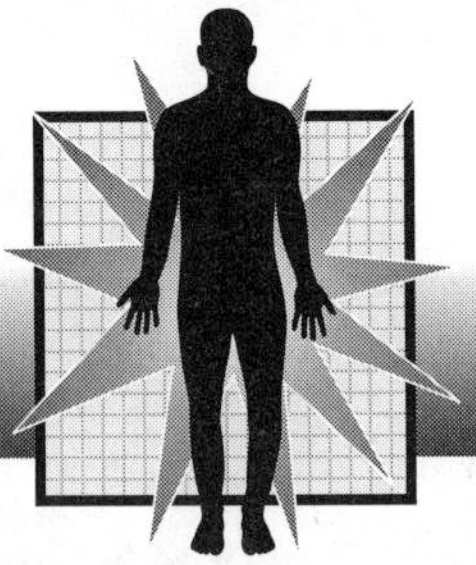

Osteoarthritis

Osteoarthritis is inflammation and pain in a joint. It generally affects older people, women more than men, and is often referred to as the wear-and-tear disease because it results from gradual deterioration of the cartilage in the joints. When cartilage is not present to protect the joints, the bones rub against each other, creating pain that can be severe.

Symptoms

Pain and progressive stiffness, without noticeable swelling, are usually indicative of osteoarthritis. Joints affected by osteoarthritis make popping or clicking noises.

Common Causes

Osteoarthritis results from chronic irritation of the joints, which could be due to injury, high intensity exercise, occupational strain, poor posture, or overweight. (For more information on Inflammation, see inset on page 81.) Obesity is a big risk factor for osteoarthritis—each pound of added body weight puts two to four pounds of extra stress on the knees and hips. And for some people, osteoarthritis is due to a substance in their gut known as solanine, which their systems cannot destroy. Instead of being sloughed off, as it is in most people, it gets absorbed into their system and causes osteoarthritis. (*See also* Bad Foods below for additional information on solanine.)

Diagnosing the Problem

X-rays are used to diagnose osteoarthritis. The joints will appear shrunken, and/or there will be obvious calcification at the ends of the bones.

Fluid from affected joints can be aspirated to see if there is an infection caused by a bacterial or viral invasion of the joints. This is known as infectious arthritis and can occur after a staph infection, TB, gonorrhea, or Lyme disease.

Conventional Treatments

- ❑ Aspirin, taken daily in large doses, alleviates pain and helps reduce inflammation.
- ❑ Bextra and Celebrex control pain.
- ❑ Codeine relieves pain.
- ❑ Cortisone, taken orally or injected into the joints, can dramatically reduce pain.
- ❑ Heat applications help ease pain.
- ❑ Hyaluronic acid injections, approved only for knee use at this time, lubricate the knee joint and help keep the bones from rubbing together, which may eventually reduce pain. (Hyaluronic acid is a lubricating fluid present in normal joints and missing in ones with arthritis.)
- ❑ Nonsteroidal anti-inflammatory drugs (NSAIDs), such as ibuprofen and naproxen, reduce inflammation.
- ❑ Phenylbutazone reduces inflammation.
- ❑ Quinine derivatives (anti-malarials) help some.
- ❑ Physical therapy can bring pain relief.
- ❑ Splints and braces reduce pressure on joints.
- ❑ Suprofen, an NSAID, can reduce inflammation.
- ❑ Surgery, including joint replacement and fusion, is performed when other treatments fail.

Problems with Some Conventional Treatments

- ❑ Cortisone weakens the adrenal glands and, if taken for long periods, it can lead to osteoporosis. It can also cause bloating, cataracts, weight gain, and a moon-faced appearance.
- ❑ NSAIDs work by blocking hormone-like substances called prostaglandins that trigger inflammation. However, prostaglandins also control the secretion of both your gastric juices and the mucous lining your stomach. This is why prolonged use of NSAIDs can eventually cause ulcers and gastric bleeding.
- ❑ The entire class of COX-2 inhibitors, including Bextra and Celebrex, may be linked to potentially damaging side effects to the heart.
- ❑ A series of hyaluronic-acid injections cost about $1200 and their effects last only about one year.
- ❑ Splints and braces restrict motion and can eventually cause joints to atrophy from lack of use.
- ❑ Suprofen can cause kidney damage.
- ❑ Surgery fails to address the true cause of the disability. Further, scar tissue attracts bacteria and fungi to the area, and they attack the tissue, causing it to become inflamed, and leading to further deterioration.

INFLAMMATION

Inflammation is a double-edged sword. Almost invariably a component of most painful conditions, it is considered beneficial as the first line of defense against injuries or infections, limiting and repairing damage to the body, cleaning and healing wounds, and even keeping people alive. But in its out-of-control negative role as silent internal inflammation, it makes continuous low-level assaults on the body's defense systems. Bacterial or viral infections, environmental pollution, free-radical damage, or poor diets cause an eventual breakdown and turn inflammation into a major culprit in chronic illnesses and the declining quality of life as we age. Our knowledge concerning inflammation's central role in chronic illness, including painful osteoarthritis, is relatively recent, and began with the discovery that it is a major predictor of heart disease—far more accurate than cholesterol levels.

In *The Inflammation Cure,* Dr. William Meggs writes that "every fever, bump, rash, or bruise" involves inflammation. While visible external inflammation generally helps lessen damage to the body, silent internal inflammation is just the opposite. As the common thread that links arthritis, cancer in some forms, diabetes, heart disease, irritable bowel syndrome, migraine headaches, and even periodontal disease, it *causes* damage.

Dr. Meggs says that, "On a microscopic level, the inflammatory response involves dozens of different chemicals, each performing a specific action." One of these, C-reactive protein (CRP)—a circulating inflammatory component of blood—is coming under increasing scrutiny as an important marker for the degree of inflammation in the body. Studies have shown that people with elevated levels of this dangerous clotting element were three to four times more likely to have heart attacks than people with low CRP levels. C-reactive protein is produced in the liver, and any source of infection, or any inflammatory condition, such as arthritis, can increase CRP levels throughout the body. It can be detected with a simple blood test that more and more practitioners are including in regular checkups.

Meat and dairy products contain arachidonic acid, a harmful eicosanoid (fatty acid) which causes inflammation, while the beneficial omega-3 eicosanoids (eicosapentaenoic acid–EPA), fatty acids found in fish oils, can help lower it. Other measures to reduce or eliminate inflammation include the dietary and lifestyle recommendations found throughout this book, and it will be to your advantage to investigate these.

SELF-HELP ALTERNATIVE TREATMENTS

The following techniques can be done at home. Since osteoarthritis is among the most widespread of all painful conditions, it could seem almost inevitable to many, but by adhering to the methods discussed here, it is possible to ward it off, or at least alleviate its symptoms without resorting to the use of harmful drugs. All herbs, homeopathic remedies, packs, and supplements mentioned in this entry are available in health food stores and, increasingly, in large drug and grocery stores, as well as on the Internet.

Aromatherapy

Apply topical applications of cajeput, camphor oil, eucalyptus oil, pine needle oil, or rosemary oil to the affected joints several times daily. They can be used singly or in combination, but be sure to dilute them in a carrier oil. (*See* AROMATHERAPY in PART 2 Treatment Section for additional information.

Castor Oil Packs

Soak a piece of white flannel in warm castor oil, wring it out and place over the inflamed area. Cover with plastic and apply a heating pad. Do this twice a day for an hour each time. (*See* COMPRESSES, PACKS, and POULTICES in PART 2 Treatment Section for additional information.)

Diet

Diet is extremely important in determining whether inflammation and other symptoms of osteoarthritis will be alleviated or exacerbated.

Good Foods

In addition to their other therapeutic benefits, the following foods can help reduce inflammation.

- ❏ Asparagus, eggs, garlic, and onions contain sulfur which helps remove metals.
- ❏ Brown rice.
- ❏ Fresh fruits that are non-acidic.

- Fresh vegetables, especially green leafy ones.
- Lentils.
- Oatmeal.
- Sardines and other oily fish.
- Whole grains.

(*See* NUTRITIONAL THERAPY in PART 2 Treatment Section for additional information.)

Bad Foods

The following foods contain elements that can cause inflammation and should be reduced or eliminated to keep symptoms of osteoarthritis from flaring up.

- Citrus fruits.
- Dairy products containing vitamin D, which can cause sore joints.
- Fatty foods, especially those containing animal fats (if not avoided altogether, these should be limited).
- Foods in the nightshade family, including eggplant, peppers, tomatoes, and white potatoes. These contain the toxin solanine, which causes inflammation in the joints.
- Sugar products.

Other Substances to Avoid

- Fluorine. Added to the water supply to strengthen teeth and bones, it also causes unneeded bone growth in arthritic joints.

Heat and Cold Therapy

Applying cold to the painful area reduces swelling and applying heat helps to increase blood flow. (*See* HEAT THERAPY/COLD THERAPY in PART 2 Treatment Section for additional information.)

Herbal Remedies

- Alfalfa increases vitality.
- Black cohosh relieves pain and inflammation.
- Boswellia has anti-inflammatory properties and acts similarly to NSAIDs without the side effects of stomach irritation or ulceration.
- Burdock root can be taken internally or applied externally to relieve painful joints.
- Cat's claw has both anti-inflammatory and antioxidant properties.
- Cayenne cream, used topically, relieves pain.
- Chaparral, also used topically, has anti-inflammatory properties.
- Devil's claw has both anti-inflammatory and analgesic actions. Take 800 mg in capsule form three times a day.
- Ginger acts as an anti-inflammatory.
- Horsetail strengthens connective tissues.
- Hydrangea acts like cortisone, but without its side effects.
- Sarsaparilla has anti-inflammatory properties.
- Turmeric helps protect your body from free radicals. Its active component is curcumin, a potent anti-inflammatory compound. Studies have shown that 400 mg of curcumin three times a day was as effective as the drug phenylbutazone, but without any side effects.
- White willow relieves inflammation and pain. Take 60–120 mg per day. Although the pain-relieving aspects are slower than aspirin, they last longer.
- Yucca reduces symptoms of osteoarthritis by blocking the release of toxins from the intestines that inhibit the normal formation of cartilage. It also helps stimulate your adrenal glands to make your body's own cortisone. You can make a tea by simmering 8 grams of the root in a pint of water for fifteen minutes, or you can use it in capsule form according to the directions on the label.

Take the above herbs as directed on label. They can also be used in teas and infusions. (*See* HERBAL REMEDIES in PART 2 Treatment Section for additional information.)

Homeopathic Remedies

You can self-treat with homeopathic remedies by selecting the one that most closely matches your symptoms. If you don't see improvement, try another, or a combination product. Follow the instructions on the label. If you do not have relief in a reasonable amount of time, consult a physician who specializes in homeopathic medicine.

Cat's Claw

Cat's claw is an herb that has been used for centuries by the indigenous people of South America to treat arthritis, gastric ulcers, inflammation, and intestinal ailments and tumors. It has both anti-inflammatory and antioxidant properties, and clinical studies have confirmed that it is an effective treatment for osteoarthritis. In Germany and Austria, standardized extract of cat's claw is being studied for its additional ability to stimulate the immune systems of cancer patients.

- ❑ Aconitum napellus eases the pain and inflammation of osteoarthritis that comes from exposure to cold.
- ❑ Apis mellifica helps acute osteoarthritis conditions accompanied by redness, tenderness and swelling.
- ❑ Arnica aids osteoarthritis where pain is worse from touch. It is also available in a gel or ointment form for external application.
- ❑ Belladonna eases sudden flare-ups of osteoarthritis accompanied by a sensation of heat and throbbing pain.
- ❑ Bryonia eases throbbing pain made worse by motion.
- ❑ Calcarea carbonica is useful for osteoarthritis when soreness is worse from cold and dampness.
- ❑ Calcarea fluorica is indicated when pain osteoarthritis is eased by heat or motion.
- ❑ Cimicifuga eases severe aching and stiffness of osteoarthritis that is accompanied by shooting pains.
- ❑ Dulcamara helps when osteoarthritis flare-up following exposure to cold damp weather.
- ❑ Kali carbonicum helps osteoarthritis when the joints thicken or become deformed and pain worsens from cold and dampness.
- ❑ Kalmia latiflora eases the intense pain of osteoarthritis that appears suddenly and is worse from motion. Pain usually starts in the joints in the upper body and works its way down.
- ❑ Ledum palustre eases the pain of osteoarthritis that starts in the joints in the lower part of the body and works its way up.
- ❑ Pulsatilla eases the pain in osteoarthritis when it moves from one joint to another.
- ❑ Rhus toxicodendron eases the pain and stiffness of osteoarthritis when they are worse in the morning and then diminish with continued motion.
- ❑ Ruta graveolens helps osteoarthritis when a feeling of great stiffness is present and symptoms worsen from cold, dampness, and exertion.

Combination remedies sometimes work more effectively than single ones. (*See* HOMEOPATHY in PART 2 Treatment Section for additional information.)

Hydrotherapy

Running hot water over a painful area while in the shower, or soaking in a hot tub can help diminish the pain. (*See* HYDROTHERAPY in PART 2 Treatment Section for additional information.)

Magnet Therapy

Magnet therapy relieves pain, accelerates healing, and reduces inflammation. Placing magnets around the sore joint brings increased blood to the area which, in turn, brings oxygen and other healing substances to reduce the pain. (*See* MAGNET THERAPY in PART 2 Treatment Section for additional information.)

Supplements

- ❑ Beta-carotene, 15,000 IU, helps neutralize free radicals.
- ❑ Boron aids calcium metabolism. Take 6 mg per day.
- ❑ Bromelain has anti-inflammatory activity, and has been reported to relieve joint swelling and impaired mobility. Take 500 mg twice daily between meals.
- ❑ Chondroitin sulfate is a major component of the lining of the joints and may help restore joint function in people with osteoarthritis. It is most advantageously used in combination with glucosamine sulfate. Take according to directions on label.
- ❑ DL-phenylalanine (DLPA), an amino acid, inhibits the enzyme that breaks down some of the body's natural painkillers. Take 250 mg three to four times a day between meals.
- ❑ Evening primrose oil controls pain and inflammation. Take two capsules twice daily.
- ❑ Fish oil contains EPA and DHA and has anti-inflammatory effects. Taking 10 grams per day delivers 3 grams of the omega-3 fatty acids EPA and DHA.
- ❑ Gamma linolenic acid (GLA) has anti-inflammatory properties. It is present in borage oil, black currant-seed oil, and evening primrose oil. Take these according to directions on label.
- ❑ Glucosamine sulfate, a nutrient derived from chitin, (a substance found in crab, shrimp, and oyster shells and broken down in a series of acids and bases until the pure glucosamine is isolated) aids in the repair of joint cartilage. Take 500 mg three times a day with meals. Although it does not provide the quick relief of NSAIDs, over time it actually helps repair joint damage.
- ❑ MSM (methylsulfonylmethane), a natural sulfur compound helps alleviate joint pain and inflammation and promotes healing. It is available in capsule, tablet, or powder form. Take according to directions on label.
- ❑ Niacinamide increases joint mobility, improves muscle strength, and decreases fatigue in those with osteoarthri-

tis. Start with 250 mg four times a day and increase the dose if your arthritis is more advanced.

- ❑ SAMe (S-adenosyl methionine) increases the formation of healthy tissue and reduces pain, stiffness and swelling. It has anti-inflammatory, pain-relieving and tissue-healing properties. Take 400 mg three times a day.
- ❑ Shark cartilage reduces inflammation and helps prevent blood vessels from invading the cartilage of your joints. Take according to directions on the label.
- ❑ SierraSil, a blend of more than sixty-five naturally occurring supplements, helps to alleviate the pain, stiffness, and inflammation of arthritis. Take according to label instructions. (*See also* Carpal Tunnel Syndrome in Conditions section.)
- ❑ Vitamin B_5 (pantothenic acid) relieves morning stiffness and pain. Take 1000 mg per day.
- ❑ Vitamin B_6 helps repair tissues by enhancing collagen production. (Collagen is present in bones, ligaments, skin, and tendons.) Take 100 mg three times a day.
- ❑ Vitamin C also helps repair tissues by enhancing collagen production. Take 1000 mg three times a day.
- ❑ Vitamin E helps osteoarthritis because it is a powerful antioxidant.
- ❑ Zinc helps repair tissues by enhancing collagen production. Take 50 mg a day.

(*See* SUPPLEMENT THERAPY in PART 2 Treatment Section for additional information.)

ASSISTED ALTERNATIVE TREATMENTS

The following techniques may require specialized training or the aid of a healthcare professional.

Acupuncture and Accupressure

Acupuncture and acupressure create a smooth flow of energy throughout the body. Acupuncture involves the insertion of extremely thin solid needles into specific points of your body to stimulate its own healing mechanism and improve blood flow to the areas affected by painful arthritis. It reduces inflammation, relieves pain, improves mobility, and there are rarely any risks or side effects. (*See* ACUPUNCTURE and ACUPRESSURE in PART 2 Treatment Section for additional information.)

Applied Kinesiology

Applied Kinesiology is excellent for reducing pain rapidly. The AK practitioner tests your muscles to determine the origin of your problem and then decides on the best course of action, choosing from a wide variety of therapeutic methods at her or his disposal. (*See* APPLIED KINESIOLOGY in PART 2 Treatment Section for additional information.)

Bee Venom Therapy

Some components of bee venom are thought to stimulate the immune system. Other components are thought to modify the transmission of pain signals within the nervous system, and the therapy has proven consistently useful for painful conditions. (*See* BEE VENOM THERAPY in PART 2 Treatment Section for additional information.)

Chiropractic

When the spinal vertebrae are misaligned they can pinch nerves, which leads to pressure, causing symptoms in various body parts. When these misaligned vertebrae (subluxations) are properly aligned, the nervous system can function properly and chronic pain can often be reversed. (*See* CHIROPRACTIC in PART 2 Treatment Section for additional information.)

Craniosacral Therapy

A trained craniosacral practitioner can feel areas where healthy tissue function is restricted, usually due to physical or emotional trauma. The theory is that physical injuries and emotional traumas are stored or frozen in the body, causing arthritis pain that can be released by this therapy. (*See* CRANIOSACRAL THERAPY in PART 2 Treatment Section for additional information.)

Exercise

Anyone with osteoarthritis should start an exercise program slowly and carefully, and it must be supervised in the beginning to avoid further damage to the affected area. Moving your joints stimulates the cartilage to absorb more nutrients. Exercise also strengthens muscles so they support the joints more effectively. If you feel stiff, take a warm bath or shower first. Stretch slowly and avoid bouncing or high-impact exercise. Good exercises for osteoarthritis are swimming, water aerobics, walking, and cycling with a low-pedal resistance. Tai chi and qigong, two gentle, highly effective forms of martial arts training that also calm and center you, are excellent exercises for those with osteoarthritis. (*See* EXERCISE, STRETCHING, and SPORTS, and TAI CHI, QIGONG, and YOGA in PART 2 Treatment Section for additional information.)

Guided Imagery and Visualization Techniques

These help to relieve stress and minimize pain. To alleviate the burning, either visualize a temperature guage set on high and then turn down the heat, or picture cool water putting out a fire. For the stiffness, visualize a tight band that you gradually loosen. (*See* GUIDED IMAGERY and VISUALIZATION in PART 2 Treatment Section for additional information.)

Massage

Massage helps relax contracted muscles and alleviate muscle tension in one area of the body, which can affect other areas. It also increases blood flow, which nourishes and oxygenates tissues. (*See* MASSAGE in PART 2 Treatment Section for additional information.)

Osteopathic Manipulation

Osteopathic manipulation can correct faulty structure and function and rebalance your body's system, enabling it to function better. (*See* OSTEOPATHIC MANIPULATION in PART 2 Treatment Section for additional information.)

Oxygen Therapy

Oxygen therapy enhances your body's ability to heal itself by encouraging its own natural production of oxygen. (*See* OXYGEN THERAPIES in PART 2 Treatment Section for additional information.)

Physical Therapy

Physical therapy increases the range of motion in your joints and corrects and improves your body's natural healing mechanism. (*See* PHYSICAL THERAPY in PART 2 Treatment Section for additional information.)

Reflexology

By helping to eliminate energy blockages, improve circulation, and relieve stress and tension, reflexology helps the body heal itself naturally. (*See* REFLEXOLOGY in PART 2 Treatment Section for additional information.)

Rolfing

Rolfing helps place your body in balance with gravity by releasing stress patterns that keep it out of alignment. It can have long-lasting effects in easing pain. (*See* ROLFING in PART 2 Treatment Section for additional information.)

Tai Chi, Qigong, and Yoga

These therapies help your body to enter a relaxed state and also increase production of endorphins, which are natural painkillers. (*See* TAI CHI, QIGONG, and YOGA in PART 2 Treatment Section for additional information.)

PRACTICAL SUGGESTIONS

- ❏ Celadrin. This natural topical ointment has been shown to significantly reduce painful symptoms of osteoarthritis.
- ❏ Copper bracelets. Users have reported surprising, effective results.
- ❏ DMSO (dimethyl sulfoxide). This industrial solvent, applied topically, has anti-inflammatory properties and relieves pain by inhibiting the pain messages transmitted by the nerves.

IONIZED BRACELETS

Ionized bracelets are said to balance the body's energy fields to bring relief from pain in the joints and muscles. Researchers at The Mayo Clinic in Jacksonville, Florida ran some tests on ionized bracelets to see if wearing them helped, but found they were no more effective at relieving a wearer's muscle and joint pain than other look-alike, non-ionized placebo bracelets. Anecdotally, however, several men wearing ionized bracelets reported that they worked very effectively, even referring to them as "wonderful."

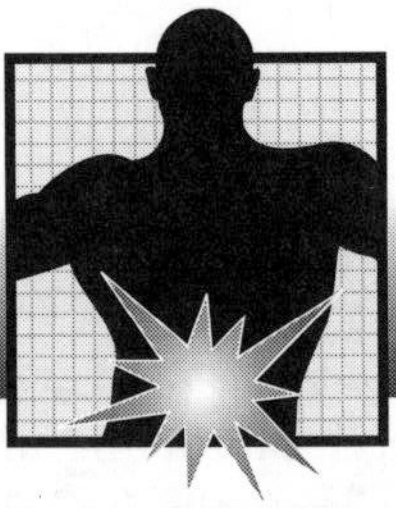

Pelvic Floor Tension Myalgia

Pelvic floor tension myalgia is a painful spasm of the pelvic floor muscles that support the bladder and rectum and, in women, also the uterus and vagina.

Symptoms

- Pelvic pain.
- Painful intercourse.
- Pressure or heaviness in lower pelvic area.
- Urinary frequency.
- Urinary urgency.

Common Causes

- Weak or overly relaxed muscles.
- Pelvic organ prolapse.
- Overly tense muscles that don't have a chance to relax and go into a spasm.
- A low-back problem, or having one leg shorter than the other.
- Pain from a bladder infection that can trigger spasms because the normal reaction to pain is to tighten muscles.
- Hemorrhoid pain that can also trigger spasms because muscles tighten as a normal reaction to pain.

Diagnosing the Problem

If, during a pelvic examination, any pressure on the muscles causes the same pain that you complain of, your problem is most likely pelvic floor tension myalgia.

Conventional Treatments

- Internal massage. A do-it-yourself type of massage that can be taught to you by your gynecologist.
- Kegel exercises. These help prevent and treat bladder, rectum, uterine, or vaginal prolapse (referred to as a cystocele if the weakness is in the anterior vaginal wall, or a rectocele if the weakness is in the posterior vaginal wall). Kegel exercises can be performed anywhere, anytime. All you have to do is contract the muscles as if you were trying to hold back the urine stream. Many women practice them while waiting for red lights to change.
- Muscle relaxants.
- Physical therapy that can help relax muscles. A physical therapist can determine if the pelvic bones are out of alignment and if the muscles attached to them are able to relax properly. (*See also* PHYSICAL THERAPY in PART 2 Treatment Section for additional information.)
- Trigger point therapy.

Problems with Some Conventional Treatments

- Muscle relaxants can make you sleepy.

SELF-HELP ALTERNATIVE TREATMENTS

The following techniques can be done at home. Although they may not work as fast as drugs or surgery, natural alternatives help the body heal itself. All herbs, homeopathic remedies, packs, and supplements discussed here are available in health food stores and, increasingly, in large drug and grocery stores, as well as on the Internet.

Aromatherapy

Aromatherapy, particularly the essential oils of bergamot, chamomile, clary sage, fennel, geranium, grapefruit, jasmine, lavender, melissa, neroli, nutmeg, palmarosa, parsley seed, rose, vetiver, and ylang ylang all help regulate hormonal balance. They also relieve spasms and help heal tissues. You can either put a few drops into a hot bath and soak, or add a few drops to vegetable oil and massage into the affected area. Do not ingest essential oils or use them full strength as they are very powerful compounds. They are available in health food stores and stores specializing in aromatherapy products, which you can find in the yellow pages. (*See* AROMATHERAPY in PART 2 Treatment Section for additional information.)

Castor Oil Packs

Dip a piece of white flannel into some warm castor oil. Wring it out and place it over your pelvic area. Cover with plastic and apply a heating pad for one hour. Do this twice daily. (*See* COMPRESSES, PACKS, and POULTICES in PART 2 Treatment Section for additional information.)

Heat Therapy/Cold Therapy

Warm baths help relax the muscles. (*See* HEAT THERAPY/COLD THERAPY, and HYDROTHERAPY in PART 2 Treatment Section for additional information.)

Meditation

Meditation helps reduce stress, which contributes to pelvic pain. (*See* MEDITATION in PART 2 Treatment Section for additional information.)

ASSISTED ALTERNATIVE TREATMENTS

The following techniques may require specialized training or the aid of a healthcare professional.

Acupuncture and Acupressure

Acupuncture involves the insertion of extremely thin solid needles into specific points of your body to stimulate its own healing mechanism and improve blood flow to the pelvic area. It also reduces inflammation and relieves pain, and there are rarely any risks or side effects. (*See* ACUPUNCTURE and ACUPRESSURE in PART 2 Treatment Section for additional information.)

Applied Kinesiology

Applied Kinesiology is excellent for reducing pain rapidly. The AK practitioner tests your muscles to determine the origin of your problem and then decides on the best course of action, choosing from a wide variety of therapeutic methods at his or her disposal. (*See* APPLIED KINESIOLOGY in PART 2 Treatment Section for additional information.)

Biofeedback

If you have pelvic floor tension myalgia, biofeedback can help you determine when the muscles are relaxed and when they are tense. (*See* BIOFEEDBACK in PART 2 Treatment Section for additional information.)

MALE PELVIC FLOOR TENSION MYALGIA HELPED BY BIOFEEDBACK

Nineteen men at Northwestern Medical School in Chicago found that bi-weekly sessions of non-invasive biofeedback measures were helpful in diminishing pelvic floor muscle spasms and their accompanying pain. Although this entry concerns only the problems that women with this condition have, it is interesting to note the positive results of this twelve-week study on men.

Chiropractic

Chiropractic theory is based on the assumption that a properly aligned spine is essential for good health, and that any misalignment of the vertebrae in the spine causes pressure on the spinal nerves, leading to pain. The chiropractor makes spinal adjustments to move misaligned vertebrae to more normal positions, which helps the nervous system to function properly. In pelvic disorders, a chiropractor can determine if the pelvic bones are out of alignment and if the muscles attached to them are able to properly relax. (*See* CHIROPRACTIC in PART 2 Treatment Section for additional information.)

Craniosacral Therapy

Craniosacral therapy is a form of energy healing that can help balance your system. It has been shown to be effective for alleviating pelvic problems. (*See* CRANIOSACRAL THERAPY in PART 2 Treatment Section for additional information.)

Exercise and Stretching

Regular aerobic exercise aids circulation, helps oxygenate the blood, and relaxes the uterus. To avoid further damage to the pelvic area, it must be carefully supervised in the beginning. (*See* EXERCISE, STRETCHING, and SPORTS in PART 2 Treatment Section for additional information.) (*See also* Kegel Exercises in Conventional Treatments above.)

Guided Imagery and Visualization Techniques

Guided imagery can help manage pelvic pain. To relieve the sensation of chronic heaviness, change the pain into a light object that you can easily handle. (*See* GUIDED IMAGERY and VISUALIZATION in PART 2 Treatment Section for additional information.)

Massage

A massage helps bring blood to the pelvic area and relieves the pain. There are many kinds of massage therapies available and you can ask your practitioner to suggest the appropriate one for your pelvic pain. (*See* MASSAGE in PART 2 Treatment Section for additional information.)

Osteopathic Manipulation

The goal of osteopathic manipulation in the treatment of pelvic pain is to reduce uterine congestion, relieve pain, and improve blood circulation. (*See* OSTEOPATHIC MANIPULATION in PART 2 Treatment Section for additional information.)

Reflexology

Reflexology massage therapy can be performed on the part of the foot or hand corresponding to the pelvic area that is in pain. (*See* REFLEXOLOGY in PART 2 Treatment Section for additional information.)

Rolfing

Rolfing can improve circulation, ease fascia tension, and promote relaxation in pelvic tension myalgia. (*See* ROLFING in PART 2 Treatment Section for additional information.)

Tai Chi, Qigong, and Yoga

These therapies induce a profoundly relaxed state and help bring healing energy to the body. (*See* TAI CHI, QIGONG, and YOGA in PART 2 Treatment Section for additional information.)

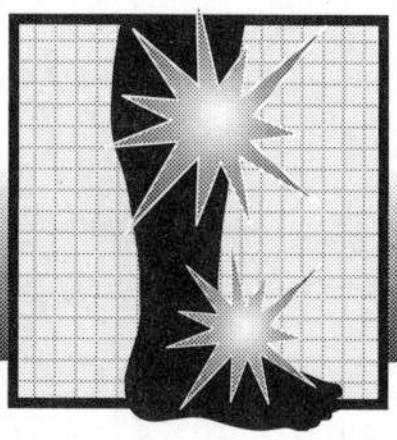

Peripheral Neuropathy

Peripheral neuropathy is a nerve disorder that damages nerves in the arms and legs. Most of the time, the feet and legs are affected before the arms. The primary cause of peripheral neuropathy is diabetes and, over time, peripheral nerve damage caused by diabetes can lead to problems with your digestive tract, heart, internal organs, and sex organs. Since we are discussing peripheral neuropathy, we will mention only briefly that these nerve-related problems can cause indigestion, dizziness, bladder infections, bowel disorders, and impotence, among other things, which do not necessarily belong in a pain book.

Symptoms

Symptoms usually start in your feet, either the full foot or just a toe. As the neuropathy progresses, symptoms move up the leg. Those with neuropathy usually feel worse at night and walking may bring some relief. Sensations include:

- ❑ Aching;
- ❑ Burning;
- ❑ Coldness;
- ❑ Electric shock-like sensations;
- ❑ Impaired function;
- ❑ Itching;
- ❑ Muscle weakness and loss of reflexes;
- ❑ Numbness, which can be serious because injuries leading to blisters and sores may not be noticed, and if not treated promptly, infection could occur and spread to the bone;
- ❑ Pins-and-needles sensations;
- ❑ Reduced temperature and lower pain level;
- ❑ Skin sensitivity in the legs and feet, even to a light touch, and contact with clothing or bedding can be painful;
- ❑ Tingling;
- ❑ Wasting of the muscles in the feet or hands.

Common Causes

High blood glucose (sugar), in the case of those with diabetic peripheral neuropathy, the most common form. When too much glucose is present in the blood, a large amount of the excess goes into the nerve cells and forms sugar alcohols. Then, when these sugar alcohols build up, they adversely affect the production of other nutrients needed by the nerve cells to function properly. The eventual result of too much glucose is permanent nerve damage.

Additional causes include:

- ❑ Alcohol, which has a harmful effect on glucose levels;
- ❑ Autoimmunity: type 1 (insulin-dependent) diabetes occurs when your body mistakenly recognizes the insulin-producing cells in your pancreas as invaders; diabetic peripheral neuropathy occurs when your body treats the nerves the same way;
- ❑ High blood pressure;
- ❑ High cholesterol levels;
- ❑ Smoking, which deprives nerve cells of oxygen, which they need to function properly.

Peripheral neuropathy may also be due to other causes, such as back problems, circulatory problems, degenerative arthritis, gout, low thyroid function, or pernicious anemia.

Diagnosing the Problem

It is important to diagnose this condition because, if you have peripheral neuropathy and don't know it, you could damage your feet without being aware of it. (*See* Numbness in symptoms section above.) Your doctor should do the following during a physical examination.

- ❑ Test reflexes with a rubber hammer. A delayed response may indicate neuropathy.
- ❑ Use a tuning fork to determine whether or not you can feel vibrations in your feet.
- ❑ Touch your feet and lower legs with a pin to see if you have any pain sensation.

Conventional Treatments

The goal of treatment is to relieve pain and prevent further tissue damage. At the present time, however, no drug has FDA approval specifically for the treatment of peripheral neuropathy. Powerful narcotic painkillers do not work well for it as they are intended for short-time use only due to the risk of addiction. Some drugs used for other conditions, such as antidepressants and anticonvulsants, in small doses, have proven effective. The most frequently recommended treatments are:

- Anticonvulsant drugs, such as carbamazepine and clonazepam, in small doses, to help relieve symptoms;
- Baclofen pumps;
- Botoxin injections;
- Capsaicin cream, which acts against the neurotransmitter, substance P, the chemical in nerves that causes pain (*see also* Herbal Remedies in this entry);
- Controlling blood glucose levels, which is crucial in order to prevent further nerve damage;
- Elastic stockings;
- Foot care (*see* foot-care details below in Practical Suggestions);
- Lidocaine, which is effective from two days to two weeks, given intravenously can help relieve symptoms temporarily;
- Mexiletine, which is similar to lidocaine, but can be taken orally;
- Muscle relaxants;
- NSAIDs, nonsteroidal anti-inflammatory drugs, which help relieve symptoms;
- Physical therapy, which helps restore function, improve mobility, and relieve pain by using conservative methods that do not involve surgery (*see also* PHYSICAL THERAPY in PART 2 Treatment Section for additional information);
- Transcutaneous electrical nerve stimulation (TENS units)—once considered alternative treatment, but now mainstream—is a device providing nerve stimulation that may help relieve pain;
- Tricyclic antidepressants, such as amitriptyline or imipramine, in small doses, may help relieve symptoms, and help you sleep;
- Trigger point therapy is similar to acupressure and rolfing but, unlike these, it is now considered conventional treatment;
- Walking on land or in water, which can help leg pain.

Problems with Some Conventional Treatments

All drugs can interact adversely with other medications.

- Anticonvulsants can cause dizziness, lack of coordination, liver toxicity, memory loss, and sleepiness.
- Antidepressants can make you sleepy.
- Muscle relaxants can cause sleepiness.
- NSAIDs can cause gastrointestinal bleeding.
- TENS units devices give only temporary relief.
- Tricyclic antidepressants can cause blurred vision, constipation, dizziness, dry mouth, and liver toxicity. Less common side effects are a sudden drop in blood pressure if you stand up too quickly from a lying or sitting position, and an irregular heart rhythm. Also, unless you are weaned off them slowly, they can have rebound effects, such as depression and insomnia.

SELF-HELP ALTERNATIVE TREATMENTS

The following techniques can be done at home. Although they may not work as fast as drugs or surgery, natural alternatives help the body heal itself. All herbs, homeopathic remedies, and supplements discussed here are available in health food stores and, increasingly, in large drug and grocery stores, as well as on the Internet.

Aromatherapy

Aromatherapy, particularly the essential oils of chamomile, ginger lavender, marjoram, peppermint, and rosemary, are useful for relieving peripheral neuropathy. They are available in health food stores and stores specializing in aromatherapy products which you can find in the yellow pages. (*See* AROMATHERAPY in PART 2 Treatment Section for additional information.)

Diet

Peripheral Neuropathy is inflammatory in nature so certain dietary modifications may be helpful.

Good Foods

A high protein, low carbohydrate diet helps control blood-sugar levels. (*See* NUTRITIONAL THERAPY in PART 2 Treatment Section for additional information.)

Bad Foods

Avoid foods that are high in fat and sugar to help keep your blood glucose levels under control.

Other Substances to Avoid

- Alcohol and smoking.
- Birth control pills affect carbohydrate metabolism in a negative manner.
- Cortisone is antagonistic to insulin.
- Diuretics (prescription) stimulate excretion of water and cause an increase in the concentration of glucose.

Heat Therapy/Cold Therapy

Heat increases blood flow to the area and cold reduces swelling. (*See* HEAT THERAPY/COLD THERAPY in PART 2 Treatment Section for additional information.)

Herbal Remedies

- ❑ Cayenne improves circulation. Sprinkle liberally on your food or take capsules according to label.
- ❑ Evening primrose oil, 6 grams per day, reduces nerve damage.
- ❑ Ginkgo biloba, 60 mg three times daily, helps prevent and treat early stage diabetic neuropathy.

Take the above herbs as directed on label. They can also be used in teas and infusions. (*See* HERBAL REMEDIES in PART 2 Treatment Section for additional information.)

Homeopathic Remedies

You can self-treat with homeopathic remedies by selecting the one that most closely matches your symptoms. If you don't see improvement, try another, or a combination product. Follow the instructions on the label. If you do not have relief in a reasonable amount of time, consult a physician who specializes in homeopathic medicine.

- ❑ Codeinum helps alleviate skin irritation.
- ❑ Phosphorus helps stabilize blood sugar.
- ❑ Syzygium is a general remedy.

Combination remedies sometimes work more effectively than single ones. (*See* HOMEOPATHY in PART 2 Treatment Section for additional information.)

Hydrotherapy

Warm baths help relieve leg pain. (*See* HYDROTHERAPY in PART 2 Treatment Section for additional information.)

Supplements

- ❑ Alpha-lipoic acid, 1000 mg daily, is a natural antioxidant that is particularly good for the nerves and the brain, and has been shown to reduce pain from peripheral nerve damage, particularly if it is caused by diabetes.
- ❑ Carnitine, one gram per day by injection, reduces pain from diabetic nerve damage.
- ❑ Inositol, 500 mg twice daily, aids normal nerve function.
- ❑ Magnesium, 500 mg twice daily, is essential in the breakdown of glucose into cell energy.
- ❑ Vitamin B_6 (especially pyridoxine alpha-ketogluterate), 1800 mg per day, improves glucose tolerance.
- ❑ Vitamin B_{12}, 500 mcg three times daily, taken orally or by injection, helps normal functioning of nerve cells. It has been shown to reduce nerve damage, especially diabetic neuropathy. Note: For balance, when taking individual Bs, be sure to supplement with a B-complex once daily, or a multivitamin containing B-complex.
- ❑ Vitamin C, 1000 mg three times daily, helps lower sorbitol, a sugar that can accumulate and damage the eyes, nerves, and kidneys of those with diabetic peripheral neuropathy.
- ❑ Vitamin E, 900 IU daily, can improve glucose tolerance. It prevents blood from clotting too fast and protects your blood vessels from damage. Note: It can take three to six months for improvement.

(*See* SUPPLEMENT THERAPY in PART 2 Treatment Section for additional information.)

ASSISTED ALTERNATIVE TREATMENTS

The following techniques may require specialized training or the aid of a healthcare professional.

Acupuncture and Acupressure

Acupuncture involves the insertion of extremely thin solid needles into specific points of your body to stimulate its own healing mechanism and improve blood flow to the affected areas. It also reduces inflammation, relieves pain, improves mobility, and there are rarely any risks or side effects. (*See* ACUPUNCTURE and ACUPRESSURE in PART 2 Treatment Section for additional information.)

Applied Kinesiology

Applied Kinesiology is excellent for reducing pain rapidly. The AK practitioner tests your muscles to determine the origin of your problem and then decides on the best course of action, choosing from a wide variety of therapeutic methods at her or his disposal. (*See* APPLIED KINESIOLOGY in PART 2 Treatment Section for additional information.)

Chiropractic

Chiropractic theory is based on the assumption that a properly aligned spine is essential for good health, and that any misalignment of the vertebrae in the spine causes pressure on the spinal nerves, leading to pain. The chiropractor makes spinal adjustments to move misaligned vertebrae to more normal positions, which helps the nervous system to function properly. According to Dr. Larry Segal, DC, chiropractic is useful for treating neuropathy because it helps get blood to the affected area, and because of the way it helps the central nervous system to work better. (*See* CHIROPRACTIC in PART 2 Treatment Section for additional information.)

Exercise

Aerobic activity reduces stress and increases the production of endorphins, which helps raise your pain threshold. To avoid further injury, it must be carefully supervised in the beginnning. (*See* EXERCISE, STRETCHING, and SPORTS in PART 2 Treatment Section for additional information.)

Guided Imagery and Visualization Techniques

Guided imagery can help manage pain. Since there are many different pain sensations associated with PN, you might want to identify whether yours is a feeling of burning, coldness, or stabbing, etc., and mentally bring in the appropriate tools to counteract the sensation. (*See* GUIDED IMAGERY and VISUALIZATION in PART 2 Treatment Section for additional information.)

Osteopathic Manipulation

The goal of osteopathic manipulation in the treatment of peripheral neuropathy is to increase range of motion, decrease muscle tension, and improve blood circulation. (*See* OSTEOPATHIC MANIPULATION in PART 2 Treatment Section for additional information.)

Oxygen Therapy

Oxygen therapy is a useful adjunct for treating peripheral neuropathy. (*See* OXYGEN THERAPIES in PART 2 Treatment Section for additional information.)

Reflexology

Reflexology massage therapy can be performed on the part of the foot or hand corresponding to the area that is in pain. (*See* REFLEXOLOGY in PART 2 Treatment Section for additional information.)

PRACTICAL SUGGESTIONS

❏ Control your blood sugar levels.

❏ Keep your cholesterol levels and blood pressure down.

❏ Don't smoke.

❏ Drink alcohol in moderation, or better yet, don't drink.

❏ Be meticulous about foot care. Keep feet clean and dry and inspect them daily for cuts, blisters, redness, swelling, or other problems. Untreated injuries increase the risk of infections that may lead to amputation. It is estimated that almost half of the 86,000 neuropathy-related amputations in the United States every year could have been prevented by proper foot care. Here are some ABCs of foot care:

- Always wear shoes or slippers to protect your feet from injury.
- Be sure your shoes fit properly.
- Check inside your shoes to be sure the lining is intact and smooth. And, always check your socks when you take them off to be sure there is no blood or fluid from a sore that you might not have noticed.

HBOT to the Rescue with Misdiagnosed Peripheral Neuropathy

In his fifties, Joe developed a major foot infection that his doctors incorrectly diagnosed, putting him on the wrong medications and augmenting the problem to the point that their only solution for him was to amputate half of his foot. Determined not to allow that, Joe went on the Internet to research his, by then, properly diagnosed peripheral neuropathy, and discovered oxygen treatments. He tracked down a practitioner in his area who immediately started him on hyperbaric oxygen therapy five days a week, two to two and a half hours at a time, to reverse his condition. It took a number of months in the chamber, but Joe's foot is still attached to his body, and the biggest aggravation he had after deciding on the oxygen treatments was with his original *misdiagnosing* HMO doctors. Luckily for him, though, when they refused to refer him for HBOT therapy (for reasons that had more to do with money than proper treatment), his excellent insurance policy allowed him to fire them and refer himself for the treatment that helped save his foot. In recounting the story, Joe takes great pleasure in saying that, no thanks to those HMO doctors, the little toe that started it all is *still there.*

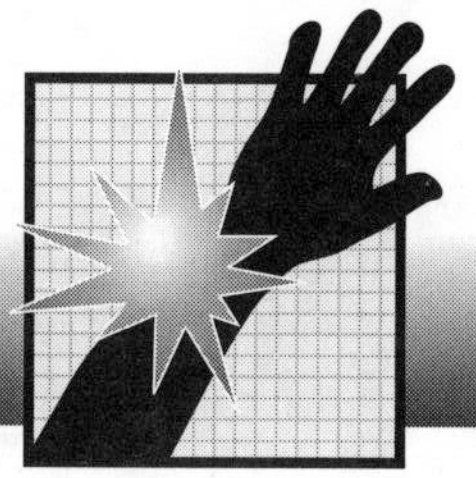

Phantom Pain

Phantom pain is the pain or sensation felt in a body part that has been amputated—an arm or a leg, for example, or in a breast following a mastectomy. Studies and articles about phantom pain go back as far as the sixteenth century. It was not until the late nineteenth century, however, that it became a regular part of the medical literature, and only recently that it was considered a serious condition and not merely something that doctors considered "just in the heads" of their patients with amputated body parts.

Symptoms

Phantom pain is experienced by almost everyone who has had an amputation. The sensations in these body parts that do not exist anymore can be feelings of heat, cold, touch, or changes of position, and the pain has been variously described as burning, cramping, piercing, stabbing, stinging, tearing, throbbing, tingling with pins and needles, or even shocking.

Causes

The cause of phantom pain is not known, but most researchers believe it is the result of faulty signals in the brain.

Diagnosing the Problem

This condition is diagnosed by observing the symptoms.

Conventional Treatments

Physical therapists recommend activities and treatments to increase blood flow to the site of the amputation because increased blood flow can often reduce the amount of pain. They consider bike riding, running, walking, and weightlifting, along with stretching, particularly effective activities (all are considered beneficial alternative therapies as well.) Physical therapists also advise how to put a prosthesis on properly to avoid pinching a nerve. (*See* EXERCISE, STRETCHING, and SPORTS and PHYSICAL THERAPY in PART 2 Treatment Section for additional information.)

SELF-HELP ALTERNATIVE TREATMENTS

As with all conditions in this book, anyone with phantom pain can benefit from proper nutrition, herbs, homeopathic remedies, and supplements. Although they may not work as fast as drugs or surgery, natural alternatives help the body heal itself. Herbs, homeopathic remedies, packs, and supplements are available in health food stores and, increasingly, in large drug and grocery stores, as well as on the Internet. (*See* HERBAL REMEDIES, HOMEOPATHY, NUTRITIONAL THERAPY, and SUPPLEMENT THERAPY in PART 2 Treatment Section for additional information.)

Baths and Compresses

Warm baths, hot tubs, and warm compresses to increase circulation are also advised. Even wrapping the stump in a warm soft towel can help to increase circulation and reduce pain. (*See* COMPRESSES, PACKS, and POULTICES, HEAT THERAPY/COLD THERAPY, and HYDROTHERAPY in PART 2 Treatment Section for additional information.)

ASSISTED ALTERNATIVE TREATMENTS

Some with phantom pain find they are helped by such techniques as acupuncture, biofeedback, chiropractic, and hypnosis that require the assistance of a healthcare professional. (*See* ACUPUNCTURE and ACUPRESSURE, BIOFEEDBACK, CHIROPRACTIC, HYPNOSIS, and OSTEOPATHIC MANIPULATION in PART 2 Treatment Section for additional information.)

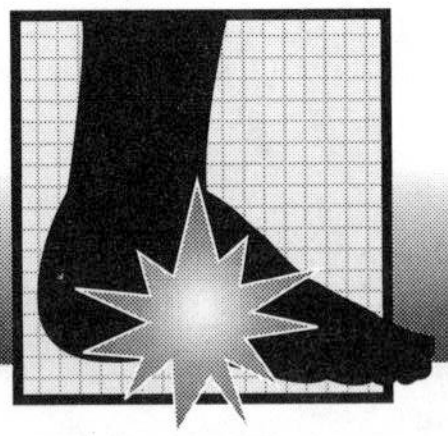

Plantar Fasciitis

The plantar fascia is a band of tissue extending from the ball of the foot to the bottom of the heel. If you overuse your feet and subject them to an unusual amount of stress, this tissue becomes inflamed and a condition called plantar fasciitis occurs.

Symptoms

The primary symptom of plantar fasciitis is an extremely painful tender heel that feels hot to the touch and is often swollen.

Common Causes

Although activities such as jogging and tennis are good for your cardiovascular system, they do have a downside. Repetitive force on the plantar fascia, either from overexercising or from being overweight, can cause tears in it where it attaches to your heel. The problem can also be caused by shoes with insufficient cushioning in the heel, so it is a good idea to make sure the shoes you wear have flexible soles, arch supports, and soft heel pads. If the resulting pain from the tear is at its worst while walking, running, or even standing for a while, you might have to give up running for some time and take up cycling instead, then ease into walking for exercise.

Diagnosing the Problem

This problem is diagnosed by observing the symptoms.

Conventional Treatments

There are no medications for healing the damaged plantar fascia, only palliative cortisone injections or painkillers. They do not make the problem disappear and they do have harmful side effects.

SELF-HELP ALTERNATIVE TREATMENTS

Using the stretching and icing remedies outlined below, which you can perform at home, may help you avoid the drastic measures of being placed in a walking cast for a period of three to six weeks, or having surgery to release the ligament.

Also, as with all conditions in this book, a person with plantar fasciitis can benefit from proper nutrition, herbs, homeopathic remedies, and supplements. Although they may not work as fast as drugs or surgery, natural alternatives help the body heal itself. Herbs, homeopathic remedies, and supplements are available in health food stores and, increasingly, in large drug and grocery stores, as well as on the Internet. (*See* HERBAL REMEDIES, HOMEOPATHY, NUTRITIONAL THERAPY, and SUPPLEMENT THERAPY in PART 2 Treatment Section for additional information.)

Exercise and Stretching

The best remedy for plantar fasciitis is stretching. While most exercises for this condition should be supervised by a trained person, such as a physical therapist, here is a simple stretch that is safe for you to try. Stand at arm's length from a wall and brace your body against it with your palms. Keep your feet flat on the floor and your knees locked. Bend your elbows and lean toward the wall until you feel a pull on your calf muscles, without feeling any pain. Hold that position for about fifteen seconds, and repeat it six times, several times a day. It is also helpful to roll a small ball, such as a golf ball, under the ball of your foot while you are sitting. (*See* EXERCISE, STRETCHING, and SPORTS in PART 2 Treatment Section for additional information.)

Ice Pack

Icing the area for twenty minutes several times a day helps, as does resting (do it while the ice is being applied). (*See* HEAT THERAPY/COLD THERAPY, and HYDRO- THERAPY in PART 2 Treatment Section for additional information.)

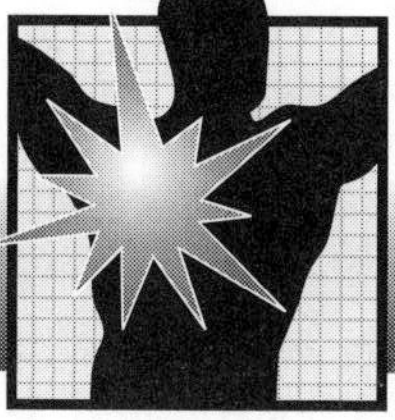

Postherpetic Neuralgia

Shingles, also known as herpes zoster, affects about one million people in the United States every year. It is an acute viral infection characterized by an inflammation of nerves, usually along just one side of the body, and is usually accompanied by a severe neuralgia (nerve pain). Postherpetic neuralgia, or PHN, is severe pain located in the area where the shingles was present. It is the most common chronic complication of shingles and appears after the shingles rash has gone. Those who have PHN say it is a shooting, stabbing pain, or it feels like their skin is on fire, and some say it is even more painful than shingles. Twenty percent, or one out of every five people with shingles, develops PHN, and the older you are, the more likely you are to get it. If you are over age seventy, you have a 75 percent chance of developing PHN if you have had shingles.

Symptoms

The primary symptom of PHN is continuing pain in the area where the shingles rash had been, covering either a smaller or a slightly larger area than the original rash. Severe itching often accompanies the sharp, piercing, burning, stabbing pain. This pain can be so severe that those experiencing it cannot even tolerate having their clothing touch the area, and something as insignificant as a mild breeze or a change in temperature can make the skin unusually sensitive. These symptoms can come to completely dominate the lives of those unlucky enough to experience PHN, almost to the point of rendering them incapable of normal everyday functioning.

Cause

Postherpetic neuralgia is a result of nerve damage caused by the varicella-zoster virus (VZV) during the shingles infection (the virus responsible for both chicken pox and shingles). You cannot get PHN unless you have had shingles, and shingles only appear in people who have had chicken pox, and thus still have the VZV in their system. This nerve damage can be very painful and can last for months or, in the worst cases, years. A delay in treating shingles with anti-viral medication when the virus first appears can lead to PHN.

Diagnosing the Problem

PHN is generally diagnosed by its obvious symptoms in those who have had shingles. If pain is present in the area where the rash appeared, if touching the skin causes pain, or if the skin is overly sensitive to the lightest touch of clothing or whiff of wind, PHN is suspected.

Conventional Treatments

At the present time there is no cure for PHN. Pain relief is the primary treatment. The antiviral drugs prescribed to treat shingles do not help PHN, but if administered early enough (within seventy-two hours) in a shingles attack, they may help prevent it.

- ❑ Anticonvulsants (drugs used to prevent seizures or convulsions) help ease pain and calm sensitive nerves that were injured by the shingles infection. The dosage used to treat PHN is much lower than that used in the treatment of epilepsy. Anticonvulsants include:
- ❑ Gabapentin (Neurontin) is currently the most prescribed and has the advantage of not interacting with other medications;
- ❑ Carbamazepine (Tegretol);
- ❑ Phenytoin (Dilantin).
- ❑ Lidocaine patch (Lidoderm) is helpful in easing the pain. It is a topical treatment that contains a 5 percent solution of lidocaine, the same analgesic used by dentists. It does not enter the bloodstream, make the skin numb, or interact with other medications. When the lidocaine comes into contact with damaged nerves under the skin, it helps make them less sensitive.
- ❑ Opioids (narcotics), such as oxycodone (Oxycontin), morphine, and combination formulas, are strong pain relievers. They include:
- ❑ Oxycodone mixed with aspirin (Percodan);
- ❑ Oxycodone mixed with acetaminophen (Percoset);
- ❑ Hydromorphine (Dilaudid);
- ❑ Hydrocodone with acetaminophen (Vicodin and Zydone).
- ❑ Transcutaneous electrical nerve stimulation (TENS units) is one of the treatments once considered alternative that is now mainstream. Electrodes are attached to the skin and the low amounts of electrical current they send to the nerves help to interrupt pain pathways.

- ❑ Tricylic antidepressants help reduce pain signals from damaged nerves. They work by their effect on neurotransmitters (hormones or proteins in the body that carry signals between nerve cells and other cells). For PHN treatment, the dosage of antidepressants is one-tenth the amount of that used to treat depression, but treatment should be continued for three to six months after there has been pain relief. Tricyclic antidepressants include:
- ❑ Amitripyline (Elavil);
- ❑ Nortriptyline (Pamelor);
- ❑ Desipramine (Norpramin).

Problems with Some Conventional Treatments

All drugs can interact adversely with other medications. Older people are more likely to have side effects from medications and, as mentioned before, most of those with PHN are elderly.

- ❑ Anticonvulsants can cause dizziness, lack of coordination, liver toxicity, memory loss, and sleepiness.
- ❑ Lidocaine patches, which sometimes cause the skin to swell or redden in the area of the patch, offer only temporary relief, lasting from four to twelve hours per application.
- ❑ Opioids can cause constipation, dizziness, or sleepiness, and can impair thinking. They can also become addictive.
- ❑ TENS units devices give only temporary relief.
- ❑ Tricyclic antidepressants can cause blurred vision, constipation, dizziness, dry mouth, and liver toxicity. Less common side effects are a sudden drop in blood pressure if you stand up too quickly from a lying or sitting position, and an irregular heart rhythm. Also, unless you are weaned off them slowly, they can have rebound effects, such as depression and insomnia.

SELF-HELP ALTERNATIVE TREATMENTS

The following techniques can be done at home. Although they may not work as fast as drugs or surgery, natural alternatives help the body heal itself. They get at the root of the problem instead of just temporarily alleviating the symptoms. All herbs, homeopathic remedies, and supplements discussed here are available in health food stores and, increasingly, in large drug and grocery stores, as well as on the Internet.

Aromatherapy

Aromatherapy is useful for PHN, particularly the essential oils of bergamot, chamomile, clary sage, jasmine, lavender, melissa, neroli, and rose. They are available in health food stores and stores specializing in aromatherapy products which you can find in the yellow pages. (*See* AROMATHERAPY in PART 2 Treatment Section for additional information.)

Diet

Postherpetic neuralgia is inflammatory in nature so certain dietary modifications may be helpful.

Good Foods

Yogurt and buttermilk help alleviate pain and promote healing. (*See* NUTRITIONAL THERAPY in PART 2 Treatment Section for additional information.)

Bad Foods

Avoid argenine-producing foods, such as chocolate, nuts, peanuts, pork, soybeans, and turkey, since they tend to deplete your body of lysine, which is needed to control the herpes virus (VZV).

Heat Therapy/Cold Therapy

Cold compresses, or ice placed on the affected area, can give short-term pain relief from PHN. (*See* HEAT THERAPY/COLD THERAPY in PART 2 Treatment Section for additional information.)

Herbal Remedies

- ❑ Catnip relaxes the nervous system.
- ❑ Cayenne capsules (containing capsaicin, the chemical that gives hot peppers their zing) relieve pain and help healing.
- ❑ Capsaicin cream. First used by alternative practitioners, capsaicin cream is now being suggested by mainstream medicines and is widely sold.
- ❑ Echinacea has antiviral and anti-inflammatory properties.
- ❑ Hops relax the nervous system.
- ❑ Licorice gel, applied topically, helps relieve PHN.
- ❑ Myrrh soothes inflammation.
- ❑ Passionflower relaxes the nervous system.
- ❑ Slippery elm bark helps your body produce its own anti-inflammatory cortisone.
- ❑ Valerian relaxes the nervous system.

Take the above herbs as directed on label. They can also be used in teas and infusions. (*See* HERBAL REMEDIES in PART 2 Treatment Section for additional information.)

Homeopathic Remedies

You can self-treat with homeopathic remedies by selecting the one that most closely matches your symptoms. If you don't see improvement, try another, or a combination product. Follow the instructions on the label. If you do not have relief in a reasonable amount of time, consult a physician who specializes in homeopathic medicine.

- ❑ Apis mellifica helps ease burning, stinging, and itching.
- ❑ Hypericum (St. John's wort) helps repair damaged nerves and is useful for any type of nerve pain.
- ❑ Ranunculus bulbosus eases itching and helps ease pain caused by contact with clothing or touch.

Combination remedies sometimes work more effectively than single ones. (*See* HOMEOPATHY in PART 2 Treatment Section for additional information.)

Hydrotherapy

Warm baths and hot tubs help relax your body and can alleviate the PHN pain. (*See* HYDROTHERAPY in PART 2 Treatment Section for additional information.)

Supplements

- ❑ Bromelain, 500 mg twice daily between meals, acts as an anti-inflammatory.
- ❑ Fish oil, two 1000 mg capsules three times daily, acts as an anti-inflammatory.
- ❑ L-Lysine, 500 mg four times daily on an empty stomach, helps fight the herpes virus.
- ❑ Magnesium citrate, 400 mg four times daily, acts as an antispasmodic that relieves pain.
- ❑ Vitamin B-complex, 100 mg twice daily, is essential for healthy nerve function.
- ❑ Vitamin B_{12}, 500 mcg sublingually twice daily, helps relieve symptoms of PHN. It is more effective if injected by a physician. For balance when taking individual Bs, be sure to supplement with a B-complex once daily, or a multivitamin containing B-complex.
- ❑ Vitamin C, 3000–5000 mg (3–5 grams) daily, will aid tissue repair. Take it to bowel tolerance. (If diarrhea occurs, reduce the dosage until normal bowel function returns.) It is preferable to take Ester-C because more of the vitamin is absorbed in this form.
- ❑ Vitamin E, 1200–1600 IU daily, aids in controlling PHN. Work up slowly to this dosage and continue for at least six months. (For this short term, these high amounts are safe.) Vitamin E oil can also be applied to your skin.

(*See* SUPPLEMENT THERAPY in PART 2 Treatment Section for additional information.)

ASSISTED ALTERNATIVE TREATMENTS

The following techniques may require specialized training or the aid of a healthcare professional.

Bee Venom Therapy

Some components of bee venom are thought to stimulate the immune system. Other components are thought to modify the transmission of pain signals within the nervous system, and the therapy has proven dramatically helpful with postherpetic neuralgia. (*See* BEE VENOM THERAPY in PART 2 Treatment Section for additional information.)

Biofeedback

Electrodes taped to the skin transmit impulses to a computer screen so you can actually see when you tense and relax your muscles. (*See* BIOFEEDBACK in PART 2 Treatment Section for additional information.)

Craniosacral Therapy

A trained craniosacral practitioner can feel areas where healthy tissue function is restricted, usually due to physical or emotional trauma. The theory is that physical injuries and emotional traumas are stored or frozen in the body until they are released. (*See* CRANIOSACRAL THERAPY in PART 2 Treatment Section for additional information.)

Cupping and Bleeding

Some of those with PHN have found relief from this ancient practice, which is now being revived as a treatment. After puncturing the skin with a needle, a cup with vacuum suction is placed over the bleeding area to stimulate circulation. (*See* CUPPING in PART 2 Treatment Section for additional information.)

Massage

Stress can lead to even more pain, and massage helps alleviate stress. (*See* MASSAGE in PART 2 Treatment Section for additional information.)

Oxygen Therapy

Hydrogen peroxide therapy (H_2O_2) and ultraviolet irradiation of blood (UVIB) can help alleviate the pain of postherpetic neuralgia. (*See* OXYGEN THERAPIES in PART 2 Treatment Section for additional information.)

Reflexology

Reflexology massage therapy performed on the specific part of the foot and/or hand that corresponds to the area affected by the PHN can be helpful. (*See* REFLEXOLOGY in PART 2 Treatment Section for additional information.)

Rolfing

Rolfing can be effective in the treatment of postherpetic neuralgia. It can have long-lasting effects. (*See* ROLFING in PART 2 Treatment Section for additional information.)

Stress Management and Relaxation Techniques

Biofeedback, guided imagery, meditation, and yoga breathing exercises, are often helpful with PHN. Reducing stress helps strengthen the immune system. (*See* BIOFEEDBACK, GUIDED IMAGERY and VISUALIZATION, MEDITATION, and TAI CHI, QIGONG, and YOGA in PART 2 Treatment Section for additional information.)

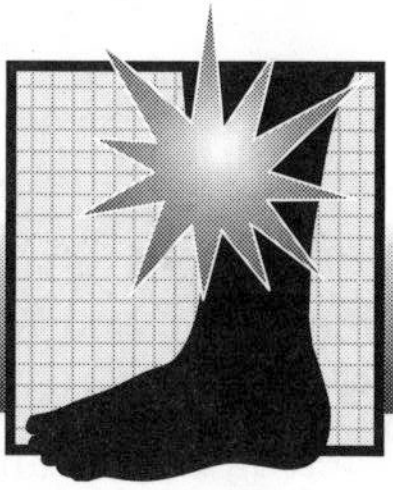

Post-Polio Syndrome

Post-polio syndrome is a combination of fatigue, muscle weakness, and pain described as a burning sensation or a deep muscle ache. It occurs between twenty and thirty years after the initial polio attack and does not appear to favor either men or women. People who recovered from polio decades before find that the long-ago affected muscles begin to progressively weaken and atrophy. The new symptoms progress very slowly, are not as severe as the original symptoms, and do not lead to total paralysis. Of the approximate 300,000 polio survivors in the United States, half may have some of the PPS symptoms, while about 20 percent have them to a significant degree.

Unlike other conditions, there is little interest in, or education about, PPS, for two reasons. First, doctors trained after the 1950s have an extremely limited knowledge of polio because the Salk and Sabin vaccines have been so effective in preventing the disease. The other reason is that most of those with PPS are over sixty-years-old and the condition will very likely be non-existent in a few years.

Although not within the scope of this book, breathing problems due to underventilation may also be evident in post-polio syndrome. If your lungs were affected by polio and you are experiencing breathing difficulties, you should be evaluated by a pulmonary specialist.

Symptoms

- ❑ New, increasing weakness and atrophy in muscles that were once paralyzed or only minimally affected.
- ❑ Unusual fatigue from normal activities.
- ❑ Intolerance to cold.
- ❑ Low back pain.
- ❑ Muscle pain described as aching, burning, or cramping.
- ❑ Numbness in fingers and toes.
- ❑ Pain that occurs at night and is worse after an active day.
- ❑ Pain and inflammation of joints, with swelling and tenderness.
- ❑ Stiffness.

In addition, poor posture due to PPS-related muscular weakness can result in neck pain and headaches in the back of the head. And, progressive weakness of the back and hip muscles can result in back pain, just as similar progressive weakness of the muscles surrounding the knee can result in knee pain.

Common Causes

The primary cause of post-polio syndrome is, of course, having had polio. But listed below are subsidiary causes that worsen the PPS.

- ❑ Overuse of nerves and muscles that were either affected or took over for those killed by the polio virus.
- ❑ Pain in the hands, shoulders, and wrists that can occur from using crutches or propelling a wheelchair. Use of canes or crutches can lead to carpal tunnel syndrome. (*See* CARPAL TUNNEL SYNDROME in PART 1 Conditions Section for additional information.)
- ❑ Premature aging and/or a wearing down of those nerve cells and/or muscles that were originally affected by polio.
- ❑ The condition can also be worsened in those who continue to push themselves despite weakness and fatigue. Use it or lose it does not apply to PPS. Overworking affected muscles can actually make them weaker and cause pain.
- ❑ If the same muscle is constantly being strained and results in intermittent pain, it could be due to PPS.

Diagnosing the Problem

Diagnosis is based on evaluating the symptoms and performing specific tests, such as an electromyographic study (EMG) and a nerve conduction study (NCS). The EMG tests how the muscles are working. It involves placing needles into the muscles and measuring what is happening to them on a screen. It can determine the cause of the injury and whether it is old or new. The NCS tests the nerves by applying surface electrodes to the skin and administering electrical impulses to them with a stimulator. The two tests are usually performed at the same time, to establish a correct diagnosis and to see if new problems are occurring.

Conventional Treatments

In general, treatments neither cure nor arrest PPS. All they can do is address some of its symptoms.

- ❑ Antidepressants, such as doxepin, elavil, imipramine, at one-third to one-half the usual dosages, work by altering some of the brain's chemical signals that are involved with pain relief. They are also helpful in promoting a good night's sleep.

- ❑ Antiseizure medications help relax muscles and stabilize the nerves.
- ❑ Injections of corticosteroids into the affected joints can alleviate pain.
- ❑ Muscle relaxants help relieve pain.
- ❑ Non-steroidal anti-inflammatory drugs (NSAIDs) help relieve pain in muscles and joints.
- ❑ Physical therapy treatments for PPS help restore function, improve mobility, and relieve pain by using conservative methods that do not involve surgery. Treatments include gentle stretching of tissues, relaxation exercises, traction, and ultrasound, which can help alleviate pain. (*See* PHYSICAL THERAPY in PART 2 Treatment Section for additional information.) (*See also* PHYSICAL THERAPY in Assisted Alternative Treatments below.)
- ❑ Quinine can help alleviate muscle spasms.
- ❑ Recommendation not to overuse muscles and joints.
- ❑ Surgical release of compressed nerves can be performed.
- ❑ Tranquilizers can help quiet the pain.
- ❑ Trigger-point injections can decrease pain and muscle spasms.
- ❑ TENS units (transcutaneous electronic nerve stimuators) help mask, alleviate, and control pain.
- ❑ Weight control. Overweight can put too much load on already overworked muscles.

Problems with Some Conventional Treatments

- ❑ Antidepressants, antiseizure medications, muscle relaxants, and tranquilizers can cause sleepiness and impair motor function.
- ❑ Corticosteroid injections give only temporary relief.
- ❑ NSAIDs can cause irritation to the lining of the gastrointestinal tract.
- ❑ Quinine has been known to cause visual problems.
- ❑ Surgical procedures are never entirely risk-free.
- ❑ Weight loss can be difficult when you are limiting exercise.

SELF-HELP ALTERNATIVE TREATMENTS

The following techniques can be done at home. Although they may not work as fast as drugs or surgery, natural alternatives help the body heal itself. All herbs, homeopathic remedies, packs, and supplements discussed here are available in health food stores and, increasingly, in large drug and grocery stores, as well as on the Internet.

Aromatherapy

Aromatherapy, particularly the essential oils of bergamot, black pepper, chamomile, clary sage, ginger, grapefruit, juniper, lavender, marjoram, and rosemary help alleviate muscle pain and spasm. Add seven to ten drops of any one, or a combination, diluted in two ounces of a carrier oil, such as sweet almond oil or apricot kernel oil, and gently rub into the affected area after a warm shower or bath. These essential oils are available in health food stores and stores specializing in aromatherapy products, which you can find in the yellow pages. (*See* AROMATHERAPY in PART 2 Treatment Section for additional information.)

Castor Oil Packs

Dip a piece of white flannel into some warm castor oil. Wring it out and place it over any particularly painful area. Cover with plastic and apply a heating pad for one hour. Do this twice daily. (*See* COMPRESSES, PACKS, and POULTICES in PART 2 Treatment Section for additional information.)

Diet

Dietary considerations are always important in determining the course of a condition.

Good Foods

- ❑ Calcium-rich foods, such as broccoli, dairy products, salmon, sardines, and tofu, are good because calcium is helpful in preventing muscle cramps.
- ❑ Season your food with cayenne red pepper, garlic, ginger, and horseradish to aid circulation.
- ❑ Tonic water contains quinine and does not have the side effects of quinine medicines.

(*See* NUTRITIONAL THERAPY in PART 2 Treatment Section for additional information.)

Bad Foods

Sugary foods and others with empty calories lead to weight gain and the proliferation of free radicals. These include sodas, candy, cookies, ice cream, and pastries.

Other Substances to Avoid

Tobacco smoke. Smoking keeps oxygen and blood from nourishing your muscles.

Heat Therapy/Cold Therapy

Cold will reduce swelling and heat increases blood flow to the area. (*See* HEAT THERAPY/COLD THERAPY in PART 2 Treatment Section for additional information.)

Herbal Remedies

- ❑ Butchers Broom helps alleviate leg cramps and relieve inflammation.
- ❑ Cayenne improves circulation.
- ❑ Cramp bark helps balance calcium, magnesium, and potassium, which alleviates muscle cramping.
- ❑ Ginger aids circulation and alleviates muscle spasms and cramps.

Take the above herbs as directed on label. They can also be used in teas and infusions. (*See* HERBAL REMEDIES in PART 2 Treatment Section for additional information.)

Homeopathic Remedies

You can self-treat with homeopathic remedies by selecting the one that most closely matches your symptoms. If you don't see improvement, try another, or a combination product. Follow the instructions on the label. If you do not have relief in a reasonable amount of time, consult a physician who specializes in homeopathic medicine.

- ❑ Bryonia relieves pain that is worse with motion.
- ❑ Hypericum soothes nerve pain.
- ❑ Kali phos is a calming nerve nutrient.
- ❑ Magnesium phosphate calms cramps and cramping-type pain.
- ❑ Rhus toxicodendron helps relieve stiffness and pain caused by overuse of the muscles.
- ❑ Spigelia relieves stabbing-type nerve pain.

Combination remedies sometimes work more effectively than single ones. (*See* HOMEOPATHY in PART 2 Treatment Section for additional information.)

Hydrotherapy

Running hot water over a painful area while in the shower, or soaking in a hot tub can help diminish the pain. (*See* HYDROTHERAPY in PART 2 Treatment Section for additional information.)

Magnet Therapy

Magnet therapy relieves pain, accelerates healing, and reduces inflammation. An increasing body of evidence is showing that magnets placed on the sore spots are effective for treating the pain associated with PPS. (*See* MAGNET THERAPY in PART 2 Treatment Section for additional information.)

Supplements

- ❑ Calcium, 1000 mg in divided doses, helps alleviate muscle cramps and has the additional advantage of preventing osteoporosis.
- ❑ Magnesium citrate, 400 mg four times daily, helps relieve muscle pain and spasms.
- ❑ Good quality multivitamin/mineral combination because most diets are inadequate in essential nutrients needed by the body for optimum health.

(*See* SUPPLEMENT THERAPY in PART 2 Treatment Section for additional information.)

ASSISTED ALTERNATIVE TREATMENTS

The following techniques may require specialized training or the aid of a healthcare professional.

Acupuncture and Acupressure

Acupuncture involves the insertion of extremely thin solid needles into specific points of your body to stimulate its own healing mechanism and improve blood flow to the affected areas. It also reduces inflammation, relieves pain, improves mobility, and there are rarely any risks or side effects. It is particularly useful in treating PPS because it stimulates the release of natural chemicals produced by the body that reduce pain sensations and help to redirect energy flow. (*See* ACUPUNCTURE and ACUPRESSURE in PART 2 Treatment Section for additional information.)

Applied Kinesiology

Applied Kinesiology is excellent for reducing pain rapidly. The AK practitioner tests your muscles to determine the origin of your problem and then decides on the best course of action, choosing from a wide variety of therapeutic methods at his or her disposal. (*See* APPLIED KINESIOLOGY in PART 2 Treatment Section for additional information.)

Chiropractic

Chiropractic theory is based on the assumption that a

properly aligned spine is essential for good health, and that any misalignment of the vertebrae in the spine causes pressure on the spinal nerves, leading to pain. The chiropractor makes spinal adjustments to move misaligned vertebrae to more normal positions, which helps the nervous system to function properly. Anyone with post-polio syndrome who has muscle weakness and decreased bone density should select a chiropractor who will not do forceful manipulations that could possibly cause further injury. (*See* CHIROPRACTIC in PART 2 Treatment Section for additional information.)

Exercise and Stretching

Gentle strengthening exercise supervised by a trainer experienced in treating people with PPS can help improve coordination, endurance, flexibility and strength. Be careful not to overdo exercises. (*See* EXERCISE, STRETCHING, and SPORTS in PART 2 Treatment Section for additional information.)

Guided Imagery and Visualization Techniques

These help to relieve stress and minimize pain. Although not likely to restore motion, a trained therapist may be able to offer techniques to help you cope with the stress and pain associated with post-polio syndrome. (*See* GUIDED IMAGERY and VISUALIZATION in PART 2 Treatment Section for additional information.)

Massage

A massage helps bring blood to the affected area to relieve the pain. There are many kinds of massage therapies available and you can ask your practitioner to suggest the appropriate one for your problem. Gentle massage can be helpful for the muscles, and it also helps you relax. (*See* MASSAGE in PART 2 Treatment Section for additional information.)

Osteopathic Manipulation

The goal of osteopathic manipulation in the treatment of post-polio syndrome is to increase range of motion, decrease muscle tension, and improve blood circulation. (*See* OSTEOPATHIC MANIPULATION in PART 2 Treatment Section for additional information.)

Oxygen Therapies

Hyperbaric oxygen therapy (HBOT) enhances your body's ability to heal itself by encouraging its own natural production of oxygen. (*See* OXYGEN THERAPIES in PART 2 Treatment Section for additional information.)

Physical Therapy

Environmentally Enhanced Physical Therapy is an unconventional form of physical therapy that we feel is worth mentioning because it has helped many of those with post-polio syndrome. It was originated by Ed Snapp, a licensed physical therapist who also has PPS. People who have taken the treatment, which consists of twelve days of (six to) eight-hour-a-day therapy, claim remarkable results, with 85 percent of them experiencing positive results that range from moderate to profound. The simple basic therapies (hydrotherapy, massage, repetitive passive exercise performed in a dark quiet room) that can produce significant positive results within twelve days are potent enough to be detrimental if improperly applied, so it is crucial to use only a therapist trained in this particular therapy. Under the theory that

No Distance Too Far for Relief

Kevin had polio as a child in England, which left his right arm paralyzed. His legs compensated for this loss and allowed him to lead a very active life of sports and adventure until, in his late fifties, his polio symptoms returned and caused a drastic deterioration in his legs, back, and stomach muscles, along with other painful symptoms of post-polio syndrome. After three years of futile visits to London's premier specialists and hospitals looking to find a treatment for his continually deteriorating situation, Kevin's daughter got on the Internet and found the Futures Unlimited post-polio clinic in Mississippi, U.S.A.

Desperate to try anything, Kevin overcame his skepticism and arrived at the clinic with his wheelchair and crutch. A short twelve days later, after daily non-invasive six-hour treatments, Kevin was able to walk short distances without even a crutch. And, as he continued to improve back home in England, he was once again able to drive his car. No matter what the distance and the expense, Kevin said it was the best trip he had ever taken because the clinic gave him back the life he thought he had lost forever.

the body will heal itself by re-establishing sensory pathways, you remain passive as the therapist works and do not actually perform any direct exercise—all treatment is done to you.

With passive treatment, the nervous system uses what it already has stored in memory to put the sensory factors in the right places, that is, in the same order they were in the person's original genetic code. The nervous system defines what was written in the genetic code by scanning its own functions in a fashion similar to a computer, and uses that information to correct everything, thus allowing a person with PPS to regain a lot of what they had after they originally recovered from polio and before they got PPS. You can get more information on this effective method by contacting Futures Unlimited at 662-327-7333, or by accessing their website at *www.futuresunlimited.com*.

Reflexology

Reflexology massage therapy can be performed on the part of the foot or hand corresponding to the area that is in pain. (*See* REFLEXOLOGY in PART 2 Treatment Section for additional information.)

Rolfing

Rolfing has been shown to be effective in treating impaired mobility. It can have long-lasting effects in easing pain. (*See* ROLFING in PART 2 Treatment Section for additional information.)

Tai Chi, Qigong, and Yoga

Tai chi, qigong, and yoga are gentle, highly effective forms of martial arts training that also calm and center you. They are excellent exercises for anyone with post-polio syndrome. (*See* TAI CHI, QIGONG, and YOGA in PART 2 Treatment Section for additional information.)

PRACTICAL SUGGESTIONS

- ❑ Join a support group.
- ❑ Get enough sleep. Try practicing relaxation techniques, such as guided imagery, meditation, and tai chi, qigong, and yoga.
- ❑ Be conscious of your posture.
- ❑ Avoid neck strain. Do not cradle the telephone between your ear and shoulder.

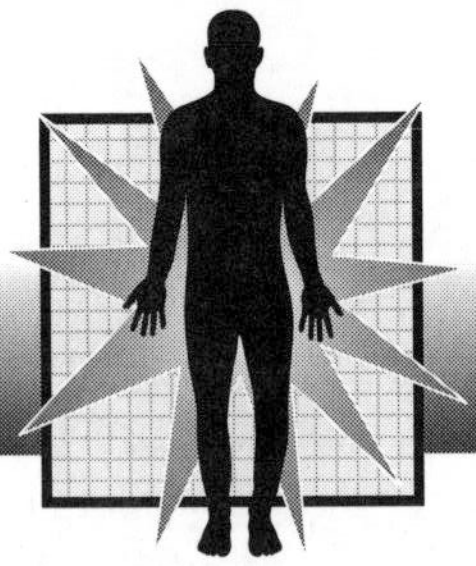

Premenstrual Syndrome (PMS)

Premenstrual syndrome (PMS) affects some women a week or two before their menstrual period begins and manifests in a wide variety of symptoms. Here we are only addressing those aspects of it that contribute to pelvic pain, including midcycle pain, also known as mittelschmerz, which occurs on one side of the lower abdomen around the time of ovulation.

Symptoms

- ❑ One-sided lower abdominal pain mid-cycle.
- ❑ Monthly pain that can switch sides and last from several minutes up to forty-eight hours.

Common Causes

- ❑ The egg follicle's growing and stretching the surface of the ovary just before ovulation can cause pain.
- ❑ When the ruptured egg follicle releases its fluid or blood at the time of ovulation, it can irritate the abdominal lining, causing pain.

Diagnosing the Problem

A pelvic examination does not usually show any abnormalities. Your gynecologist may order an ultrasound study to rule out potentially serious ovarian problems.

Conventional Treatments

- ❑ Birth control pills. They prevent ovulation, thereby preventing pain.
- ❑ Physical therapy treatments. They help restore function, improve mobility, and relieve pain by using conservative methods that do not involve surgery. (*See also* PHYSICAL THERAPY in PART 2 Treatment Section for additional information.)

Problems with Some Conventional Treatments

- ❑ Birth control pills can cause abdominal bloating, ankle swelling, deep vein thrombosis, and sore breasts.

SELF-HELP ALTERNATIVE TREATMENTS

The following techniques can be done at home. Although they may not work as fast as drugs or surgery, natural alternatives help the body heal itself. All herbs, homeopathic remedies, packs, and supplements discussed here are available in health food stores and, increasingly, in large drug and grocery stores, as well as on the Internet.

Aromatherapy

Aromatherapy, particularly the essential oils of bergamot, chamomile, clary sage, fennel, geranium, grapefruit, jasmine, lavender, melissa, neroli, nutmeg, palmarosa, parsley seed, rose, vetiver, and ylang ylang all help regulate hormonal balance. They also relieve spasms and help heal tissues. You can either put a few drops into a hot bath and soak, or add a few drops to vegetable oil and massage into the affected area. Do not ingest essential oils or use them full strength as they are very powerful compounds. They are available in health food stores and stores specializing in aromatherapy products, which you can find in the yellow pages. (*See* AROMATHERAPY in PART 2 Treatment Section for additional information.)

Castor Oil Packs

Dip a piece of white flannel into some warm castor oil. Wring it out and place it over your pelvic area. Cover with plastic and apply a heating pad for one hour. Do this twice daily. (*See* COMPRESSES, PACKS, and POULTICES in PART 2 Treatment Section for additional information.)

Diet

What you eat can play a role in PMS so certain dietary modifications can be helpful.

Good Foods

Try to get most of your protein from organic chicken, turkey, and fish. Low thyroid function can be a cause of PMS, so foods that stimulate the thyroid should be added to your diet. These include:

- ❑ Apples;
- ❑ Kelp;
- ❑ Mushrooms;
- ❑ Sesame seeds.

(*See* NUTRITIONAL THERAPY in PART 2 Treatment Section for additional information.)

Bad Foods

It's a good idea to avoid the following foods as they can worsen your symptoms.

- ❑ Dairy products, eggs, and meat from non-organic sources because most animals are raised on hormones which can affect your system.
- ❑ Dried fruits, fermented foods, overripe fruits, and sugars all cause yeast proliferation.
- ❑ Estrogen-producing foods, such as alfalfa, carrots, endive, legumes, liver, oatmeal, wheat germ, and yams (except for wild Mexican yams).
- ❑ Fatty foods because hormones store in fatty tissue.

Other Substances to Avoid

- ❑ Dioxin Exposure. Use only unbleached tampons and sanitary napkins.
- ❑ Do not use an IUD for contraception because it increases menstrual flow.
- ❑ PABA produces estrogen, so be sure your multivitamin does not contain it. Do not use sunscreens containing PABA because it can be absorbed through the skin.

Heat Therapy/Cold Therapy

Warm baths ease cramping. (*See* HEAT THERAPY/COLD THERAPY,and HYDROTHERAPY in PART 2 Treatment Section for additional information.)

Herbal Remedies

- ❑ Blessed thistle helps balance hormones.
- ❑ Cayenne improves circulation.
- ❑ Dandelion leaf is a diuretic herb that eases bloating.
- ❑ Dong quai is known as the queen of all herbs for women. It has a tranquilizing effect on the nervous system and relieves pain and bloating.
- ❑ Raspberry leaves relax uterine spasms.
- ❑ Sarsaparilla helps regulate hormones.

Take the above herbs as directed on label. They can also be used in teas and infusions. (*See* HERBAL REMEDIES in PART 2 Treatment Section for additional information.)

Homeopathic Remedies

You can self-treat with homeopathic remedies by selecting the one that most closely matches your symptoms. If you don't see improvement, try another, or a combination product. Follow the instructions on the label. If you do not have relief in a reasonable amount of time, consult a physician who specializes in homeopathic medicine.

- ❑ Cimicifuga helps relieve cramps in the pelvic area.
- ❑ Lilium tigrinum helps relieve rectal pressure.
- ❑ Nux vomica helps relieve pain in the rectal and/or tailbone area.

Combination remedies sometimes work more effectively than single ones. (*See* HOMEOPATHY in PART 2 Treatment Section for additional information.)

Meditation

Meditation helps reduce stress, which contributes to pelvic pain. (*See* MEDITATION in PART 2 Treatment Section for additional information.)

Supplements

- ❑ Calcium citrate, 500 mg twice daily, helps reduce PMS symptoms.
- ❑ Magnesium citrate, 400 mg three times daily, helps slow heavy bleeding and reduce muscle spasms.
- ❑ Vitamin A from fish liver oil, 25,000 IU twice daily, and from beta-carotene (a vitamin-A precursor), 25,000 IU twice daily, reduces PMS symptoms.
- ❑ Vitamin B_1, 100 mg twice daily, relieves muscle cramping.
- ❑ Vitamin B_6, 250 mg twice daily, acts as a diuretic. Note: For balance, when taking individual Bs, be sure to supplement with a B-complex once daily, or a multivitamin containing Bs.
- ❑ Vitamin C, 1000 mg three times daily, acts as a natural diuretic.
- ❑ Vitamin E helps balance hormones. Start with 400 IU once daily and work up gradually to twice daily.

Note: Several PMS combinations are available. If you use them with any of the above supplements, check labels carefully so you don't double dose. (*See* SUPPLEMENT THERAPY in PART 2 Treatment Section for additional information.)

ASSISTED ALTERNATIVE TREATMENTS

The following techniques may require specialized training or the aid of a healthcare professional.

Acupuncture and Acupressure

Acupuncture involves the insertion of extremely thin solid needles into specific points of your body to stimulate its own healing mechanism and improve blood flow to the pelvic area. It also reduces inflammation and relieves pain, and there are rarely any risks or side effects. (*See* ACUPUNCTURE and ACUPRESSURE in PART 2 Treatment Section for additional information.)

Applied Kinesiology

Applied Kinesiology is excellent for reducing pain rapidly. The AK practitioner tests your muscles to determine the origin of your problem and then decides on the best course of action, choosing from a wide variety of therapeutic methods at his or her disposal. (*See* APPLIED KINESIOLOGY in PART 2 Treatment Section for additional information.)

Bee Venom Therapy

Some components of bee venom are thought to stimulate the immune system. Other components are thought to modify the transmission of pain signals within the nervous system, and the therapy has proven consistently useful for painful conditions. (*See* BEE VENOM THERAPY in PART 2 Treatment Section for additional information.)

Biofeedback

Electrodes taped to the skin transmit impulses to a computer screen so you can actually see when you tense and relax your muscles. (*See* BIOFEEDBACK in PART 2 Treatment Section for additional information.)

Chiropractic

Chiropractic theory is based on the assumption that a properly aligned spine is essential for good health, and that any misalignment of the vertebrae in the spine causes pressure on the spinal nerves, leading to pain. The chiropractor makes spinal adjustments to move misaligned vertebrae to more normal positions, which helps the nervous system to function properly. In pelvic disorders, a chiropractor can determine if the pelvic bones are out of alignment and if the muscles attached to them are able to properly relax. (*See* CHIROPRACTIC in PART 2 Treatment Section for additional information.)

Craniosacral Therapy

Craniosacral therapy is a form of energy healing that can help balance your system. It has been shown to be effective for alleviating pelvic problems. (*See* CRANIOSACRAL THERAPY in PART 2 Treatment Section for additional information.)

Exercise and Stretching

Regular aerobic exercise aids circulation, helps oxygenate the blood, and relaxes the uterus. To avoid damage, it must be carefully supervised in the beginning. (*See* EXERCISE, STRETCHING, and SPORTS in PART 2 Treatment Section for additional information.)

Guided Imagery and Visualization Techniques

Guided imagery can help manage pelvic pain. To relieve the sensation of chronic heaviness, change the pain into a light object that you can easily handle. (*See* GUIDED IMAGERY and VISUALIZATION in PART 2 Treatment Section for additional information.)

Massage

A massage helps bring blood to the pelvic area and relieves the pain. There are many kinds of massage therapies available and you can ask your practitioner to suggest the appropriate one for your pelvic pain. (*See* MASSAGE in PART 2 Treatment Section for additional information.)

Osteopathic Manipulation

The goal of osteopathic manipulation in the treatment of pelvic pain is to reduce uterine congestion, relieve pain, and improve blood circulation. (*See* OSTEOPATHIC MANIPULATION in PART 2 Treatment Section for additional information.)

Reflexology

Reflexology massage therapy can be performed on the part of the foot or hand corresponding to the pelvic area that is in pain. (*See* REFLEXOLOGY in PART 2 Treatment Section for additional information.)

Tai Chi, Qigong, and Yoga

These therapies induce a profoundly relaxed state and help bring healing energy to the body. (*See* TAI CHI, QIGONG, and YOGA in PART 2 Treatment Section for additional information.)

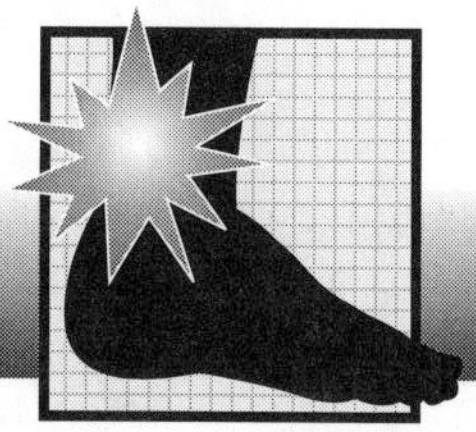

Reflex Sympathetic Dystrophy Syndrome

Reflex sympathetic dystrophy syndrome (RSDS) is a disorder that usually develops following a traumatic injury to the limbs, such as a fracture or a sprain in the foot or hand that can involve nerve damage. The condition is known by several additional names, including complex regional pain syndrome (CRPS), shoulder-hand syndrome, or its most common name, posttraumatic syndrome. Its original name, causalgia (hot pain), was coined by Dr. Silas Weir Mitchell, who discovered the condition among the injured soldiers he treated during the Civil War. It currently affects more than 6 million people, about 80 percent of them women now, and not many doctors are familiar with it. Although age is not a factor—RSDS can strike anyone, from less than a year old to the aged—the condition is generally contracted by people in their thirties to forties. It starts out in an acute stage, characterized by burning spontaneous pain. Six or more months after the original injury, the joints often become fixed, the muscles and tendons contract, the bones demineralize, and ultimately the muscles waste and atrophy. Early diagnosis is critical because, if this highly destructive condition is treated early enough, the chances of reversing it are very high.

Symptoms

The symptoms usually occur near the area of an injury that could have been either major or minor, and can affect either one, two, three, or all four extremities, often spreading from one to another. Symptoms may also appear in the back, face, or shoulders, and are usually localized at first, but can spread over time. They include:

❑ Burning, searing pain that is constant;

❑ Decreased hair growth;

❑ Depression;

❑ Difficulty concentrating;

❑ Emotional disturbances;

❑ Inflammation;

❑ Increased sensitivity to temperature and touch;

❑ Insomnia;

❑ Joint tenderness and reduced flexibility;

❑ Memory problems (short-term memory);

❑ Prolonged pain more severe than the original injury, that gets worse rather than better over time;

❑ Sensitivity to touch, even contact with clothing or the sheet on your bed, or a breeze blowing over the affected area;

❑ Skin changes and discoloration—the skin is warm, red, and shiny at first, then becomes cool and bluish;

❑ Spasms of the muscles and blood vessels, in the arms and legs particularly;

❑ Swelling;

❑ Sweating;

❑ Vision problems, such as blurriness.

Common Causes

RSDS is usually caused by an injury to a body part that has multiple nerve endings, such as a hand or foot. The injury can be as minor as a pinprick, or as severe as an accident, a stab wound, a burn, frostbite, or surgery. RSDS can also be caused by diseases that affect the internal organs, or by nerve damage in either the sympathetic or the central nervous system—among other things, these systems regulate the diameter of blood vessels, and the smaller, constricted blood vessels can add to the pain of RSDS. The damaged nerves send inappropriate signals to the brain, and these interfere with normal information about sensations. In addition to affecting the nerves and blood vessels, the disorder also affects the bones, and skin. Some specific causes include:

❑ Arthritis;

❑ Cancer;

❑ Infections;

❑ Myocardial infarction;

❑ Neurological disorders involving the spinal cord and nerves;

❑ Trauma from accidents, or reactions to certain medical procedures, such as tight casts, scars from surgery, peripheral nerve damage from injections, or forceful manipulation;

❑ Tumors;

❑ Weather changes can exacerbate the existing condition. A drop in barometric pressure causes an increase in pain in 75 percent of those with RSDS.

Note: Not every injury will result in RSDS. Most injuries heal normally, and only a very small percentage of them are ever affected by RSDS.

Diagnosing the Problem

Diagnosis is usually made by observing the symptoms and it is preferable to go to a doctor knowledgeable about RSDS because there is no single test to show or rule out the presence of the condition. A combination of tests has to be performed, including:

- ❑ Bone scans to determine the progress of bone density loss;
- ❑ Color-coded thermograms to show an altered blood supply to the painful area;
- ❑ Thermography to determine any variations in heat emitted from the body, and any changes in body temperature that are common in RSDS;
- ❑ X-rays to show bone changes.

Conventional Treatments

- ❑ Anticonvulsants help to dilate blood vessels.
- ❑ Antidepressants help block nerve-induced pain and have the added benefit of easing insomnia.
- ❑ Anti-inflammatory drugs help reduce pain.
- ❑ Capsaicin, applied topically, relieves pain. (*See* HERBAL REMEDIES in PART 2 Treatment Section for additional information.)
- ❑ Corticosteroids relieve inflammation.
- ❑ Nerve Blocks. Local anesthesia can be injected in appropriate sites, depending on which body part is affected.
- ❑ Neurostimulation. An implanted lead (a flexible insulated wire) powered by an implanted battery or receiver is placed near the spinal cord to send electrical impulses that block pain messages to the brain. Also used for chronic back or leg pains, neuropathies, and spinal stenosis, among other chronic pain conditions, when drugs or surgery have failed.
- ❑ Physical therapy treatments help restore function, improve mobility, and relieve pain by using conservative methods that do not involve surgery. Lack of motion leads to muscle deterioration and frozen joints. That is why it is crucial for someone with RSDS to keep the affected limbs mobile. (*See* PHYSICAL THERAPY in PART 2 Treatment Section for additional information.)
- ❑ Surgery (sympathectomy). Cutting or burning the nerves with chemicals to eliminate the pain.
- ❑ TENS units (transcutaneous electrical nerve stimulation). Pulses of electricity applied to the nerve endings under the skin can help someone in chronic pain.
- ❑ Vasodilators improve circulation.

Problems with Some Conventional Treatments

- ❑ Nerve blocks are more effective when RSDS is in its early stages, but since pain relief lasts only as long as the anesthetic keeps working, people with RSDS require either repeated injections or continuous infusions of the pain-relieving agents.
- ❑ Neurostimulation is an invasive procedure, and, as such, can invite complications.
- ❑ Physical therapy must be administered by a practitioner skilled in treating RSDS because she or he must take care to insure that the affected areas are not overstressed. Improper treatment can lead to setbacks, injuries, and the spread of the RSDS.
- ❑ Sympathectomies, while effective in the short term, can lead to the spread of RSDS and even more pain after a year or more. And, although cutting the nerves can eliminate pain, the procedure also destroys other sensations. There is a high failure rate, up to 70 percent, and the procedure can cause the condition to spread or worsen.

SELF-HELP ALTERNATIVE TREATMENTS

The following techniques can be done at home. Although they may not work as fast as drugs or surgery, natural alternatives help the body heal itself. All herbs, homeopathic remedies, and supplements discussed here are available in health food stores and, increasingly, in large drug and grocery stores, as well as on the Internet.

Aromatherapy

Aromatherapy, particularly the essential oils of black pepper, blue gum, cardamom, chamomile, eucalyptus, ginger, lavender, marjoram, pine, and rosemary can alleviate the symptoms of RSDS. You can put a few drops into a warm bath and soak, or add a few drops to vegetable oil and gently massage this mix into the affected area, but do not ingest essential oils or use them full strength as they are very powerful compounds. They are available in health food stores and stores specializing in aromatherapy products, which you can find in the yellow pages. (*See* AROMATHERAPY in PART 2 Treatment Section for additional information.)

Diet

Since RSDS is inflammatory in nature, it is important to eat pure foods and avoid foods and beverages that lead to inflammation.

Good Foods

In addition to their other therapeutic benefits, the following foods can help reduce inflammation:

- Asparagus, eggs, garlic, and onions;
- Brown rice;
- Fresh fruits that are non-acidic;
- Fresh vegetables, especially green leafy ones;
- Lentils;
- Oatmeal;
- Sardines and other oily fish;
- Whole grains.

(*See* NUTRITIONAL THERAPY in PART 2 Treatment Section for additional information.)

Bad Foods

The following foods contain elements that can cause inflammation and they should be reduced or eliminated to keep RSDS symptoms from flaring up:

- Citrus fruits;
- Dairy products containing vitamin D, which can cause sore joints;
- Fatty foods, especially those containing animal fats (if not avoided altogether, these should be limited);
- Sugar products.

(*See* NUTRITIONAL THERAPY in PART 2 Treatment Section for additional information.)

Other Substances to Avoid

Tobacco smoke. By constricting blood vessels, smoking keeps oxygen and blood from nourishing your system, which can increase the pain of RSDS.

Herbal Remedies

- Alfalfa increases vitality.
- Black cohosh relieves pain and inflammation.
- Boswellia has anti-inflammatory properties and acts similarly to NSAIDs without the side effects of stomach irritation or ulceration.
- Chaparral, used topically, has anti-inflammatory properties.
- Devil's claw has both anti-inflammatory and analgesic (painkilling) actions. Take 800 mg in capsule form three times a day.
- Digestive enzymes taken between meals act as anti-inflammatories.
- Ginger acts as an anti-inflammatory.
- Horsetail strengthens connective tissues.
- Hydrangea acts like cortisone, but without its side effects.
- Sarsaparilla has anti-inflammatory properties.
- Turmeric helps protect your body from free radicals.
- White willow relieves inflammation and pain. Take 60–120 mg per day. Although the pain-relieving aspects are slower than aspirin, they last longer.
- Yucca helps stimulate your adrenal glands to make your body's own cortisone. You can make a tea by simmering 8 grams of the root in a pint of water for fifteen minutes, or you can use it in capsule form according to the directions on the label.

Take the above herbs as directed on label. They can also be used in teas and infusions. (*See* HERBAL REMEDIES in PART 2 Treatment Section for additional information.)

Homeopathic Remedies

You can self-treat with homeopathic remedies by selecting the one that most closely matches your symptoms. If you don't see improvement, try another, or a combination product. Follow the instructions on the label. If you do not have relief in a reasonable amount of time, consult a physician who specializes in homeopathic medicine.

- Aconitum napellus eases pain and inflammation that comes from exposure to cold.
- Apis mellifica helps conditions accompanied by redness, tenderness, and swelling.
- Arnica aids RSDS, especially when pain is worse from touch. It is also available in gel or ointment form for external application.
- Bryonia eases throbbing pain made worse by motion.
- Calcarea carbonica is useful when soreness is worse from cold and dampness.
- Dulcamara helps relieve pain following exposure to cold damp weather.
- Kali carbonicum helps when the joints thicken or become deformed and pain worsens from cold and dampness.

- ❑ Rhododendron is useful when pain flares up before a storm or lowering barometric presssure.
- ❑ Ruta graveolens helps when symptoms worsen from cold, dampness, and exertion.

Combination remedies sometimes work more effectively than single ones. (*See* HOMEOPATHY in PART 2 Treatment Section for additional information.)

Hydrotherapy

Due to heightened sensations in people with RSDS, only warm, not hot, water should be used. And, while ice is often the treatment of choice for inflammation, it can make this condition worsen, or spread, and should not be used. Contrast baths of warm, not hot, and cold, not ice, water are recommended for RSDS. (*See* HEAT THERAPY/COLD THERAPY and HYDROTHERAPY in PART 2 Treatment Section for additional information.)

Magnet Therapy

Magnet therapy relieves pain, accelerates healing, and reduces inflammation. Placing magnets on and around sore places brings increased blood to the area which, in turn, brings oxygen and other healing substances to reduce the pain. (*See* MAGNET THERAPY in PART 2 Treatment Section for additional information.)

Supplements

- ❑ Beta-carotene helps neutralize free radicals. Take 15,000 IU daily.
- ❑ Boron aids calcium metabolism. Take 6 mg per day.
- ❑ Bromelain has anti-inflammatory activity, and has been reported to relieve joint swelling and impaired mobility. Take 500 mg twice daily between meals.
- ❑ DL-phenylalanine (DLPA), an amino acid, inhibits the enzyme that breaks down some of the body's natural painkillers. Take 250 mg three to four times a day between meals.
- ❑ Evening primrose oil controls pain and inflammation. Take per instructions on label.
- ❑ Fish oil contains the omega-3 fatty acids EPA and DHA, which have anti-inflammatory effects. Take ten grams per day, which delivers three grams of each fatty acid.
- ❑ Gamma linolenic acid (GLA) has anti-inflammatory properties. It is present in black current seed oil, borage oil, and evening primrose oil. Take according to directions on label.
- ❑ MSM (methylsulfonylmethane), a natural sulfur compound, helps alleviate inflammation and promotes healing. It is available in capsule, tablet, or powder form. Take according to directions on label.
- ❑ Niacinamide increases joint mobility, improves muscle strength, and decreases fatigue. Take 250 mg four times a day.
- ❑ SAMe (S-adenosyl methionine) increases the formation of healthy tissue and reduces pain, stiffness, and swelling. It has anti-inflammatory, pain-relieving, and tissue-healing properties. Take 400 mg three times a day.
- ❑ Vitamin B_5 (pantothenic acid) relieves morning stiffness and pain. Take 1000 mg per day.
- ❑ Vitamin B_6 helps repair tissues by enhancing collagen production which helps strengthen bones, ligaments, skin, and tendon). Take 100 mg three times a day. Note: For balance, when taking individual Bs, be sure to supplement with a B-complex once daily, or a multivitamin containing Bs.
- ❑ Vitamin C (Ester-C) also helps repair tissues by en-hancing collagen production. Take 1000 mg three times a day.
- ❑ Zinc, too, helps repair tissues by enhancing collagen production. Take 50 mg a day.

(*See* SUPPLEMENT THERAPY in PART 2 Treatment Section for additional information.)

ASSISTED ALTERNATIVE TREATMENTS

The following techniques may require specialized training or the aid of a healthcare professional.

Acupuncture and Acupressure

Acupuncture involves the insertion of extremely thin solid needles into specific points of your body to stimulate its own healing mechanism and improve blood flow to the affected areas. It also reduces inflammation, relieves pain, improves mobility, and there are rarely any risks or side effects. (*See* ACUPUNCTURE and ACUPRESSURE in PART 2 Treatment Section for additional information.)

Applied Kinesiology

Applied Kinesiology is excellent for reducing pain rapidly. The AK practitioner tests your muscles to determine the origin of your problem and then decides on the best course of action, choosing from a wide variety of therapeutic methods at her or his disposal. (*See* APPLIED KINESIOLOGY in PART 2 Treatment Section for additional information.)

Biofeedback

One of the things biofeedback can do is teach someone with RSDS to control body temperature. This can be very useful since the temperature in the extremities tends to fluctuate. (*See* BIOFEEDBACK in PART 2 Treatment Section for additional information.)

Chiropractic

Chiropractic theory is based on the assumption that a properly aligned spine is essential for good health, and that any misalignment of the vertebrae in the spine causes pressure on the spinal nerves, leading to pain. The chiropractor makes spinal adjustments to move misaligned vertebrae to more normal positions, which helps the nervous system to function properly. (*See* CHIROPRACTIC in PART 2 Treatment Section for additional information.)

Exercise and Stretching

Exercises and stretching can be helpful for RSDS, but they must be carefully supervised in order not to overstress the body. (*See* EXERCISE, STRETCHING, and SPORTS in PART 2 Treatment Section for additional information.)

Guided Imagery

Guided imagery can help you manage stress and reduce your pain. With practice, you can develop specific techniques to cool the burning, and reduce the sensitivity associated with RSDS. (*See* GUIDED IMAGERY and VISUALIZATION in PART 2 Treatment Section for additional information.)

Osteopathic Manipulation

The goal of osteopathic manipulation in the treatment of RSDS is to increase range of motion, decrease muscle tension, and improve blood circulation. (*See* OSTEOPATHIC MANIPULATION in PART 2 Treatment Section for additional information.)

Oxygen Therapy

Oxygen Therapy is a useful adjunct for treating people with reflex sympathetic dystrophy syndrome. (*See* OXYGEN THERAPIES in PART 2 Treatment Section for additional information.)

HBOT FOR RSDS

A forty-four-year-old woman with many physical problems and an intolerance for most drugs was treated for smoke inhalation and RSDS of the left foot and ankle at the Hyperbaric Medicine Department of the University of Baltimore's Medical Center. After only one treatment with hyperbaric oxygen, which she tolerated well, she reported that her foot was "pinker than it's been in years," and that she was completely free of pain, and remained so for eighteen hours following treatment. Subsequent HBOT treatments continued to improve her condition and the duration of her pain-free periods continued to increase.

Physical Therapy

Physical therapy helps correct and improve your body's natural healing mechanism. It increases the range of motion in the joints. (*See* PHYSICAL THERAPY in PART 2 Treatment Section for additional information.)

Reflexology

Reflexology massage therapy can be performed on the part of the foot or hand corresponding to the area that is in pain. (*See* REFLEXOLOGY in PART 2 Treatment Section for additional information.)

Rolfing

Rolfing has long-lasting effects in easing pain. (*See* ROLFING in PART 2 Treatment Section for additional information.)

PRACTICAL SUGGESTIONS

- ❑ Regular, gentle exercise is important to keep your muscles strong and your joints flexible, but do not overdo.
- ❑ Do not slouch.
- ❑ If you have to sit for long periods of time, take breaks to get up and stretch gently.

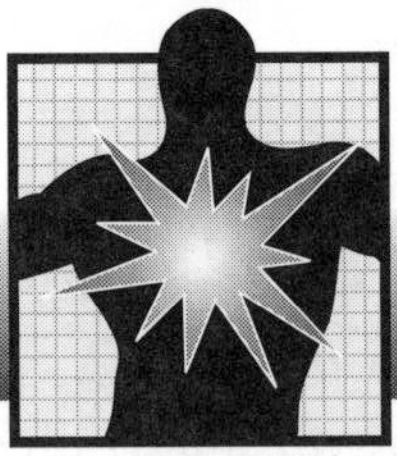

Rheumatoid Arthritis

Arthritis is inflammation and pain in a joint. Its most common forms are rheumatoid arthritis and osteoarthritis and, of the two, rheumatoid is the more serious because it is more crippling. Considered an autoimmune disease, it is a chronic inflammatory condition that affects the entire body because it attacks the membranes surrounding the lubricating fluid in the joints. Scar tissue replaces this damaged membrane tissue, causing the joint spaces to narrow and eventually fuse together. Three times as many women as men are affected by this form of arthritis, which usually starts between the ages of twenty and forty-five.

Symptoms

Painful swelling, accompanied by inflammation and stiffness in the extremities, is usually a sign of rheumatoid arthritis. Joints affected by rheumatoid arthritis make a sound similar to that of crinkling cellophane. (For more information on Inflammation, see inset on page 81.)

Common Causes

Rheumatoid arthritis is an autoimmune system disorder in which the immune system attacks the joints. One theory is that it may originate from a viral or bacterial infection. Food allergies may also be a cause of rheumatoid arthritis, as well as a lack of certain nutrients, such as folic acid and zinc.

Diagnosing the Problem

For rheumatoid arthritis, blood tests can be performed to see if antibodies called rheumatoid factors are present.

Fluid from affected joints can be aspirated to see if there is an infection caused by a bacterial or viral invasion of the joints. This is known as infectious arthritis and can occur after a staph infection, TB, gonorrhea, or Lyme disease.

Conventional Treatments

- ❑ Aspirin, taken daily in large doses, alleviates pain and helps reduce inflammation.
- ❑ Bextra and Celebrex control pain.
- ❑ Codeine relieves pain.
- ❑ Cortisone, taken orally or injected into the joints, can dramatically reduce pain.
- ❑ Gold salts are effective for some with rheumatoid arthritis, but not all.
- ❑ Heat applications help ease pain.
- ❑ Hyaluronic acid injections, approved only for knee use at this time, lubricate the knee joint and help keep the bones from rubbing together, which may eventually reduce pain. (Hyaluronic acid is a lubricating fluid present in normal joints and missing in ones with arthritis.)
- ❑ Indomethacin, a prescription NSAID, can relieve pain of moderate to severe rheumatoid arthritis.
- ❑ Nonsteroidal anti-inflammatory drugs (NSAIDs), such as ibuprofen and naproxen, reduce inflammation.
- ❑ Penicillamine helps some who do not respond to other rheumatoid arthritis treatments.
- ❑ Phenylbutazone reduces inflammation.
- ❑ Quinine derivatives (anti-malarials) help some.
- ❑ Physical therapy can bring pain relief.
- ❑ Splints and braces reduce pressure on joints.
- ❑ Suprofen, an NSAID, can reduce inflammation.
- ❑ Surgery, including joint replacement and fusion, is performed when other treatments fail.

New drugs are being developed for rheumatoid arthritis. Known as DMARDs (disease-modifying anti-rheumatic drugs), these drugs address the underlying problem instead of merely treating the symptoms. They include:

- ❑ Hydroxychloroquine (Plaquenil)
- ❑ Leflunomide (Arava)
- ❑ Methotrexate (Rheumatrex and Trexall)

Problems with Some Conventional Treatments

- ❑ Cortisone weakens the adrenal glands and, if taken for long periods, it can lead to osteoporosis. It can also cause bloating, cataracts, weight gain, and a moon-faced appearance.
- ❑ DMARDs can cause anemia and damage the liver,

lungs, and other organs. They can also lead to bleeding because they reduce the number of white cells and platelets.

- ❏ Gold therapy can cause a disruption of cell metabolism.
- ❏ NSAIDs work by blocking hormone-like substances called prostaglandins that trigger inflammation. However, prostaglandins also control the secretion of both your gastric juices and the mucous lining your stomach. This is why prolonged use of NSAIDs can eventually cause ulcers and gastric bleeding.
- ❏ The entire class of COX-2 inhibitors, including Bextra and Celebrex, may be linked to potentially damaging side effects to the heart.
- ❏ A series of hyaluronic acid injections costs about $1200 and their effects last only about one year.
- ❏ Splints and braces restrict motion and can eventually cause joints to atrophy from lack of use.
- ❏ Suprofen can cause kidney damage.
- ❏ Surgery fails to address the true cause of the disability. Further, scar tissue attracts bacteria and fungi to the area, and they attack the tissue, causing it to become inflamed, and leading to further deterioration.

SELF-HELP ALTERNATIVE TREATMENTS

The following techniques can be done at home. Although rheumatoid arthritis is a widespread painful condition, by adhering to the methods discussed here, it is possible to alleviate its symptoms without resorting to the use of harmful drugs. All herbs, homeopathic remedies, packs, and supplements mentioned in this entry are available in health food stores and, increasingly, in large drug and grocery stores, as well as on the Internet.

Aromatherapy

Apply topical applications of cajeput, camphor oil, eucalyptus oil, pine needle oil, or rosemary oil to the affected joints several times daily. They can be used singly or in combination, but be sure to dilute them in a carrier oil. (*See* AROMATHERAPY in PART 2 Treatment Section for additional information.

Castor Oil Packs

Soak a piece of white flannel in warm castor oil, wring it out and place over the inflamed area. Cover with plastic and apply a heating pad. Do this twice a day for an hour each time. (*See* COMPRESSES, PACKS, and POULTICES in PART 2 Treatment Section for additional information.)

Diet

Diet is extremely important in determining whether arthritis symptoms will be alleviated or exacerbated.

Good Foods

The following foods can help reduce inflammation, in addition to their other therapeutic benefits.

- ❏ Asparagus, eggs, garlic, and onions contain sulfur which helps remove metals.
- ❏ Brown rice.
- ❏ Fresh fruits that are non-acidic.
- ❏ Fresh vegetables, especially green leafy ones.
- ❏ Lentils.
- ❏ Oatmeal.
- ❏ Sardines and other oily fish.
- ❏ Whole grains.

(*See* NUTRITIONAL THERAPY in PART 2 Treatment Section for additional information.)

Bad Foods

The following foods contain elements that can cause inflammation and should be reduced or eliminated to keep arthritis symptoms from flaring up.

- ❏ Citrus fruits.
- ❏ Dairy products containing vitamin D, which can cause sore joints.
- ❏ Fatty foods, especially those containing animal fats (if not avoided altogether, these should be limited).
- ❏ Foods in the nightshade family, including eggplant, peppers, tomatoes, and white potatoes. These contain the toxin solanine, which causes inflammation in the joints.
- ❏ Sugar products.

Other Substances to Avoid

- ❏ Allergy-causing foods, particularly for anyone with rheumatoid arthritis.
- ❏ Fluorine. Added to the water supply to strengthen teeth and bones, it also causes unneeded bone growth in arthritic joints.

Heat and Cold Therapy

Applying cold to the painful area reduces swelling and applying heat helps to increase blood flow. (*See* HEAT THERAPY/COLD THERAPY in PART 2 Treatment Section for additional information.)

Herbal Remedies

- ❑ Alfalfa increases vitality.
- ❑ Black cohosh relieves pain and inflammation.
- ❑ Boswellia has anti-inflammatory properties and acts similarly to NSAIDs without the side effects of stomach irritation or ulceration.
- ❑ Burdock root can be taken internally or applied externally to relieve painful joints.
- ❑ Cat's claw has both anti-inflammatory and antioxidant properties.
- ❑ Cayenne cream, used topically, relieves pain.
- ❑ Chaparral, also used topically, has anti-inflammatory properties.
- ❑ Devil's claw has both anti-inflammatory and analgesic actions. Take 800 mg in capsule form three times a day.
- ❑ Ginger acts as an anti-inflammatory.
- ❑ Horsetail strengthens connective tissues.
- ❑ Hydrangea acts like cortisone, but without its side effects.
- ❑ Sarsaparilla has anti-inflammatory properties.
- ❑ Turmeric helps protect your body from free radicals. Its active component is curcumin, a potent anti-inflammatory compound. Studies have shown that 400 mg of curcumin three times a day was as effective as the drug phenylbutazone, but without any side effects.
- ❑ White willow can relieve inflammation and pain. Take 60–120 mg per day. Although the pain-relieving aspects are slower than aspirin, they last longer.

Take the above herbs as directed on label. They can also be used in teas and infusions. (*See* HERBAL REMEDIES in PART 2 Treatment Section for additional information.)

Homeopathic Remedies

You can self-treat with homeopathic remedies by selecting the one that most closely matches your symptoms. If you don't see improvement, try another, or a combination product. Follow the instructions on the label. If you do not have relief in a reasonable amount of time, consult a physician who specializes in homeopathic medicine.

- ❑ Arnica aids rheumatoid arthritis where pain is worse from touch. It is also available in a gel or ointment form for external application.
- ❑ Bryonia eases throbbing pain made worse by motion. Calcarea carbonica is useful when soreness is worse from cold and dampness.
- ❑ Calcarea fluorica is indicated when pain is eased by heat or motion.
- ❑ Dulcamara helps when flare-up of rheumatoid arthritis follows exposure to cold damp weather.
- ❑ Kali carbonicum helps when the joints thicken or become deformed and pain worsens from cold and dampness.
- ❑ Kalmia latiflora eases the intense pain of rheumatoid arthritis that appears suddenly and is worse from motion. Pain usually starts in the joints in the upper body and works its way down.
- ❑ Ledum palustre eases the pain of rheumatoid arthritis that starts in the joints in the lower part of the body and works its way up.
- ❑ Pulsatilla eases the pain in rheumatoid arthritis when it moves from one joint to another.
- ❑ Rhododendron is for when the pain and stiffness of rheumatoid arthritis flares up before a storm.
- ❑ Rhus toxicodendron eases the pain and stiffness of rheumatoid arthritis when they are worse in the morning and then diminish with continued motion.
- ❑ Ruta graveolens helps rheumatoid arthritis when a feeling of great stiffness is present and symptoms worsen from cold, dampness, and exertion.

Combination remedies sometimes work more effectively than single ones. (*See* HOMEOPATHY in PART 2 Treatment Section for additional information.)

Hydrotherapy

Running hot water over a painful area while in the shower, or soaking in a hot tub can help diminish the pain. (*See* HYDROTHERAPY in PART 2 Treatment Section for additional information.)

Magnet Therapy

Magnet therapy relieves pain, accelerates healing, and reduces inflammation. Placing magnets around the sore joint brings increased blood to the area which, in turn, brings oxygen and other healing substances to reduce the pain. (*See* MAGNET THERAPY in PART 2 Treatment Section for additional information.)

Supplements

- ❑ Betaine HCL, per label, helps increase stomach acidity,

necessary for proper digestion. This helps to reduce food-allergy reactions in those with low stomach acid, a condition often found in rheumatoid arthritis.

- ❑ Beta-carotene, 15,000 IU, helps neutralize free radicals.
- ❑ Boron aids calcium metabolism. Take 6 mg per day.
- ❑ Bromelain has anti-inflammatory activity, and has been reported to relieve joint swelling and impaired mobility. Take 500 mg twice daily between meals.
- ❑ DL-phenylalanine (DLPA), an amino acid, inhibits the enzyme that breaks down some of the body's natural painkillers. Take 250 mg three to four times a day between meals.
- ❑ Evening primrose oil controls pain and inflammation. Take two capsules twice daily.
- ❑ Fish oil contains EPA and DHA and has anti-inflammatory effects. Take 10 grams per day, which delivers 3 grams of the omega-3 fatty acids EPA and DHA.
- ❑ Gamma linolenic acid (GLA) has anti-inflammatory properties. It is present in borage oil, black currant-seed oil, and evening primrose oil. Take these according to directions on label.
- ❑ Glucosamine sulfate, a nutrient derived from chitin, (a substance found in crab, shrimp, and oyster shells and broken down in a series of acids and bases until the pure glucosamine is isolated) aids in the repair of joint cartilage. Take 500 mg three times a day with meals. Although it does not provide the quick relief of NSAIDs, over time it actually helps repair joint damage.
- ❑ MSM (methylsulfonylmethane), a natural sulfur compound helps alleviate joint pain and inflammation and promotes healing. It is available in capsule, tablet, or powder form. Take according to directions on label.
- ❑ Niacinamide increases joint mobility and improves muscle strength. Start with 250 mg four times a day and increase the dose if your arthritis is more advanced.
- ❑ SAMe (S-adenosyl methionine) increases the formation of healthy tissue and reduces pain, stiffness and swelling. It has anti-inflammatory, pain-relieving and tissue-healing properties. Take 400 mg three times a day.
- ❑ Shark cartilage reduces inflammation and helps prevent blood vessels from invading the cartilage of your joints. Take according to directions on the label.
- ❑ SierraSil, a blend of more than sixty-five naturally occurring supplements, helps to alleviate the pain, stiffness, and inflammation of arthritis. Take according to label instructions. (*See also* CARPAL TUNNEL SYNDROME in PART 1 Conditions Section.)
- ❑ Vitamin B_5 (pantothenic acid) relieves morning stiffness and pain. Take 1000 mg per day.
- ❑ Vitamin B_6 helps repair tissues by enhancing collagen production. (Collagen is present in bones, ligaments, skin, and tendons). Take 100 mg three times a day.
- ❑ Vitamin C (Ester-C) also helps repair tissues by enhancing collagen production. Take 1000 mg three times a day.
- ❑ Vitamin E has a beneficial effect on those with rheumatoid arthritis. Start by taking 400 IU daily and gradually build up to as much as 1800 IU per day. This amount should be under the supervision of a nutritionally oriented physician.
- ❑ Zinc helps repair tissues by enhancing collagen production. Take 50 mg a day.

(*See* SUPPLEMENT THERAPY in PART 2 Treatment Section for additional information.)

ASSISTED ALTERNATIVE TREATMENTS

The following techniques may require specialized training or the aid of a healthcare professional.

Acupuncture and Accupressure

Acupuncture and acupressure create a smooth flow of energy throughout the body. Acupuncture involves the insertion of extremely thin solid needles into specific points of your body to stimulate its own healing mechanism and improve blood flow to the areas affected by painful arthritis. It reduces inflammation, relieves pain, improves mobility, and there are rarely any risks or side effects. (*See* ACUPUNCTURE and ACUPRESSURE in PART 2 Treatment Section for additional information.)

Applied Kinesiology

Applied Kinesiology is excellent for reducing pain rapidly. The AK practitioner tests your muscles to determine the origin of your problem and then decides on the best course of action, choosing from a wide variety of therapeutic methods at his or her disposal. (*See* APPLIED KINESIOLOGY in PART 2 Treatment Section for additional information.)

Bee Venom Therapy

Some components of bee venom are thought to stimulate the immune system. Other components are thought to modify the transmission of pain signals within the nervous system, and the therapy has proven consistently useful for painful conditions. (*See* BEE VENOM THERAPY in PART 2 Treatment Section for additional information.)

Chiropractic

When the spinal vertebrae are misaligned they can pinch nerves, which leads to pressure, causing symptoms in various body parts. When these misaligned vertebrae (subluxations) are properly aligned, the nervous system can function properly and chronic pain can often be reversed. (*See* CHIROPRACTIC in PART 2 Treatment Section for additional information.)

Craniosacral Therapy

A trained craniosacral practitioner can feel areas where healthy tissue function is restricted, usually due to physical or emotional trauma. The theory is that physical injuries and emotional traumas are stored or frozen in the body, causing arthritis pain that can be released by this therapy. (*See* CRANIOSACRAL THERAPY in PART 2 Treatment Section for additional information.)

Exercise

Moving your joints stimulates the cartilage to absorb more nutrients. Exercise also strengthens muscles so they support the joints more effectively. Anyone with arthritis should start an exercise program slowly and with careful supervision at the beginning. If you feel stiff, take a warm bath or shower first. Stretch slowly and avoid bouncing or high-impact exercise. Good exercises for arthritis are swimming, water aerobics, walking, and cycling with a low pedal resistance. Tai chi and qigong, two gentle, highly effective forms of martial arts training that also calm and center you, are excellent exercises for those with arthritis. (*See* EXERCISE, STRETCHING, and SPORTS, and TAI CHI, QIGONG, and YOGA in PART 2 Treatment Section for additional information.)

Guided Imagery and Visualization Techniques

These help to relieve stress and minimize pain. To alleviate the burning, either visualize a temperature guage set on high and then turn down the heat, or picture cool water putting out a fire. For the stiffness, visualize a tight band that you gradually loosen. (*See* GUIDED IMAGERY and VISUALIZATION in PART 2 Treatment Section for additional information.)

Massage

Massage helps relax contracted muscles and alleviate muscle tension in one area of the body, which can affect other areas. It also increases blood flow, which nourishes and oxygenates tissues. (*See* MASSAGE in PART 2 Treatment Section for additional information.)

Osteopathic Manipulation

Osteopathic manipulation can correct faulty structure and function and rebalance your body's system, enabling it to function better. (*See* OSTEOPATHIC MANIPULATION in PART 2 Treatment Section for additional information.)

Oxygen Therapy

Oxygen therapy enhances your body's ability to heal itself by encouraging its own natural production of oxygen. (*See* OXYGEN THERAPIES in PART 2 Treatment Section for additional information.)

Physical Therapy

Physical therapy increases the range of motion in your joints and corrects and improves your body's natural healing mechanism. (*See* PHYSICAL THERAPY in PART 2 Treatment Section for additional information.)

Reflexology

By helping to eliminate energy blockages, improve circulation, and relieve stress and tension, reflexology helps the body heal itself naturally. (*See* REFLEXOLOGY in PART 2 Treatment Section for additional information.)

Rolfing

Rolfing helps place your body in balance with gravity by releasing stress patterns that keep it out of alignment. It can have long-lasting effects in easing pain. (*See* ROLFING in PART 2 Treatment Section for additional information.)

Tai Chi, Qigong, and Yoga

By helping you achieve a profoundly relaxed state, these therapies are useful for relieving your pain and boosting your general health. (*See* TAI CHI, QIGONG, and YOGA in PART 2 Treatment Section for additional information.)

PRACTICAL SUGGESTIONS

- ❑ Celadrin. This natural topical ointment has been shown to significantly reduce painful arthritis symptoms.
- ❑ Copper bracelets. Users have reported surprising, effective results.
- ❑ DMSO (dimethyl sulfoxide). This industrial solvent, applied topically, has anti-inflammatory properties and relieves pain by inhibiting the pain messages transmitted by the nerves.
- ❑ NAET. The Nambudripad Allergy Elimination Therapy is primarily used for allergy relief, and many with rheumatoid arthritis find relief through allergy-elimination techniques. For this and other such methods, a nutritionally oriented physician or NAET practitioner should be consulted.

IONIZED BRACELETS

Ionized bracelets are said to balance the body's energy fields to bring relief from pain in the joints and muscles. Researchers at The Mayo Clinic in Jacksonville, Florida ran some tests on ionized bracelets to see if wearing them helped, but found they were no more effective at relieving a wearer's muscle and joint pain than other look-alike, non-ionized placebo bracelets. Anecdotally, however, several men wearing ionized bracelets reported that they worked very effectively, even referring to them as "wonderful."

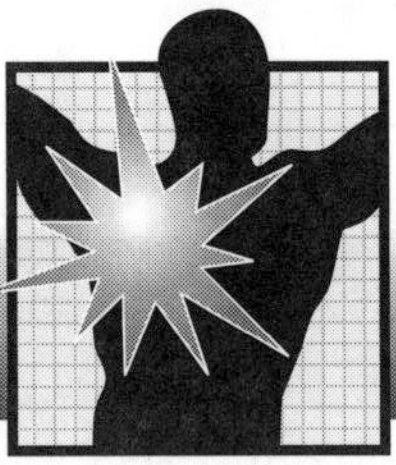

Rotator Cuff Tendonitis

Rotator cuff tendonitis, also referred to as shoulder impingement syndrome, or in sports terms, as pitcher's shoulder or tennis shoulder, is an inflammation of the tendons in the shoulder (tendons are the fibrous cords of tissue that connect muscles to bones). Although aging makes any tendon more susceptible to injury, young people who are athletic, or anyone who performs repetitive motions, can also develop tendonitis.

Symptoms

The pain of tendonitis is aggravated by activity, movement, or pressure, and often occurs at night. The skin over the tendon may feel hot and appear red, and there is visible swelling of the tendon sheaths. Symptoms specific to shoulder tendonitis include pain with arm movement, difficulty reaching behind the back, and night pain in the arm. There is tenderness over the head of the upper arm bone, the humerus, and in specific positions the shoulder is weak.

Causes

Athletic activities are the main ways to develop this tendonitis. If overdone or done improperly, pitching a ball, swimming, or weightlifting, especially lifting weights over the head, can all lead to rotator cuff tendonitis.

Diagnosing the Problem

An MRI will show inflammation and the presence of a tear, and x-rays can show bone spurs.

Conventional Treatments

- ❑ Arthroscopic surgery.
- ❑ Avoiding the offending activities.
- ❑ Cortisone injections.
- ❑ Physical therapy.

Problems with Some Conventional Treatments

- ❑ The recovery period following surgery can take up to nine months and the outcome depends on the size and duration of the tear.
- ❑ The surgical treatment may not improve the symptoms.

SELF-HELP ALTERNATIVE TREATMENTS

The following techniques can be done at home. Although they may not work as fast as drugs or surgery, natural alternatives help the body heal itself. All herbs, homeopathic remedies, packs, and supplements discussed here are available in health food stores and, increasingly, in large drug and grocery stores, as well as on the Internet.

Aromatherapy

Aromatherapy can help relieve the pain of tendonitis, particularly the essential oils of clove bud, marjoram, rosemary, and pine. Add a few drops to vegetable oil and massage into the affected area. Apply gently twice daily to the affected area. Do not use a vigorous massage over any swollen joint. Essential oils are available in health food stores and stores specializing in aromatherapy products, which you can find in the yellow pages. (*See* AROMATHERAPY in PART 2 Treatment Section for additional information.)

Castor Oil Packs

Dip a piece of white flannel into some warm castor oil. Wring it out and place it over the affected shoulder area. Cover with plastic and apply a heating pad for one hour. Do this twice daily. (*See* COMPRESSES, PACKS, and POULTICES in PART 2 Treatment Section for additional information.)

Diet

Tendonitis is inflammatory in nature so certain dietary modifications may be helpful.

Good Foods

All the foods listed below help to reduce inflammation.

- ❑ Foods that contain B vitamins, such as complex carbohydrates, fruits, nuts, seeds, vegetables, and whole grains.
- ❑ Fish, particularly wild salmon.
- ❑ Flaxseed meal.
- ❑ Fresh vegetables and fruits, preferably organically raised. Dark green vegetables contain antioxidants, which help scavenge and neutralize the free radicals that are causing the inflammation.
- ❑ Garlic.

(*See* NUTRITIONAL THERAPY in PART 2 Treatment Section for additional information.)

Bad Foods

Avoid the following foods, which can all trigger an inflammatory reaction in your body.

- ❑ Alcohol.
- ❑ Processed foods and fast foods.
- ❑ Saturated fats, as found in meats and dairy products.
- ❑ Spicy foods.
- ❑ Sugary-type foods.
- ❑ White flour products, such as pasta and bread.

Heat Therapy/Cold Therapy

Applying cold to the painful area reduces swelling, and heat helps increase blood flow. (*See* HEAT THERAPY/COLD THERAPY in PART 2 Treatment Section for additional information.)

Herbal Remedies

- ❑ Black currant oil relieves pain and inflammation.
- ❑ Boswellia has anti-inflammatory properties and acts similarly to NSAIDs without the side effects of stomach irritation or ulceration.
- ❑ Cayenne ointment, applied topically, relieves pain.
- ❑ Coltsfoot and comfrey, used externally in soaks or poultices, reduce fluid retention. (Note: Comfrey taken internally has the potential to cause liver damage and should be used only under careful supervision.)
- ❑ Evening primrose oil relieves pain and inflammation.
- ❑ Ginger stimulates circulation.
- ❑ Hydrangea acts like cortisone.
- ❑ Watercress reduces fluid retention.
- ❑ White willow bark relieves inflammation and pain. Take 60–120 mg per day. Although its pain-relieving aspects are slower than aspirin, they last longer.
- ❑ Yucca is a precursor of synthetic cortisone. It enables your adrenal glands to produce and release their own cortisone into your system.

Take the above herbs as directed on label. They can also be used in teas and infusions. (*See* HERBAL REMEDIES in PART 2 Treatment Section for additional information.)

Homeopathic Remedies

You can self-treat with homeopathic remedies by selecting the one that most closely matches your symptoms. If you don't see improvement, try another, or a combination product. Follow the instructions on the label. If you do not have relief in a reasonable amount of time, consult a physician who specializes in homeopathic medicine.

- ❑ Arnica soothes inflammation. It is also available in cream and ointment form for external application.
- ❑ Calcarea phosphorica eases pain and stiffness.
- ❑ Hypericum eases nerve pain.
- ❑ Ruta graveolens helps ease stiffness and weakness.

Take the above remedies as indicated on label. Combination remedies sometimes work more effectively than single ones. (*See* HOMEOPATHY in PART 2 Treatment Section for additional information.)

Hydrotherapy

Running hot water over a painful area while in the shower or soaking in a hot tub can help diminish the pain. (*See* HYDROTHERAPY in PART 2 Treatment Section for additional information.)

Magnet Therapy

Magnet therapy relieves pain, accelerates healing, and reduces inflammation. (*See* MAGNET THERAPY in PART 2 Treatment Section for additional information.)

Supplements

- ❑ Bromelain is a digestive enzyme if taken with meals, but acts as an anti-inflammatory when taken on an empty stomach. Take 400 mg 3 times a day between meals.
- ❑ Flaxseed oil, 1–2 teaspoons daily.
- ❑ Magnesium citrate, 500 mg three times daily, acts as a muscle antispasmodic.
- ❑ Manganese, 25–100 mg twice a day during the acute phase. Then take 10–15 mg twice a day.
- ❑ Proteolytic enzymes taken between meals can reduce pain and swelling and help speed up the healing process. Take per instruction on label.
- ❑ Selenium, 100–200 mcg daily.
- ❑ Vitamin B_6 aids the normal function of nerve cells and

helps reduce swelling because it has a natural ability to eliminate water retention. Dr. Edward M. Wagner, ND, recommends 200 mg three times a day. He says it is more effective to use the pyrodoxal #5 phosphate form of B_6, which has a higher assimilation rate than plain pyrodoxine.

- ❑ Vitamin B_{12}, sublingual, helps prevent nerve damage. Take 500 mcg twice daily. Note: For balance when taking individual Bs, be sure to supplement with a B-complex once daily, or a multivitamin containing Bs.
- ❑ Vitamin C (Ester-C), 1000 mg three times daily, is a general overall antioxidant.
- ❑ Vitamin E, 400 IU daily.

(*See* SUPPLEMENT THERAPY in PART 2 Treatment Section for additional information.)

ASSISTED ALTERNATIVE TREATMENTS

The following techniques may require specialized training or the aid of a healthcare professional.

Acupuncture and Acupressure

Acupuncture involves the insertion of extremely thin solid needles into specific points of your body to stimulate its own healing mechanism and improve blood flow to the affected areas. It also reduces inflammation, relieves pain, improves mobility, and there are rarely any risks or side effects. (*See* ACUPUNCTURE and ACUPRESSURE in PART 2 Treatment Section for additional information.)

Applied Kinesiology

Applied Kinesiology is excellent for reducing pain rapidly. The AK practitioner tests your muscles to determine the origin of your problem and then decides on the best course of action, choosing from a wide variety of therapeutic methods at her or his disposal. (*See* APPLIED KINESIOLOGY in PART 2 Treatment Section for additional information.)

Chiropractic

Chiropractic theory is based on the assumption that a properly aligned spine is essential for good health, and that any misalignment of the vertebrae in the spine causes pressure on the spinal nerves, leading to pain. The chiropractor makes spinal adjustments to move misaligned vertebrae to more normal positions, which helps the nervous system to function properly. (*See* CHIROPRACTIC in PART 2 Treatment Section for additional information.)

Exercise and Stretching

Exercise and stretching can be helpful, but it must be carefully supervised in order not to further damage the affected area.

Do shoulder shrugs slowly, first with no weights, then gradually with very light weights. Raise and lower the affected arm, slowly at first and without weights, then gradually add light weights. Move your arm slowly and carefully in a circular motion. For this maneuver, do not add weights unless you are under supervision. (*See* EXERCISE, STRETCHING, and SPORTS in PART 2 Treatment Section for additional information.)

Guided Imagery

Guided imagery is a useful adjunct to help you manage your pain. In your mind, picture the affected shoulder area as an object and bring in the appropriate tools. If the pain is burning, picture a cool stream of water soothing it. If it is stabbing, picture a pliers removing what is stabbing. (*See* GUIDED IMAGERY and VISUALIZATION in PART 2 Treatment Section for additional information.)

Massage

A massage helps bring blood to the affected area and relieve the pain. There are many kinds of massage therapies available and you can ask your practitioner to suggest the appropriate one for your tendonitis. (*See* MASSAGE in PART 2 Treatment Section for additional information.)

Osteopathic Manipulation

The goal of osteopathic manipulation in the treatment of tendonitis is to increase range of motion, decrease muscle tension, and improve blood circulation. (*See* OSTEOPATHIC MANIPULATION in PART 2 Treatment Section for additional information.)

Physical Therapy

Physical therapy increases the range of motion in your joints and corrects and improves your body's natural healing mechanism. (*See* PHYSICAL THERAPY in PART 2 Treatment Section for additional information.)

Reflexology

Reflexology massage therapy can be performed on the part of the foot or hand corresponding to the shoulder area that is in pain. (*See* REFLEXOLOGY in PART 2 Treatment Section for additional information.)

Rolfing

Rolfing helps place your body in balance with gravity by releasing stress patterns that keep it out of alignment. It can have long-lasting effects in easing pain. (*See* ROLFING in PART 2 Treatment Section for additional information.)

PRACTICAL SUGGESTIONS

- ❏ Don't let your arm dangle. Keep it supported. Keep your hand in a pocket or rest your elbow on the arm of a chair.
- ❏ DMSO (dimethylsulfoxide), applied topically, may relieve pain.
- ❏ If you are just starting to exercise, be sure to stretch properly, then start out slowly and increase your activity gradually.
- ❏ Keep your body in a balanced alignment and change positions frequently.
- ❏ Keep your shoulder warm. When you are in bed, sleep with your arm under the covers.
- ❏ Try not to overuse any one joint.

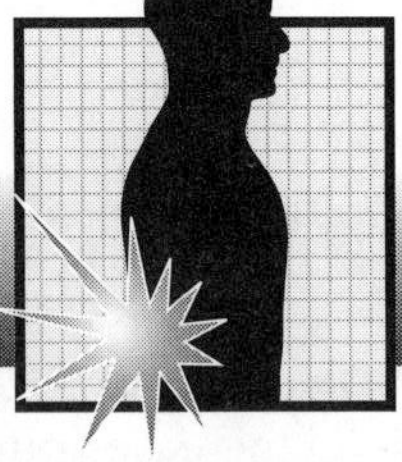

Sciatica

The sciatic nerve, the largest and longest nerve in the body, is about as thick as your thumb. It originates in the lumbar region of the back, passes between the vertebrae, runs through the pelvic bones and hip joint, then down the back and side of the leg all the way to the foot. When it becomes compressed, inflamed, or irritated, the severe pain known as sciatica occurs. During some time in life, about 40 percent of the population experiences some degree of sciatica.

Symptoms

The pain of sciatica is usually described as sharp and shooting, sometimes as an electrical wave of pain that runs down the thigh and the outside of the leg to the little toe, each becoming worse when you move your leg. The area is extremely sensitive to touch and can be accompanied by a burning feeling, numbness, tingling, and weakness.

Common Causes

A compression of the sciatic nerve occurs when the intervertebral disc shifts position, or is damaged from some injury or disease, and the shifted tissue or vertebra impinges on the nerve. Additional reasons for sciatica include:

- ❑ Emotional stress, causing muscles to contract;
- ❑ Inflammation of the sciatic nerve;
- ❑ Muscle strain;
- ❑ Piriformis syndrome (this occurs when the piriformis muscle, located in the hip joint close to the sciatic nerve, is injured or goes into spasm, putting pressure on the sciatic nerve and compressing it);
- ❑ A ruptured intervertebral disc, also referred to as a herniated disc;
- ❑ Sports that incorporate a twisting motion, especially golf and tennis;
- ❑ Wallet-itis (this occurs when you keep your wallet in the hip pocket of your trousers and sit on it, thereby causing an irritation of the sciatic nerve);
- ❑ Weak muscles resulting from a sedentary lifestyle.

Diagnosing the Problem

There are several diagnostic procedures to determine if the pain you are experiencing is sciatica, which is normally felt on only one side of your body. First, you can have an evaluation of your symptoms made, then to back it up, you can have a CAT scan and/or x-ray studies done.

Conventional Treatments

A variety of treatments have been developed by Western medicine for this widespread ailment.

- ❑ Anti-inflammatories, prescribed and over-the-counter.
- ❑ Baclofen pump therapy. Baclofen is an antispasmodic pain controller. A small titanium disc, about three inches in diameter and one-inch thick, is implanted into the intrathecal spaces in the spine and delivers Baclofen on a long-term basis to help control severe spasticity. It is particularly useful for those who do not respond to oral doses of Baclofen.
- ❑ Bed rest, with the proper supports, was formerly recommended, but some doctors now believe it takes two weeks to get back in shape for every week spent in bed.
- ❑ Botoxin Injections. Botoxin is basically a poison but, in minute doses, it is used for muscle relaxation and helps with pain.
- ❑ Epidural steroid injections and nerve blocks (similar to epidural steroid injections). A mixture of corticosteroids and local anesthesia is injected into the epidural space (the same area injected into women for epidural anesthesia during childbirth) of the spine.
- ❑ Morphine to control pain.
- ❑ Muscle relaxers.
- ❑ Nerve blocks. These are similar to epidural steroid injections.
- ❑ Physical therapy. Treatments help restore function, improve mobility, and relieve pain by using conservative methods that do not involve surgery. Performed by a professional physical therapist or a physiatrist (a doctor who specializes in physical medicine; they refer to themselves as "orthopedists withoput scalpels"), treatment includes electrostimulation, hot and cold applications, massage, muscle-strengthening and stretching exercises, and ultrasound therapy. If you do not know a physiatrist, you have to be referred to a

physical therapist by your regular doctor. (*See* PHYSICAL THERAPY in PART 2 Treatment Section for additional information.)

- ❑ Surgery.
- ❑ TENS units. This is one of the treatments once considered alternative that is now mainstream. Pads connected to the unit by a wire are put over the painful area and a mild current is applied.
- ❑ Traction.
- ❑ Trigger point injections. A local anesthetic in a saline solution that is injected directly into the muscle, enabling it to relax.

Effective Conventional Treatments

Laser Disc Decompression is a useful, minimally invasive method for treating those with slightly bulging, but not fully herniated, discs. A specially trained neurosurgeon or orthopedic surgeon places a needle into the disc and attaches a laser, which transmits energy into the disc. This decreases pressure on the disc and shrinks it, which results in pulling the bulge off the sciatic nerve.

Fentanyl patches or Lidoderm patches are also considered effective conventional treatments. They are easy to use, transdermal, non-invasive medications that are applied the same way that nitroglycerine patches are (although for a different purpose).

Problems with Some Conventional Treatments

- ❑ Anti-inflammatories can cause gastrointestinal bleeding and stomach upset.
- ❑ Bed rest for more than two days can make your muscles tighten and lead to a loss of strength and flexibility. It is now believed that, for every week spent in bed, it can take two weeks to get back in shape.
- ❑ Epidural steroid injections offer only temporary relief, anywhere from a few weeks to three months. However, in many cases this may be enough time for people with sciatica to have relief. They should not be used by anyone with bleeding disorders, or anyone who has fluid-retention problems. There is also a risk of long-term headaches if the membrane around the spinal cord is punctured.
- ❑ Morphine can be addictive.
- ❑ Muscle relaxants can cause drowsiness.
- ❑ Surgery always has a degree of risk, both from the procedure and the anesthesia.
- ❑ Traction produces a high level of discomfort.

SELF-HELP ALTERNATIVE TREATMENTS

The following techniques can be done at home. Alternative/complementary solutions are always preferable to drugs with their potentially harmful side effects. All herbs, homeopathic remedies, packs, and supplements discussed here are available in health food stores and, increasingly, in large drug and grocery stores, as well as on the Internet.

Aromatherapy

Aromatherapy, particularly the essential oils of chamomile, clary sage, lavender, and sweet marjoram, help reduce inflammation and muscle spasms, and relieve nervous tension. (*See* AROMATHERAPY in PART 2 Treatment Section for additional information.)

Castor Oil Packs

Dip a piece of white flannel into some warm castor oil. Wring it out and place it over the affected area. Cover with plastic and apply a heating pad for one hour. Do this twice daily. (*See* COMPRESSES, PACKS, and POULTICES in PART 2 Treatment Section for additional information.)

Diet

Sciatica is inflammatory in nature so certain dietary modifications may be helpful.

Good Foods

Water. Many report relief within minutes if they drink two glasses of pure water as soon as the pain starts. Your body needs a minimum of sixty-four ounces of water daily to avoid dehydration, which can be a cause of muscle aches and back pain. (*See* NUTRITIONAL THERAPY in PART 2 Treatment Section for additional information.)

Bad Foods

Meats and other animal protein products are not recommended because they contain uric acid which puts a strain on the kidneys, and this can this can add to low back pain and sciatica.

Other Substances to Avoid

Tobacco smoke. Smoking keeps oxygen and blood from getting to your back.

Exercise

This is a very good exercise for the relief of sciatic pain.

1. Lie on your back, knees bent, feet flat on the floor.

2. Press the small of your back into the floor.
3. Tighten your buttocks and lift your pelvis a few inches.
4. Repeat five times. Do this three or four times a day or more.

Swimming and walking are good exercises to strengthen back muscles. (*See* EXERCISE, STRETCHING, and SPORTS in PART 2 Treatment Section for additional information.)

Herbal Remedies

- ❑ Birch bark relieves inflammation. You can make a tea by placing a handful of leaves in two cups of boiling water and steeping them for ten minutes.
- ❑ Butcher's broom relieves inflammation.
- ❑ Capsicum (red pepper) contains the pain-relieving chemical capsaicin. Used as a topical analgesic, it is available in commercial creams, or you can make some yourself by mashing some red pepper and mixing it with cold cream. Note: Keep your hands away from your eyes, and be sure to wash your hands thoroughly after applying it, as it can be extremely irritating to your eyes or other sensitive areas.
- ❑ Cardamom, rosemary, and sage all help relax muscles. You can make a tea of any of these by placing a handful of leaves in two cups of boiling water and steeping them for ten minutes.
- ❑ Chamomile relieves muscle cramps and pain and relaxes the body.
- ❑ Fenugreek and juniper berries relieve inflammation.
- ❑ Valerian root, a relaxant, is available as a tea. You might prefer taking it in capsule form, however, as many people think the tea tastes terrible. Take according to the label.
- ❑ White willow bark is a natural form of aspirin. You can make a tea by placing a handful of leaves in two cups of boiling water and steeping them for ten minutes.
- ❑ Yucca is an anti-inflammatory. Take according to the label.

Take the above herbs as directed on label. They can also be used in teas and infusions. (*See* HERBAL REMEDIES in PART 2 Treatment Section for additional information.)

Homeopathic Remedies

You can self-treat with homeopathic remedies by selecting the one that most closely matches your symptoms. If you don't see improvement, try another, or a combination product. Follow the instructions on the label. If you do not have relief in a reasonable amount of time, consult a physician who specializes in homeopathic medicine.

- ❑ Aesculus relieves dull pain that worsens after walking or stooping.
- ❑ Arnica soothes muscles and aches and helps overcome severe pain. It is also available in a gel or ointment for external use.
- ❑ Bryonia helps when movement causes pain.
- ❑ Dulcanwa is useful for pain that is worse in damp or cold weather and is relieved by heat.
- ❑ Rhus toxicodendron aids morning stiffness.

(*See* HOMEOPATHIC REMEDIES in PART 2 Treatment Section for additional information.)

Hydrotherapy

When a sciatic attack begins, applying ice or cold compresses to the painful area helps to reduce swelling and relieve pain. After forty-eight hours, gentle stretching and conditioning exercises in warm water help alleviate muscle stiffness and relax the entire body. (*See* HYDROTHERAPY in PART 2 Treatment Section for additional information.)

Meditation

As little as fifteen minutes a day spent meditating can help reduce stress, which contributes to pain. (*See* MEDITATION in PART 2 Treatment Section for additional information.)

Supplements

- ❑ Bromelain, 500 mg twice daily, acts as an anti-inflammatory.
- ❑ DL-phenylalanine (DLPA), 500 mg four times daily, on an empty stomach releases endorphins, the body's own natural painkillers. It can take up to seven days to be effective. After the pain is relieved, cut down on the dosage.
- ❑ Pantothene, 500 mg twice daily, acts as an anti-inflammatory.
- ❑ Vitamin B_1 (thiamine), 250 mg twice daily, acts as a muscle relaxant.
- ❑ Vitamin B_{12} sublingual, 1000 mcg twice daily, helps prevent nerve damage.

(*See* SUPPLEMENT THERAPY in PART 2 Treatment Section for additional information.)

ASSISTED ALTERNATIVE TREATMENTS

The following techniques may require specialized training or the aid of a healthcare professional.

Acupuncture and Acupressure

Acupuncture and acupressure help restore an even flow of chi (life energy) that aids the body's natural healing ability. Acupuncture involves the insertion of extremely thin solid needles into specific points of your body to stimulate its own healing mechanism and improve blood flow to the affected areas. It can reduce inflammation and relieve sciatica pain, and there are rarely any risks or side effects. (*See* ACUPUNCTURE and ACUPRESSURE in PART 2 Treatment Section for additional information.)

Applied Kinesiology

Applied Kinesiology is excellent for reducing pain rapidly. The AK practitioner tests your muscles to determine the origin of your problem and then decides on the best course of action, choosing from a wide variety of therapeutic methods at his or her disposal. (*See* APPLIED KINESIOLOGY in PART 2 Treatment Section for additional information.)

Chiropractic

Chiropractic theory is based on the assumption that a properly aligned spine is essential for good health, and that any misalignment of the vertebrae in the spine causes pressure on the spinal nerves, leading to pain. The chiropractor makes spinal adjustments to move misaligned vertebrae to more normal positions, which helps the nervous system to function properly. (*See* CHIROPRACTIC in PART 2 Treatment Section for additional information.)

Craniosacral Therapy

A trained craniosacral practitioner can feel areas where healthy tissue function is restricted, usually due to physical or emotional trauma. The theory is that physical injuries and emotional traumas are stored or frozen in the body until they are released. (*See* CRANIOSACRAL THERAPY in PART 2 Treatment Section for additional information.)

Cupping

Cupping increases circulation, bringing blood to the cells. It helps promote energy flow and reduces swelling and pain. (*See* CUPPING in PART 2 Treatment Section for additional information.)

Guided Imagery and Visualization Techniques

These techniques help you relieve stress and manage your pain. Since the pain is described as an electrical sensation, mentally bring in an electrician to shut off the power. (*See* GUIDED IMAGERY and VISUALIZATION in PART 2 Treatment Section for additional information.)

Hypnosis

Hypnosis helps you relax, and relaxation alleviates stress, which contributes to pain. (*See* HYPNOSIS in PART 2 Treatment Section for additional information.)

SCIATICA AND DEEP TISSUE MASSAGE

Linda was an active fifty-year-old woman who played tennis twice a week and worked out five times a week. Following a three-hour dental procedure, she developed a severe pain in her thigh, which the doctors thought was most likely from being in a bad position during the surgery. They thought the analgesics given her for the post-op pain would also help her leg, but the thigh pain became so severe, she couldn't sit or stand up straight. She walked in a bent-over position, and when she had to eat on her hands and knees from a tray on the arm of the sofa, her husband said he was going to feed her out of a dog bowl.

Doctors diagnosed her with a severe case of sciatica and recommended prescription anti-inflammatories, which did not help. When they told her that back surgery to relieve the pressure on the nerve was her only option, she began looking for another solution, and a friend recommended a massage therapist who did deep-tissue work. This was not a relaxing massage. In fact, her treatments were painful, but after seeing the therapist twice a week for three weeks, she began to get relief. The therapist explained that he was taking pressure off the nerve, and after six weeks of this therapy, Linda was able to start working out and playing tennis again. She now sees the therapist for tune-ups about every six weeks, but the excruciating pain has never returned.

Massage

Massage helps reduce pain due to muscle spasms. (*See* MASSAGE in PART 2 Treatment Section for additional information.)

Osteopathic Manipulation

The goal of osteopathic manipulation is to increase range of motion, decrease muscle tension, and improve blood circulation, which can help to relieve sciatic pain. (*See* OSTEOPATHIC MANIPULATION in PART 2 Treatment Section for additional information.)

Physical Therapy

Physical therapy aids the pain of sciatica by correcting and improving your body's natural healing mechanism and increasing the range of motion in the joints. (*See* PHYSICAL THERAPY in PART 2 Treatment Section for additional information.)

Reflexology

Reflexology treatment for sciatica helps to open blocked sciatic nerve pathways. It also helps remove accumulated waste products from the muscles. The reflexologist will massage the reflex points located in the center of the heel and the area around the outside anklebone. (*See* REFLEXOLOGY in PART 2 Treatment Section for additional information.)

Rolfing

Rolfing can have long-lasting effects in easing the pain of sciatica. (*See* ROLFING in PART 2 Treatment Section for additional information.)

Tai Chi, Qigong, and Yoga

These treatments induce a profound relaxed state, which is beneficial for easing the pain of sciatica. (*See* TAI CHI, QIGONG, and YOGA in PART 2 Treatment Section for additional information.)

PRACTICAL SUGGESTIONS

- ❑ Be careful how you lift. Use your hips and legs, not your back, and keep whatever you are lifting close to you.
- ❑ Don't slump.
- ❑ Don't sit for long periods. Get up and move around.
- ❑ Don't keep your wallet in your hip pocket.

(*See also* BACK PAIN in PART 1 Conditions Section.)

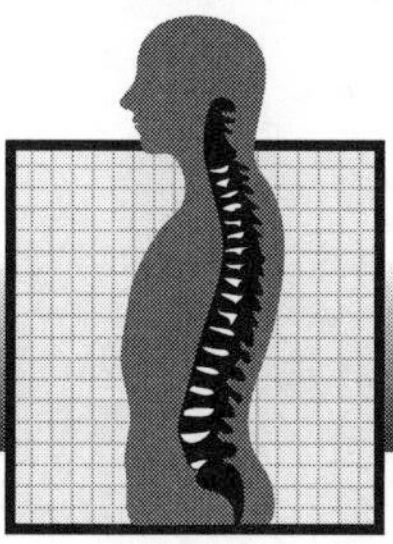

Spinal Stenosis

Your spinal canal is a narrow passage about as wide as your thumb that surrounds the entire length of your spinal cord, from your brain to the tip of your lower spine. It is the function of the vertebral bones that comprise the backbone (the vertebrae) to surround the canal and protect the spinal cord. If, however, the spinal canal becomes pinched, usually because one of the discs between the vertebrae bulges out and creates pressure on it, a condition known as spinal stenosis can develop, primarily in the lumbar (lower back) region of the spine.

Symptoms

Although many imaging studies show spinal stenosis in people who have no symptoms, most people with this problem do have symptoms, which can include back pain, and a feeling of burning, numbness, pain, or weakness in both legs. The pain gets worse when walking, standing up straight, or leaning backward.

Causes

With age, the normal wear and tear on the spine can cause arthritis or bulging discs, most often in the lumbar spine, and over time these changes can narrow the lumbar spinal canal and lead to the condition.

Diagnosing the Problem

X-rays can determine the narrowing in the lumbar region of the spinal canal. MRIs are also used to diagnose the condition.

Conventional Treatments

Mild cases of stenosis may be helped by physical therapy (being careful to avoid activities that put stress on the back), or aerobic activity, such as cycling, or by lying down with your knees drawn up to your chest to flex your spine. Bending forward or sitting increases the space in the spinal canal and can lead to significant pain relief. (All of these treatments are considered beneficial alternative therapies as well.) (*See* EXERCISE, STRETCHING, and SPORTS, and PHYSICAL THERAPY in PART 2 Treatment Section for additional information.)

SELF-HELP ALTERNATIVE TREATMENTS

As with all conditions in this book, anyone with spinal stenosis can benefit from proper nutrition, herbs, homeopathic remedies, and supplements. Although they may not work as fast as drugs or surgery, natural alternatives help the body heal itself. Herbs, homeopathic remedies, and supplements are available in health food stores and, increasingly, in large drug and grocery stores, as well as on the Internet. (*See* HERBAL REMEDIES, HOMEOPATHY, NUTRITIONAL THERAPY, and SUPPLEMENT THERAPY in PART 2 Treatment Section for additional information.)

Tarsal Tunnel Syndrome

Tarsal tunnel syndrome (TTS) is a painful condition of the foot, heel, and arch that is usually associated with repetitive stress injuries. It affects the inside part of the ankle and can be difficult to diagnose.

Symptoms

This painful condition produces burning, tingling, and weakness. The pain radiates to the lower leg and the toes, and does not ease up when you stop bearing weight. The burning or tingling gets worse with motion and eases with rest.

Common Causes

- A cyst in the area can cause compression on the nerve of the tibia (shin bone), which can adversely affect the lower leg and ankle.
- Flat feet can cause tarsal tunnel syndrome because a flattened arch can lead to compression of the tibial nerve.
- Inflammation of the posterior tibial nerve can result from abnormal pressure, arthritis, or excessive pronation (turning the foot inward and downward), and this can lead to a narrowing of the tarsal tunnel.
- Obesity can put extra pressure on the tibial nerve.
- Pregnancy can cause the canal to become smaller due to fluid retention, but this disappears after delivery in most cases.
- Prolonged standing compresses the tarsal tunnel, which contains nerves and blood vessels. Dancers, dentists, flight attendants, hairdressers, restaurant servers, and surgeons are especially susceptible.
- Rheumatoid arthritis causes the bones to thicken, leading to a narrowing of the canal.
- Tenosynovitis causes a chronic inflammation of the membranes around the tendon.
- Thyroid problems, diabetes, and injuries can lead to TTS, possibly because they can cause an increase of swelling in the tunnel, or interfere with circulation to the nerve.
- Trauma. After an ankle fracture heals, an overly large amount of scar tissue may form, which can eventually restrict movement in the tarsal tunnel and entrap the posterior tibial nerve.

Diagnosing the Problem

Tarsal tunnel syndrome is suspected when burning, pain, and tingling are present on the sole of the foot, and the pain gets worse later in the day. There are tests that can be performed to determine whether this condition is present or not.

- Tinel's sign is a test done to see if tingling, accompanied by a feeling of electric shocks, occurs when the doctor taps the skin over the tibial nerve in the leg.
- A nerve-conduction-velocity test measures how fast the nerve impulses travel along the nerve. If the test shows the impulses are traveling slowly, it confirms a diagnosis of tarsal tunnel syndrome.
- X-rays can rule out arthritis and see if old fractures exist.

Conventional Treatments

The condition can be treated conservatively if diagnostic studies show no nerve injury is present. If there is no response to conservative treatment, surgery may have to be considered. The most frequently used treatments are:

- Anti-inflammatories;
- Arch supports;
- Cortisone injections;
- Ice;
- Immobilization in a cast or walking boot;
- Orthotics and other special foot devices;
- Physical therapy;
- Reduction of repetitive foot motions;
- Surgery for TTS relieves pressure on the posterior tibial nerve; if the problem is a cyst impinging on the nerve, removing it can relieve the pressure.

Problems with Some Conventional Treatments

- Anti-inflammatories can cause gastrointestinal problems and bleeding.
- Casts and splints tend to weaken other areas of the leg muscles.
- Surgery treats only the symptoms, but does not address the cause of tarsal tunnel syndrome.

SELF-HELP ALTERNATIVE TREATMENTS

Although they may not work as fast as drugs or surgery, natural alternatives help the body heal itself. They get at the root of the problem instead of just temporarily alleviating the symptoms. All herbs, homeopathic remedies, packs, and supplements discussed here are available in health food stores and, increasingly, in large drug and grocery stores, as well as on the Internet.

Compresses, Packs, and Poultices

Soak a cloth or towel in cold water, warm herbal tea, or the appropriate aromatherapy oils (diluted). Apply the soaked cloth to the affected area, cover with a towel to retain the heat or the cold, and leave in place for twenty to thirty minutes. (*See* COMPRESSES, PACKS, and POULTICES IN PART 2 Treatment Section for additional information.)

Diet

Tarsal tunnel syndrome is inflammatory in nature so certain dietary modifications may be helpful.

Good Foods

Eat foods that contain B-vitamins, such as complex carbohydrates, fruits, nuts, seeds, vegetables, and whole grains. (*See* NUTRITIONAL THERAPY in PART 2 Treatment Section for additional information.)

Bad Foods

Alcohol, fast food, processed meats, saturated fats, simple sugars, and spicy foods can all trigger an inflammatory reaction in your body.

Exercises

- ❏ Keep a tennis or golf ball in front of your chair or under your desk and roll your foot over it periodically.
- ❏ Flex your foot back and forth and make circles with your ankle.
- ❏ After exercising, shake your foot and ankle for a few seconds. Do this periodically at work as well.

Exercise and stretching can be helpful, but it must be carefully supervised to avoid further damage to the affected area. (*See* EXERCISE, STRETCHING, and SPORTS in PART 2 Treatment Section for additional information.)

Herbal Remedies

- ❏ Coltsfoot and comfrey, used externally in soaks or poultices, reduce fluid retention. (Note: Comfrey taken internally has the potential to cause liver damage and should be used only under careful supervision.)
- ❏ Hydrangea acts like cortisone.
- ❏ Watercress reduces fluid retention.
- ❏ Yucca is a precursor to cortisone. It enables your adrenal glands to produce and release their own cortisone into your system.

Take the above herbs as directed on label. They can also be used in teas and infusions. (*See* HERBAL REMEDIES in PART 2 Treatment Section for additional information.)

Homeopathic Remedies

You can self-treat with homeopathic remedies by selecting the one that most closely matches your symptoms. If you don't see improvement, try another, or a combination product. Follow the instructions on the label. If you do not have relief in a reasonable amount of time, consult a physician who specializes in homeopathic medicine.

- ❏ Arnica soothes inflammation. It is also available in cream and ointment form for external application.
- ❏ Calcarea phosphorica eases pain and stiffness.
- ❏ Causticum helps those who have had the condition for a long time.
- ❏ Hypericum eases nerve pain.
- ❏ Rhus toxicodendron is useful for stiffness and pain that eases with motion.
- ❏ Ruta graveolens helps ease stiffness and weakness.

Take the above remedies as indicated on label. Combination remedies sometimes work more effectively than single ones. (*See* HOMEOPATHY in PART 2 Treatment Section for additional information.)

Hydrotherapy

Use ice packs for twenty-minutes at a time as long as the area is inflamed. After the inflammation has gone, when the joint no longer feels warm or appears red, then use moist heat for twenty-minute periods. Always wait until the inflammation has gone before using heat. Running hot water over the painful spots while in the shower can alleviate the pain. (*See* HYDROTHERAPY in PART 2 Treatment Section for additional information.)

Supplements

- ❏ Bromelain acts as an anti-inflammatory. Take 500 mg twice daily on an empty stomach.

- ❏ Magnesium citrate, 500 mg three times daily, acts as a muscle antispasmodic.
- ❏ Vitamin B_6 aids the normal function of nerve cells and helps reduce swelling because it has a natural ability to eliminate water retention. Dr. Edward M. Wagner, ND, recommends 200 mg three times a day. He says it is more effective to use the pyrodoxal #5 phosphate form of B_6, which has a higher assimilation rate than plain pyrodoxine.
- ❏ Vitamin B_{12}, sublingual, helps prevent nerve damage. Take 500 mcg twice daily. Note: For balance when taking individual Bs, be sure to supplement with a B-complex once daily, or a multivitamin containing B-complex.
- ❏ Vitamin C (Ester-C), 1000 mg three times daily, is a general overall antioxidant.

(*See* SUPPLEMENT THERAPY in PART 2 Treatment Section for additional information.)

Additional Self-Help Treatments

- ❏ Heat Therapy/Cold Therapy.
- ❏ Magnet Therapy.

For information on these therapies, refer to individual entries in PART 2 Treatment Section.

ASSISTED ALTERNATIVE TREATMENTS

The following techniques may require specialized training or the aid of a healthcare professional.

Acupuncture and Acupressure

Acupuncture and acupressure create a smooth flow of vibratory energy throughout the body that can help alleviate the symptoms of tarsal tunnel syndrome. (*See* ACUPUNCTURE and ACUPRESSURE in PART 2 Treatment Section for additional information.)

Applied Kinesiology

Applied Kinesiology is excellent for reducing pain rapidly. The AK practitioner tests your muscles to determine the origin of your problem and then decides on the best course of action, choosing from a wide variety of therapeutic methods at his or her disposal. (*See* APPLIED KINESIOLOGY in PART 2 Treatment Section for additional information.)

Chiropractic

By adjusting misaligned vertebrae (subluxations), the nervous system can function at its optimum level, which enhances healing. (*See* CHIROPRACTIC in PART 2 Treatment Section for additional information.)

Reflexology

Reflexology helps your body heal itself by eliminating energy blockages, improving circulation, and relieving stress and tension. (*See* REFLEXOLOGY in PART 2 Treatment Section for additional information.)

Tai Chi, Qigong, and Yoga

These therapies help you relax and direct healing energy where it is needed in your ankles and feet. (*See* TAI CHI, QIGONG, and YOGA in PART 2 Treatment Section for additional information.)

Additional Assisted Treatments

- ❏ Guided Imagery and Visualizations.
- ❏ Massage.
- ❏ Osteopathic Manipulation.
- ❏ Physical Therapy.
- ❏ Rolfing.

For information on these therapies, refer to individual entries in PART 2 Treatment Section.

PRACTICAL SUGGESTIONS

- ❏ Something as simple as wearing wider shoes might be enough to relieve pressure on the tarsal nerve.

(*See also* CARPAL TUNNEL SYNDROME in PART 1 Conditions Section for additional information.)

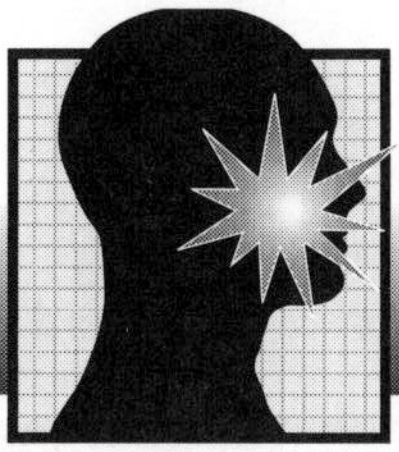

Temporomandibular Joint (TMJ) Pain

TMJ is caused by painful muscle spasms around the jaw joint. It is often more bothersome at night when you are trying to sleep because more blood goes to your head when you lie down and that causes pressure. The word temporomandibular is derived from tempero, which refers to the bones in the temple area, and mandible (your jawbone). The pain of TMJ can last from a few seconds to several hours, and comes and goes without warning. Symptoms are usually mild and frequently go away without therapy, but about 5 percent of those with TMJ may have disabling symptoms that are severe enough to warrant surgery. TMJ disorders affect more women than men, usually between the ages of fifteen and forty-five.

Symptoms

- ❏ A dull ache that gets worse after eating or yawning.
- ❏ Clicking and/or popping noises that occur while chewing.
- ❏ Difficulty opening the mouth.
- ❏ Pain that occurs while eating, usually on one cheek only, in front of the ear. Pain may also be present in the neck and shoulder muscles.

Common Causes

- ❏ Arthritis in the joint.
- ❏ Chewing.
- ❏ Clenching or grinding the teeth.
- ❏ Exposure to the elements, such as cold air or wind.
- ❏ Malocclusion (faulty bite) of the teeth.
- ❏ Misaligned bones in the temporomandibular joint.
- ❏ Muscle spasms.
- ❏ Opening the mouth too wide to bite into a large sandwich, or yawning.
- ❏ Stress.
- ❏ Tension.

Diagnosing the Problem

Diagnosis is based on history and symptoms. The dentist may examine the temperomandibular area and listen to the joint with a stethoscope while you open and close your mouth. He or she may also take impressions of your upper and lower teeth to see if they are meeting properly. Arthrography may be performed. This is a test involving the injection of an opaque dye into the joint, which is then viewed with a fluoroscope.

Conventional Treatments

- ❏ Cortisone injections into the joint.
- ❏ Dental procedures to correct improper occlusion. Some teeth may be built up with crowns and others may be ground down.
- ❏ Hot compresses.
- ❏ Missing teeth may have to be replaced.
- ❏ Muscle relaxants, such as diazepam (Valium).
- ❏ Night guards to prevent grinding or clenching while sleeping.
- ❏ Non-steroidal anti-inflammatories (NSAIDs).
- ❏ Surgery (arthroscopic) to repair, reposition, or remove a cervical disc.

Problems with Some Conventional Treatments

- ❏ Cortisone injections can give temporary relief, but they do not cure the condition.
- ❏ NSAIDs can cause gastrointestinal bleeding.
- ❏ Valium can become addictive.
- ❏ Surgery performed arthroscopically is a relatively new procedure for TMJ dysfunction. Arthroscopic surgery has been performed on larger joints, such as knees and shoulders, for some time, but much smaller instruments have to be used for TMJ surgery. If you have exhausted all other treatment plans, make sure the surgeon is highly qualified to do this procedure.

SELF-HELP ALTERNATIVE TREATMENTS

The following techniques can be done at home. Although they may not work as fast as drugs or surgery, natural alternatives help the body heal itself. They get at the root of the problem instead of just temporarily alleviating the symptoms. All herbs, homeopathic remedies, packs, and supplements discussed here are available in health food stores and, increasingly, in large drug and grocery stores, as well as on the Internet.

Aromatherapy

Aromatherapy, particularly the essential oils of cinnamon, fennel, peppermint, sage, spearmint, and thyme, are antibacterial and help to stimulate blood flow to the jaw. They are available in health food stores and stores specializing in aromatherapy products which you can find in the yellow pages. (*See* AROMATHERAPY in PART 2 Treatment Section for additional information.)

Castor Oil Packs

Dip a piece of white flannel into some warm castor oil. Wring it out and place it over the affected jaw area. Cover with plastic and apply a heating pad for one hour. Do this twice daily. (*See* COMPRESSES, PACKS, and POULTICES in PART 2 Treatment Section for additional information.)

Diet

Jaw pain has an inflammatory component so certain dietary modifications may be helpful.

Good Foods

All the foods listed below help to reduce inflammation.

- ❏ Foods that contain B vitamins, such as complex carbohydrates, fruits, nuts, seeds, vegetables, and whole grains.
- ❏ Fish, particularly wild salmon.
- ❏ Flaxseed meal.
- ❏ Fresh vegetables and fruits, preferably organically raised. Dark green vegetables contain antioxidants that help scavenge and neutralize the free radicals that are causing the inflammation.
- ❏ Garlic.

(*See* NUTRITIONAL THERAPY in PART 2 Treatment Section for additional information.)

Bad Foods

Avoid foods and drinks that stimulate the nervous system, such as caffeinated beverages and sugary-type foods and drinks, because these foods can exacerbate your pain.

Also avoid the following foods, which can all trigger an inflammatory reaction in your body.

- ❏ Alcohol.
- ❏ Processed foods and fast foods.
- ❏ Saturated fats, as found in meats and dairy products.
- ❏ Spicy foods.
- ❏ White flour products, such as pasta and bread.

Heat Therapy/Cold Therapy

Applying cold in the form of a cloth soaked in ice water, or rubbing the painful area of the jaw with an ice cube will help reduce swelling. Heat will increase blood flow to the area and aid healing after the swelling is gone. (*See* HEAT THERAPY/COLD THERAPY in PART 2 Treatment Section for additional information.)

Herbal Poultice

Chamomile used as a poultice reduces pain and swelling and is useful for TMJ Dysfunction. (*See* COMPRESSES, PACKS, and POULTICES in PART 2 Treatment Section for additional information.)

Herbal Remedies

The following herbs help your body heal itself when you have TMJ problems.

- ❏ Black cohosh relieves cramps in the jaw or neck. Note: Do not use if you are pregnant.
- ❏ Chamomile tea helps you relax.
- ❏ Hops, passionflower, and skullcap relieve muscle cramps, pain, and stress.
- ❏ Valerian root, a relaxant, is available as a tea or in capsule form.

Take the above herbs as directed on label. They can also be used in teas and infusions. (*See* Herbal Remedies in PART 2 Treatment Section for additional information.

Homeopathic Remedies

You can self-treat with homeopathic remedies by selecting the one that most closely matches your symptoms. If you don't see improvement, try another, or a combination product. Follow the instructions on the label. If you do not have relief in a reasonable amount of time, consult a physician who specializes in homeopathic medicine.

- ❏ Ammonium carbonica relieves pain that occurs while chewing.
- ❏ Belladonna is useful for those who grind their teeth.
- ❏ Causticum is useful for jaw pain that occurs when opening the mouth.
- ❏ Heper sulphuris eases pain in the jaw caused by opening the mouth.

- ❑ Kreosotum eases pain in the facial bones.
- ❑ Rhamnus californica eases TMJ pain.
- ❑ Xerophyllum eases TMJ pain.

Combination remedies sometimes work more effectively than single ones. (*See* HOMEOPATHY in PART 2 Treatment Section for additional information.)

Magnet Therapy

Magnet therapy relieves pain, accelerates healing, and reduces inflammation. (*See* MAGNET THERAPY in PART 2 Treatment Section for additional information.)

Meditation

Meditation helps alleviate stress, which contributes to pain. (*See* MEDITATION in PART 2 Treatment Section for additional information.)

Supplements

- ❑ Bromelain, 500 mg twice daily between meals, acts as an anti-inflammatory.
- ❑ Calcium, 1500–2000 mg, is necessary for strong bones and teeth, and also helps prevent muscle cramps. For better absorption, take calcium in divided doses throughout the day and at bedtime.
- ❑ Coenzyme Q_{10}, 30 mg daily, protects the body from stress.
- ❑ Magnesium citrate, 400 mg four times daily, acts as an antispasmodic that relieves pain.
- ❑ Vitamin B-complex, 100 mg 3 times daily, helps relieve stress.
- ❑ Vitamin B_1, 250 mg twice daily, acts as a muscle relaxant.
- ❑ Vitamin B_5, 100 mg twice daily, helps your body produce its own cortisone.
- ❑ Vitamin B_6 has anti-inflammatory properties. Take 200 mg three times a day. Note: For balance, when taking individual Bs, be sure to supplement with a B-complex once daily, or a multivitamin containing Bs.
- ❑ Vitamin C, 3000–5000 mg daily, aids tissue repair. Take to bowel tolerance (if diarrhea occurs, reduce the dosage until normal bowel function returns). It is preferable to take Ester-C because more of the vitamin is absorbed in this form.

(*See* SUPPLEMENT THERAPY in PART 2 Treatment Section for additional information.)

ASSISTED ALTERNATIVE TREATMENTS

The following techniques may require specialized training or the aid of a healthcare professional.

Acupuncture and Acupressure

Acupuncture involves the insertion of extremely thin solid needles into specific points of your body to stimulate its own healing mechanism and improve blood flow to the affected mouth and jaw areas. It also reduces inflammation, relieves pain, improves mobility, and there are rarely any risks or side effects. (*See* ACUPUNCTURE and ACUPRESSURE in PART 2 Treatment Section for additional information.)

Applied Kinesiology

Applied Kinesiology is excellent for reducing pain rapidly. The AK practitioner tests your muscles to determine the origin of your dental problem and then decides on the best course of action, choosing from a wide variety of therapeutic methods at his or her disposal. (*See* APPLIED KINESIOLOGY in PART 2 Treatment Section for additional information.)

Biofeedback

Electrodes taped to the skin in the TMJ area transmit impulses to a computer screen so you can actually see when you tense and relax your muscles. (*See* BIOFEEDBACK in PART 2 Treatment Section for additional information.)

Chiropractic

Chiropractic theory is based on the assumption that a properly aligned spine is essential for good health, and that any misalignment of the vertebrae in the spine causes pressure on the spinal nerves, leading to pain. The chiropractor makes spinal adjustments to move misaligned vertebrae to more normal positions, which helps the nervous system to function properly, and can help relieve TMJ pain. (*See* CHIROPRACTIC in PART 2 Treatment Section for additional information.)

Craniosacral Therapy

A trained craniosacral practitioner can feel areas in the jaw where healthy tissue function is restricted, usually due to physical or emotional trauma. The theory is that physical injuries and emotional traumas are stored or frozen in the body until they are released. (*See* CRANIOSACRAL THERAPY in PART 2 Treatment Section for additional information.)

Cupping

Cupping increases circulation, bringing blood to the cells. It helps promote energy flow and reduces swelling and pain. (*See* CUPPING in PART 2 Treatment Section for additional information.)

Guided Imagery and Visualization Techniques

These help to relieve stress and minimize pain in the jaw areas. The technique of changing your pain into an object you can manipulate can be helpful for treating TMJ pain. (*See* GUIDED IMAGERY and VISUALIZATION in PART 2 Treatment Section for additional information.)

Osteopathic Manipulation

Osteopathic manipulation can correct faulty structure and function and rebalance your body's system, enabling it to function better, and easing the jaw pain. (*See* OSTEOPATHIC MANIPULATION in PART 2 Treatment Section for additional information.)

Physical Therapy

Physical therapy increases the range of motion in your joints and corrects and improves your body's natural healing mechanism. A therapist can get blood flowing to the affected area of your jaw. Proper massaging and stretching can alleviate some of your painful symptoms. (*See* PHYSICAL THERAPY in PART 2 Treatment Section for additional information.)

Reflexology

Reflexology massage therapy performed on the specific part of the foot and/or hand that corresponds with the jaw can be helpful. (*See* REFLEXOLOGY in PART 2 Treatment Section for additional information.)

Rolfing

Rolfing is helpful for conditions caused by compressed nerves. (*See* ROLFING in PART 2 Treatment Section for additional information.)

PRACTICAL SUGGESTIONS

- ❏ Cut your food into small pieces so you don't have to open your mouth too wide.
- ❏ Do not chew gum.
- ❏ Do not chew ice.
- ❏ Do not clench your teeth.
- ❏ Do not eat any hard or tough foods.
- ❏ Replace missing teeth in a timely manner to avoid malocclusion.
- ❏ Wear mouth guards during athletic activities.

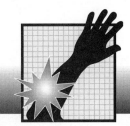

Tennis Elbow

Tennis elbow is an inflammation of the muscles, tendons, bursa, membranes (periosteum) and bony projections on the inside and outside of the elbow. Although tennis is the primary cause of tennis elbow, you do not necessarily have to play the game to have the problem. It can occur in any sport or occupational activity that requires you to twist your hand, wrist, or forearm.

Symptoms

The main symptoms of tennis elbow are pain and tenderness over either of the two bony projections (epicondyles) on your elbow that increase if you attempt to grip something, or try to rotate your wrist or forearm. Trying to twist a cap off a jar, brush your hair or teeth, or even hold a cup of coffee or tea can cause excruciating pain. Pain may radiate down your forearm, and it can be difficult to extend your arm.

Common Causes

Repeated forceful contraction of the wrist muscles causes microscopic tears in them that lead to inflammation. Activities that cause the wrist muscles to contract include bowling, gardening, golf, hammering, tennis and other racquet sports, shaking hands excessively (politicians beware!), using a screwdriver, or wringing out clothes.

Diagnosing the Problem

Tennis elbow is diagnosed by its obvious symptoms. It is not particularly helpful to take x-rays because they do not show soft tissue. This simple test can show if you have forehand or backhand tennis elbow. Place your hand and arm, palm up, on a flat surface, such as a desk or table. Bend your wrist and try to raise your fist. If that motion hurts, then your forehand stroke is probably the cause of the problem. If you feel pain when attempting to raise your fist with your palm down, it is most likely that your backhand is causing the problem.

Conventional Treatments

- ❑ Cortisone injections.
- ❑ Ice.
- ❑ NSAIDs (non-steroidal anti-inflammatory drugs).
- ❑ Physical therapy.
- ❑ Rest from the activity causing the problem.
- ❑ Splints.
- ❑ Surgery (rare) can be performed to release the tendon at the epicondyle.
- ❑ TENS units.
- ❑ Trigger point therapy.
- ❑ Ultrasound.

Problems with Some Conventional Treatments

- ❑ Cortisone injections can give temporary relief, but they do not cure tennis elbow.
- ❑ More than three cortisone injections can weaken the tendon.
- ❑ NSAIDs can cause internal bleeding, and even though they help you feel better in the short term, they do not fix the problem.
- ❑ It is difficult to convince avid tennis players that it is necessary to rest the elbow. They believe they can play through the pain.

SELF-HELP ALTERNATIVE TREATMENTS

The following techniques can be done at home. Although they may not work as fast as drugs or surgery, natural alternatives help the body heal itself. All herbs, homeopathic remedies, packs, and supplements discussed here are available in health food stores and, increasingly, in large drug and grocery stores, as well as on the Internet.

Aromatherapy

Aromatherapy can help relieve the pain of tennis elbow; particularly the essential oils of clove bud, marjoram, rosemary, and pine. Apply gently twice daily to the affected area. Do not use a vigorous massage over any swollen joint. Essential oils are available in health food stores and stores specializing in aromatherapy products, which you can find in the yellow pages. (*See* AROMATHERAPY in PART 2 Treatment Section for additional information.)

Castor Oil Packs

Dip a piece of white flannel into some warm castor oil.

Wring it out and place it over the affected area. Cover with plastic and apply a heating pad for one hour. Do this twice daily. (*See* COMPRESSES, PACKS, and POULTICES in PART 2 Treatment Section for additional information.)

Diet

Tennis elbow is inflammatory in nature so certain dietary modifications may be helpful.

Good Foods

Eat foods that contain B vitamins, such as complex carbohydrates, fruits, nuts, seeds, vegetables, and whole grains. Dark green vegetables contain antioxidants, which help scavenge and neutralize the free radicals that are causing the inflammation.

- ❏ Fish, particularly wild salmon, helps reduce inflammation.
- ❏ Garlic also reduces inflammation.

(*See* NUTRITIONAL THERAPY in PART 2 Treatment Section for additional information.)

Bad Foods

Alcohol, fast food, processed meats, saturated fats, simple sugars, and spicy foods can all trigger an inflammatory reaction in your body.

Exercise and Stretching

Lifting weights can strengthen the wrist tendon. Start with light weights and progressively increase the weight.

1. Sit at a table with a one-pound weight in your hand. Rest your arm on the table and extend your hand and the weight beyond the edge of the table. If you have backhand tennis elbow, turn your palm down. If you have forehand tennis elbow, turn it up.
2. Raise and lower the weight slowly by bending and straightening your wrist.
3. Lift 10 times, rest 10 seconds, and repeat two more times. If you feel any pain, stop.
4. Do this every other day, and as your arm gets stronger, gradually increase the weight.

If you play a lot of tennis, this exercise could prevent tennis elbow from occurring.

The following exercises are also useful to work the forearm muscles.

1. Spread your fingers as wide as you can and then close them. As you get stronger, you can add resistance by placing a rubber band around your fingertips.
2. With your palm down, bend your wrist toward your thumb and then toward your pinky.
3. Squeeze a ball.
4. Grasp your arm lightly above your elbow and rotate your forearm from a palm up to a palm down position.

(*See* EXERCISE, STRETCHING, and SPORTS in PART 2 Treatment Section for additional information.)

Heat Therapy/Cold Therapy

Use ice or cold compresses until the swelling goes down. Then alternate hot and cold. Use heat before performing exercises, and when you are finished, ice the elbow.(*See* HEAT THERAPY/COLD THERAPY and HYDROTHERAPY in PART 2 Treatment Section for additional information.)

Herbal Remedies

- ❏ Black currant oil relieves pain and inflammation.
- ❏ Boswellia has anti-inflammatory properties and acts similarly to NSAIDs without the side effects of stomach irritation or ulceration.
- ❏ Cayenne ointment, applied topically, relieves pain.
- ❏ Coltsfoot and comfrey, used externally in soaks or poultices, reduce fluid retention. (Note: Comfrey taken internally has the potential to cause liver damage and should be used only under careful supervision.)
- ❏ Evening primrose oil relieves pain and inflammation.
- ❏ Ginger stimulates circulation.
- ❏ Hydrangea acts like cortisone.
- ❏ Watercress reduces fluid retention.
- ❏ White willow bark relieves inflammation and pain. Take 60–120 mg per day. Although its pain-relieving aspects are slower than aspirin, they last longer.
- ❏ Yucca is a precursor of cortisone. It enables your adrenal glands to produce and release their own cortisone into your system.

Take the above herbs as directed on label. They can also be used in teas and infusions. (*See* HERBAL REMEDIES in PART 2 Treatment Section for additional information.)

Homeopathic Remedies

You can self-treat with homeopathic remedies by selecting the one that most closely matches your symptoms. If you don't see improvement, try another, or a combination product. Follow the instructions on the label. If you do not have relief in a reasonable amount of time, consult a physician who specializes in homeopathic medicine.

- ❑ Arnica soothes inflammation. It is also available in cream and ointment form for external application.
- ❑ Calcarea phosphorica eases pain and stiffness.
- ❑ Hypericum eases nerve pain.
- ❑ Ruta graveolens helps ease stiffness and weakness.

Take the above remedies as indicated on label. Combination remedies sometimes work more effectively than single ones. (*See* HOMEOPATHY in PART 2 Treatment Section for additional information.)

Magnet Therapy

Magnet Therapy relieves pain, accelerates healing, and reduces inflammation. A magnetic band around your elbow can help relieve pain. (*See* MAGNET THERAPY in PART 2 Treatment Section for additional information).

Supplements

- ❑ Bromelain acts as an anti-inflammatory. Take 500 mg twice daily on an empty stomach.
- ❑ Magnesium citrate, 500 mg three times daily, acts as a muscle antispasmodic.
- ❑ Vitamin B_6 aids the normal function of nerve cells and helps reduce swelling because it has a natural ability to eliminate water retention. Dr. Edward M. Wagner, ND, recommends 200 mg three times a day. He says it is more effective to use the pyrodoxal #5 phosphate form of B_6, which has a higher assimilation rate than plain pyrodoxine.
- ❑ Vitamin B_{12}, sublingual, helps prevent nerve damage. Take 500 mcg twice daily. Note: For balance when taking individual Bs, be sure to supplement with a B-complex once daily, or a multivitamin containing Bs.
- ❑ Vitamin C (Ester-C), 1000 mg three times daily, is a general overall antioxidant.

(*See* SUPPLEMENT THERAPY in PART 2 Treatment Section for additional information.)

ASSISTED ALTERNATIVE TREATMENTS

The following techniques may require specialized training or the use of a professional.

Acupuncture and Acupressure

Acupuncture involves the insertion of extremely thin solid needles into specific points of your body to stimulate its own healing mechanism and improve blood flow to the affected areas. It also reduces inflammation, relieves pain, improves mobility, and there are rarely any risks or side effects. Acupuncture treatments, as few as four, have a high success rate in the treatment of tennis elbow. (*See* ACUPUNCTURE and ACUPRESSURE in PART 2 Treatment Section for additional information.)

Applied Kinesiology

Applied Kinesiology is excellent for reducing pain rapidly. The AK practitioner tests your muscles to determine the origin of your problem and then decides on the best course of action, choosing from a wide variety of therapeutic methods at her or his disposal. (*See* APPLIED KINESIOLOGY in PART 2 Treatment Section for additional information.)

Bee Venom Therapy

Some components of bee venom are thought to stimulate the immune system. Other components are thought to modify the transmission of pain signals within the nervous system, and the therapy has proven consistently useful for painful conditions. (*See* BEE VENOM THERAPY in PART 2 Treatment Section for additional information.)

Guided Imagery

Guided imagery is useful for helping you manage the pain of tennis elbow. The technique of changing your pain into an object that you can shrink has been very effective in treating tennis elbow. (*See* GUIDED IMAGERY and VISUALIZATION in PART 2 Treatment Section for additional information.)

Osteopathic Manipulation

The goal of osteopathic manipulation in the treatment of tennis elbow is to increase range of motion, decrease muscle tension, and improve blood circulation. (*See* OSTEOPATHIC MANIPULATION in PART 2 Treatment Section for additional information.)

Physical Therapy

Physical therapy increases the range of motion in your elbow and corrects and improves your body's natural healing mechanism. (*See* PHYSICAL THERAPY in PART 2 Treatment Section for additional information.)

Reflexology

Reflexology massage therapy can be performed on the part of the foot or hand corresponding to the elbow area that is in pain. (*See* REFLEXOLOGY in PART 2 Treatment Section for additional information.)

Rolfing

Rolfing can be effective in the treatment of tennis elbow. It can have long-lasting effects. (*See* ROLFING in PART 2 Treatment Section for additional information.)

PRACTICAL SUGGESTIONS

- ❑ Try using a different size or type of tennis racquet or tool.
- ❑ Take tennis lessons from a qualified professional, who can correct your swing (usually the backhand) and prevent further injury.
- ❑ Try a midsize racquet rather than an oversize one. The larger racquets have increased torque (a turning or twisting force) if you hit a ball off-center.
- ❑ Don't have your racquet strung too tight. Even though tighter strings give better ball control, they increase torque and vibration.
- ❑ Buy your racquet in a good pro shop where your proper grip size can be determined. If the grip is too large or too small, you will have too much wrist movement.
- ❑ Special braces and bands that can help prevent reinjury are available in pro shops.

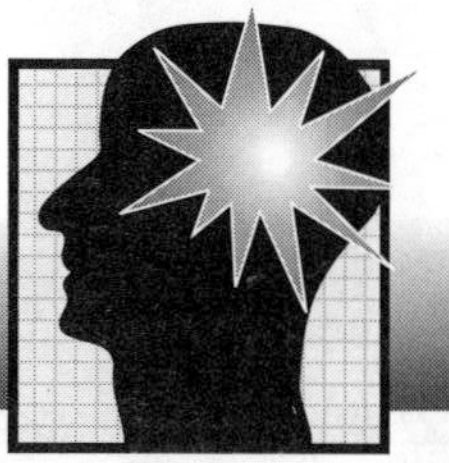

Tension Headaches

Headaches are symptoms of underlying conditions, not diseases in themselves, and are almost universal. Each year, more than forty million Americans seek treatment for relief of their headache pain. If you have a headache accompanied by breathing problems, fever, or a stiff neck, or if it occurs after a head injury or respiratory infection, you should seek medical help immediately because it could be a symptom of a life-threatening condition. Medical help should also be sought if you have headaches that: occur daily; do not respond to simple pain relievers; become progressively worse; are caused by exertion from coughing, sneezing or exercise; or are accompanied by numbness, loss of consciousness, or hallucinations. (For more information on the overall problem of headaches, see inset, THE SILENT EPIDEMIC, on page 34.)

Symptoms

Tension headaches are the most common type of headache. They usually affect both sides of the head, and the pain is described as moderate to mild, dull rather than throbbing. These headaches are accompanied by a feeling of tightness in the face, neck, shoulders, and scalp; some say it feels as though they had a vise across their temples. Tension headaches affect slightly more men than women and can start at any age, although they usually start later in life than migraines.

Common Causes

Besides tension, there are many factors that can trigger a headache. Some of the most common are:

- Air pollution;
- Alcohol consumption;
- Bruxism (grinding of teeth);
- Change in altitude;
- Clenching the jaw;
- Constipation;
- Dehydration;
- Eye problems, or improper eyeglass prescriptions;
- Glare from fluorescent lights;
- Hormonal changes;
- Imbalance in brain chemicals and nerve pathways;
- Insomnia or too much sleep;
- Low barometric pressure;
- Low levels of fresh air, as found in airplane cabins or poorly ventilated buildings;
- Low serotonin levels;
- Narrowing of the blood vessels going into the brain, muscles, and tissues of the neck and scalp;
- Overexposure to sun;
- Side effects of prescribed medications, including hormone replacement therapy, nitroglycerin (taken for angina), and some asthma drugs;
- Smoking and second-hand tobacco smoke;
- Stress;
- TMJ misalignment;
- Video display terminals and television screens.

Diagnosing the Problem

Before any treatment can begin, a proper diagnosis is essential in order to rule out the possibility of brain tumors, intracranial pressure changes, or meningeal inflammation, an inflammation of the membranes surrounding the brain and spinal cord.

Once a potentially serious condition has been ruled out, the type of headache can be determined by its symptoms, which have been described above.

Conventional Treatments

Some medications prevent the onset of headaches; others relieve them after they've begun. The following are the most frequently used medications.

- Analgesics (painkillers). These reduce or relieve pain without addressing its cause.
- Antidepressants. They help soothe a tension headache.
- Anti-inflammatory drugs. They reduce the inflammation that contributes to the pain.
- Beta-blockers and calcium channel blockers. They stabilize blood vessels.
- Oxygen. Breathing in pure oxygen helps the blood get rid of toxic material that arteries are producing, and this helps them constrict and dilate in a normal fash-

BOTOX AS A PAINKILLER?

Botulinum toxin (botox) may be a poison, but it is also an organic product derived from a common bacterium that is taking its place alongside other natural poisons with medicinal uses. Researchers all over the world are now testing it, often successfully, for a wide variety of treatments, including migraine headaches and back pain, with one researcher even comparing it to penicillin for its versatility.

ion. (*See also* OXYGEN THERAPIES in PART 2 Treatment Section.)

- ❑ Stadol. Inhaled through the nose, this spray helps relieve chronic tension headaches.

Problems with Some Conventional Treatments

- ❑ At first, caffeine constricts blood vessels, easing the pain of a tension headache, but when it wears off, rebound swelling occurs, and that can ultimately worsen the pain.
- ❑ Overuse of analgesics can be counterproductive by causing the blood vessels to become less sensitive to the medication. When this happens, higher doses are needed, setting up a vicious cycle.
- ❑ In connection with this, over-the-counter analgesics (painkillers), even used as infrequently as five times a week, can turn periodic headaches into chronic rebound headaches.
- ❑ Long-term use of nonsteroidal anti-inflammatory drugs (NSAIDs) may cause kidney, liver, or stomach problems.
- ❑ Side effects of beta-blockers can be dimished circulation to the brain and impotence.
- ❑ Calcium channel blockers can cause fatigue, flushing, heartburn, and swelling of the abdomen, ankles, or feet.
- ❑ Stadol is potentially addictive and subject to abuse.

SELF-HELP ALTERNATIVE TREATMENTS

The following techniques for alleviating tension headaches can be done at home. Although they may not work as fast as drugs or surgery, natural alternatives help the body heal itself. All herbs, homeopathic remedies, packs, and supplements discussed here are available in health food stores and, increasingly, in large drug and grocery stores, as well as on the Internet.

Aromatherapy

Aromatherapy is useful for headaches, particularly the essential oils of basil, cajeput, eucalyptus, lavender, niaouli, peppermint, and rosemary. They are available in health food stores and stores specializing in aromatherapy products listed in the yellow pages. (*See* AROMATHERAPY in PART 2 Treatment Section for additional information.)

Compresses, Packs, and Poultices

Alternate hot and cold compresses. Use heat for three minutes and cold for one minute and keep switching for about fifteen minutes. Castor oil packs have also been recommended for headaches. Soak a piece of white flannel in warm castor oil, wring it out and place it over the headache area. Cover with plastic and apply a heating pad. Do this twice a day for an hour each time. (*See* COMPRESSES, PACKS, and POULTICES, HEAT THERAPY/COLD THERAPY, and HYDROTHERAPY in PART 2 Treatment Section for additional information.)

Diet

Knowing which foods to eat and which to avoid can help ameliorate or even ward off tension headaches.

Good Foods

Caffeinated beverages taken in small amounts raise serotonin levels and help constrict dilated blood vessels, but sometimes, when caffeine wears off, a rebound effect occurs, causing swelling of the blood vessels. Do not overdo the caffeine. If a small amount helps, more will not necessarily be better.

(*See* NUTRITIONAL THERAPY in PART 2 Treatment Section for additional information.)

Bad Foods

The following list of substances can bring on, or worsen, a headache.

- ❑ Aged cheese.
- ❑ Alcohol.
- ❑ Aspartame—an artificial sweetener.
- ❑ Avocados.
- ❑ Bananas.
- ❑ Chicken livers.
- ❑ Chocolate.

- ❑ Cured meats.
- ❑ Fermented foods, such as sour cream and yogurt.
- ❑ Herring.
- ❑ Hot dogs.
- ❑ Monosodium glutamate (MSG).
- ❑ Nuts.
- ❑ Onions.
- ❑ Red wine.
- ❑ Salami.
- ❑ Vinegar.
- ❑ Wheat.

Other Substances to Avoid

Aftershave lotion, molds, perfume, and tobacco can all bring on headaches.

Herbal Remedies

- ❑ Burdock root helps purify the blood.
- ❑ Cayenne aids circulation.
- ❑ Feverfew makes your body less responsive to the chemicals that cause spasms in the muscles surrounding your brain.
- ❑ Goldenseal has anti-inflammatory properties.
- ❑ Lobelia is a relaxant.
- ❑ Mint helps relieve nausea.
- ❑ Peppermint helps oxygenate the bloodstream.
- ❑ White willow bark has an effect similar to aspirin.

Take according to label instructions. (*See* HERBAL REMEDIES in PART 2 Treatment Section for additional information.)

Homeopathic Remedies

You can self-treat with homeopathic remedies by selecting the one that most closely matches your symptoms. If you don't see improvement, try another, or a combination product. Follow the instructions on the label. If you do not have relief in a reasonable amount of time, consult a physician who specializes in homeopathic medicine.

- ❑ Belladonna relieves headaches that start at the back of the head or upper neck.
- ❑ Bryonia helps relieve splitting headaches that settle over one eye.
- ❑ Cimicifuga relieves headaches with throbbing pain that worsens with motion.
- ❑ Ignatia helps headaches caused by emotional upsets or grief.
- ❑ Spigelia relieves left-sided throbbing headaches accompanied by pain above or through the eyeball.

Instructions for use are usually printed on the label. (*See* HOMEOPATHY in PART 2 Treatment Section for additional information.)

Magnet Therapy

Magnet therapy can help relieve head pain. Placing magnets on the area of the head that is in pain brings increased amounts of blood to the area which, in turn brings oxygen and other healing substances to ease the pain. (*See* MAGNET THERAPY in PART 2 Treatment Section for additional information.)

Meditation

Meditation helps reduce stress, which contributes to head pain. (*See* MEDITATION in PART 2 Treatment Section for additional information.)

Supplements

- ❑ Calcium. Take 1500 mg daily to help transmission of nerve impulses.
- ❑ Fish Oil. Take 1 gram per pound of body weight. Fish oil modifies prostaglandins, hormone-like substances made by the body that may cause headaches.
- ❑ 5-HTP. This amino acid helps raise serotonin levels. Take per instructions on label.
- ❑ Potassium. 100 mg daily aids in proper sodium and potassium balance, necessary to avoid fluid retention, which may put pressure on the brain.
- ❑ SAMe (S-adenosyl-L-methionine) is a mood stabilizer and helps regenerate nerves. Take per instructions on label.
- ❑ Vitamin B-complex. 50 mg taken twice daily relieves stress.
- ❑ Vitamin E. 400 IU taken twice a day aids circulation.

(*See* SUPPLEMENT THERAPY in PART 2 Treatment Section for additional information.)

ASSISTED ALTERNATIVE TREATMENTS

The following techniques may require specialized training or the aid of a healthcare professional.

Acupuncture and Acupressure

Acupuncture and acupressure create a smooth flow of vibratory energy throughout the body. Practitioners aim to move the energy away from the head. For self-treatment, knead the area between your thumb and index finger. Tension headaches can be relieved by pinching the skin above each eyebrow in three places—the area near the nose, the center, and the area near the temple. (*See* ACUPUNCTURE and ACUPRESSURE in PART 2 Treatment Section for additional information.)

Applied Kinesiology

Applied Kinesiology can help reduce headache pain. The AK practitioner tests your muscles to determine the origin of your problem and then decides on the best course of action, choosing from a wide variety of therapeutic methods at his or her disposal. (*See* APPLIED KINESIOLOGY in PART 2 Treatment Section for additional information.)

Biofeedback

Biofeedback works by reducing stress and the physical responses, such as a tension headache, associated with it. (*See* BIOFEEDBACK in PART 2 Treatment Section for additional information.)

Chiropractic

Poor vertebral alignment, often the result of wearing high heels or having flat feet, may reduce blood flow to the brain, which can cause headaches. Chiropractic manipulation can help correct this situation. (*See* CHIROPRACTIC in PART 2 Treatment Section for additional information.)

Craniosacral Therapy

Headaches caused by the pressure of cranial fluid can be eased by gently manipulating the cranial bones. (*See* CRANIOSACRAL THERAPY in PART 2 Treatment Section for additional information.)

Cupping

Cupping can ease headaches that are caused by a lack of oxygen in the cells. It helps promote energy flow and reduces swelling and pain. (*See* CUPPING in PART 2 Treatment Section for additional information.)

Exercise

Aerobic activity reduces stress and increases the production of endorphins, which helps to raise the pain threshold. To avoid further damage, it must be carefully supervised at the beginning. (*See* EXERCISE, STRETCHING, and SPORTS in PART 2 Treatment Section for additional information.)

Guided Imagery and Visualization Techniques

Guided imagery can help manage headache pain. Since most headaches are described as vise-like, or as a feeling of tightness, picture a tool that can loosen the vise. (*See* GUIDED IMAGERY and VISUALIZATION in PART 2 Treatment Section for additional information.)

Hypnosis

Hypnosis helps you relax and relaxation alleviates stress, which contributes to the pain of tension headaches. (*See* HYPNOSIS in PART 2 Treatment Section for additional information.)

Massage

A massage can help your body relax, thereby reducing head pain caused by stress. There are many kinds of massage therapies available and you can ask your practitioner to suggest the appropriate one for your headache problem. Many conventional doctors are now extolling the benefits of massage. (*See* MASSAGE in PART 2 Treatment Section for additional information.)

Osteopathic Manipulation

Osteopathic manipulation can help decrease muscle tension, which is a contributing factor in tension headaches. (*See* OSTEOPATHIC MANIPULATION in PART 2 Treatment Section for additional information.)

Oxygen Therapy

Oxygen therapy, also listed in conventional therapies in this entry (which underscores its dual role as a therapy), is a useful adjunct for treating headaches. (*See* OXYGEN THERAPIES in PART 2 Treatment Section for additional information.)

Physical Therapy

Physical therapy helps correct and improve your body's natural healing mechanisms and can help prevent the return of symptoms. (*See* PHYSICAL THERAPY in PART 2 Treatment Section for additional information.)

Reflexology

Reflexology massage therapy performed on the specific part of the foot and/or hand that corresponds with the head can be helpful. (*See* REFLEXOLOGY in PART 2 Treatment Section for additional information.)

Tai Chi, Qigong, and Yoga

These therapies induce a profoundly relaxed state and help bring healing energy to the body. Relaxation techniques and concentrating on your breathing can relieve tension. One technique is to take six deep breaths, counting to four as you inhale and as you exhale. (*See* TAI CHI, QIGONG, and YOGA in PART 2 Treatment Section for additional information.)

Pass the Oxygen

Dr. Nancy Snyderman told millions of listeners to *Good Morning America* that pure oxygen is the most popular treatment for stopping headaches, and that it is safer than others, which can have powerful side effects.

PRACTICAL SUGGESTIONS

- ❑ Stay hydrated. Drink eight to ten glasses of water a day, and if your indoor air is dry, use a humidifier.
- ❑ Improve the quality of your indoor air. A negative ion generator or HEPA filter will remove unhealthy particles. If you live in an unpolluted area, open your windows at least fifteen minutes a day. Houseplants also filter indoor pollution from the air.
- ❑ Use incandescent bulbs. The flickering in fluorescent light tubes may not be noticeable, but it can be enough to bring on a headache.

Thoracic Outlet Syndrome

The thoracic outlet is a passageway at the top of the rib cage (the base of the neck), which allows the esophagus, trachea, major blood vessels, many nerves, and other structures to pass between the neck and the chest. It is a very crowded area and when its blood vessels or nerves get compressed between the overlying muscle and a rib, thoracic outlet syndrome, a nerve disorder in the passageway at the top of the rib cage, can occur.

Symptoms

Thoracic outlet syndrome causes pain and a feeling of pins and needles in the shoulders, arms, and hands. It can make the muscles of your hands weak and impair your grip, and it may make your arm turn pale when you lift it.

Common Causes

An extra cervical rib in the neck area can cause it, or the fibrous band that connects the rib to the vertebra may be abnormally tight. It could also be caused by an injury or a blockage in one of the arteries under the clavicle (collarbone) that supplies blood to the arm. If you have a long neck and droopy shoulders, or if you are overweight, you could be putting extra pressure on the nerves and blood vessels. Poor posture could also be a contributing factor.

Diagnosing the Problem

Diagnosis of thoracic outlet syndrome can be made with x-rays and MRIs, and by observing the clinical symptoms.

Conventional Treatments

In severe cases, surgery can be performed to remove the cervical rib or cut the fibrous band. A few patients with nerve-conduction disorders benefit, but some find their symptoms only worsen after surgery.

Physical therapy, a non-invasive alternative, can be used to help strengthen the shoulder muscles, and the therapist can recommend exercises that will improve your posture because, when you stand and sit straighter, there is less pressure on your nerves and blood vessels. (These treatments are considered beneficial alternative therapies as well.) It is also a good idea to avoid carrying anything particularly heavy, including shoulder bags. (*See* EXERCISE, STRETCHING, and SPORTS, and PHYSICAL THERAPY in PART 2 Treatment Section for additional information.)

SELF-HELP ALTERNATIVE TREATMENTS

As with all conditions in this book, anyone with thoracic outlet syndrome can benefit from proper nutrition, herbs, homeopathic remedies, and supplements. Although they may not work as fast as drugs or surgery, natural alternatives help the body heal itself. Herbs, homeopathic remedies, and supplements are available in health food stores and, increasingly, in large drug and grocery stores, as well as on the Internet. (*See* HERBAL REMEDIES, HOMEOPATHY, NUTRITIONAL THERAPY, and SUPPLEMENT THERAPY in PART 2 Treatment Section for additional information.)

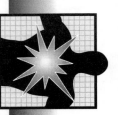

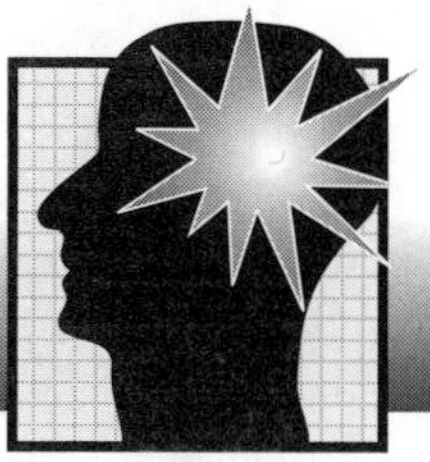

Trigeminal Neuralgia

Trigeminal Neuralgia, also known as tic douloureux, is a malfunction of the facial trigeminal nerve that causes severe pain on one side of the face. One of the largest nerves in the cranium, it is the fifth of twelve that lead from the brain to the head. It sends impulses of pain, pressure, touch, and temperature to the brain from the forehead, gums, and jaw areas, and has three branches, any one of which can be affected. If the neuralgia is in the first branch, pain occurs around the eyes and over the forehead. Neuralgia in the second branch causes pain in the cheek, nose, and upper lip, and in the third branch, pain will be on the side of the tongue and the lower lip. More women than men are affected by trigeminal neuralgia, and it seldom strikes anyone under fifty. Some with trigeminal neuralgia live in fear of initiating an attack merely by brushing their teeth, chewing and swallowing, applying makeup, or shaving. Most of those with trigeminal neuralgia try to avoid touching their faces or mouths. The pain is excruciating, but the condition is not fatal.

Symptoms

Pain in the areas of the face served by the trigeminal nerve is an indication of this condition. The pain comes in sudden spasms and is flashing and stabbing. Quick bursts occur in clusters and last several seconds. Then there are periods of sharp painful spasms that sometimes last for hours. The condition usually increases in severity and medical treatment becomes less and less effective. Sometimes attacks occur frequently, followed by periods of time with no symptoms. Unfortunately the intensity of the pain gets more severe over time, with fewer pain-free periods in between, and the pain tends to spread from the immediate area of the nerve to larger areas of the face.

Common Causes

- A malfunctioning of the portion of the trigeminal nerve that transfers impulses.
- Abnormalities of the protective lining around the nerve.
- Abnormal firing of the nerve.
- Hyper-excitability of the trigeminal nerve. Increased electrical impulses traveling through the nerve activate pain regions in the brain.
- Dental procedures. Many people with trigeminal neuralgia say their pain started shortly after dental work. Dental surgeons respond that their procedures do not cause trigeminal neuralgia, but may trigger it in those who are predisposed to it.
- Genetic predisposition. A small percentage of people with trigeminal neuralgia have a family history of the condition. It usually occurs on the same side of the face and starts at a younger age.
- Injury to the myelin sheath (the covering of the nerve fibers). This can be caused by an aneurysm, a malformation of the vessels, multiple sclerosis, pressure from a tumor, or viral infections.
- Multiple sclerosis.

Diagnosing the Problem

At the present time, there are no specific tests for diagnosing trigeminal neuralgia. Diagnosis is made by the described symptoms after other causes of facial pain, such as aneurysms, sinusitis, tooth problems, or tumors, have been ruled out. An MRI scan of the brain can rule out aneurysms and tumors. Doctors should carefully question whether massaging the painful area, or using heat or cold, relieves or exacerbates the problem.

Conventional Treatments

- Anticonvulsant medications, including baclofen (Lioresal), carbamazepine (Tegretol), neurontin (Gabapentin), clonazapam (Klonopin), lamotrigine (Lamictal), phenytoin (Dilantin).
- Botoxin injections.
- Capsaicin cream used three times a day has been shown to ease, and in many cases end, the pain.
- Gamma knife (high intensity, highly focused radiation).
- Injections of lidocaine and streptomycin.
- NSAIDs.
- Opioids.
- Percutaneous procedures, such as balloon compression, glycerol injections, and radio frequency rhizotomy, attempt to keep the pain site from being recognized by the brain.
- Sodium channel blockers, such as carbamazepine, may help disrupt impulses that are perceived as pain.

- ❑ Surgery, including microvascular decompression and cutting the nerve.
- ❑ Trigger point therapy.

Problems with Some Conventional Treatments

- ❑ Botoxin injections have to be administered by an experienced professional in order to avoid over-paralyzing an area. For instance, they can cause an eye to droop. Also, they are not a permanent solution.
- ❑ Capsaicin cream has to be applied near the eyes very carefully because it can burn, sting, and possibly cause damage.
- ❑ Carbamazepine can cause dizziness, fatigue, memory problems, and nausea. It can also lead to potentially serious blood conditions, such as agranulocytosis and aplastic anemia.
- ❑ Cutting the nerve can cause further discomfort in the face.
- ❑ Injections of lidocaine and streptomycin have not been shown to be helpful, and they cause irritation and inflammation at the injection site.
- ❑ Microvascular decompression is temporary and symptoms can return within three to six months.
- ❑ Numbness can occur following percutaneous procedures. Most of it goes away after several weeks, and some say it is preferable to the pain.
- ❑ MS symptoms in people with both trigeminal neuralgia and MS have made them more sensitive to medications, which may worsen their MS symptoms.
- ❑ NSAIDs can cause internal bleeding and are not particularly helpful.
- ❑ Opiates are addictive and, like NSAIDs, are not particularly helpful.

SELF-HELP ALTERNATIVE TREATMENTS

The following techniques can be done at home. Although they may not work as fast as drugs or surgery, natural alternatives help the body heal itself. All herbs, homeopathic remedies, packs, and supplements discussed here are available in health food stores and, increasingly, in large drug and grocery stores, as well as on the Internet.

Aromatherapy

Aromatherapy, particularly the essential oils of chamomile, ginger, lavender, marjoram, peppermint, and rosemary, can be effective. They are available in health food stores and stores specializing in aromatherapy products, which you can find in the yellow pages. (*See* AROMATHERAPY in PART 2 Treatment Section for additional information.)

Compresses, Packs, and Poultices

Chamomile used as a poultice reduces pain and swelling. (*See* COMPRESSES, PACKS, and POULTICES in PART 2 Treatment Section for additional information.)

Diet

Trigeminal neuralgia is inflammatory in nature so certain dietary modifications may be helpful.

Good Foods

- ❑ Stay hydrated. Water is essential to transport nutrients through your body and carry waste material out of it.
- ❑ Eat foods that produce B vitamins necessary for healthy nerve function. Good sources are whole grains, fruits, vegetables, nuts, seeds, and complex carbohydrates. Foods high in B_{12} are needed to prevent nerve damage. These include cheese, especially blue cheese, dairy products, organ meats, and seafood.
- ❑ Eggs and soybeans are good sources of lecithin, which is beneficial.
- ❑ Papayas and pineapples are good sources of enzymes and have anti-inflammatory properties.

(*See* NUTRITIONAL THERAPY in PART 2 Treatment Section for additional information.)

Bad Foods

- ❑ Caffeinated beverages in excess have a negative impact on the nervous system.
- ❑ Refined sugar products can cause overstimulation of electrical activity in the nervous system.

Other Substances to Avoid

Tobacco smoke keeps oxygen and blood from nourishing your tissues.

Heat Therapy/Cold Therapy

Gently apply a hot moist compress over the painful area and at the same time place an ice bag over the carotid artery. The hot compress will divert the blood from the nerve to the skin, and the ice bag decreases the amount of the blood reaching the head. (*See* HEAT THERAPY/COLD THERAPY in PART 2 Treatment Section for additional information.)

Herbal Remedies

- ❑ Chamomile relieves pain and relaxes the body.
- ❑ Catnip relaxes the nervous system.
- ❑ Cayenne capsules relieve pain.
- ❑ Fenugreek relieves inflammation.
- ❑ Hops relax the nervous system.
- ❑ Juniper relieves inflammation.
- ❑ Myrrh soothes inflammation.
- ❑ Passionflower relaxes the nervous system.
- ❑ Slippery elm bark helps your body produce its own anti-inflammatory cortisone.
- ❑ Valerian is a relaxant.
- ❑ Yucca is an anti-inflammatory.

Take the above herbs as directed on label. They can also be used in teas and infusions. (*See* HERBAL REMEDIES in PART 2 Treatment Section for additional information.)

Homeopathic Remedies

You can self-treat with homeopathic remedies by selecting the one that most closely matches your symptoms. If you don't see improvement, try another, or a combination product. Follow the instructions on the label. If you do not have relief in a reasonable amount of time, consult a physician who specializes in homeopathic medicine.

- ❑ Hypericum (St. John's wort) relieves shooting, radiating pain and numbness.
- ❑ Kali phos is a calming nerve nutrient and restorer
- ❑ Magnesium phos aids spasmodic conditions.
- ❑ Spigelia is particularly helpful for neuralgia of the fifth cranial nerve. It aids violent, burning, needle-like pains.
- ❑ Urtica urens soothes stinging pains.

Combination remedies sometimes work more effectively than single ones. (*See* HOMEOPATHY in PART 2 Treatment Section for additional information.)

Meditation

Meditation helps alleviate stress, which contributes to pain. (*See* MEDITATION in PART 2 Treatment Section for additional information.)

Supplements

- ❑ Bromelain 500 mg, twice daily, or proteolytic enzymes (digestive aids) taken between meals, per label, act as anti-inflammatories.
- ❑ Lecithin, 500 mg daily, helps protect cells from damage by oxidation.
- ❑ Magnesium citrate, 400 mg four times daily, acts as an antispasmodic that relieves pain.
- ❑ Pantothene, 500 mg twice daily, acts as an anti-inflammatory.
- ❑ Vitamin B complex, 100 mg twice daily, is essential for healthy nerve function. Note: For balance, when taking individual Bs, be sure to supplement with a B-complex once daily, or a multivitamin containing Bs.
- ❑ Vitamin B_3 (niacin), 100 mg three times daily, helps the nervous system function properly.
- ❑ Vitamin B_{12}, 500 mcg sublingually twice daily, helps strengthen nerves and prevent nerve damage. It is more effective when injected by a healthcare professional.

(*See* SUPPLEMENT THERAPY in PART 2 Treatment Section for additional information.)

ASSISTED ALTERNATIVE TREATMENTS

The following techniques may require specialized training or the aid of a healthcare professional.

Acupuncture and Acupressure

Acupuncture involves the insertion of extremely thin solid needles into specific points of your body to stimulate its own healing mechanism and improve blood flow to the affected areas. It also reduces inflammation, relieves pain, improves mobility, and there are rarely any risks or side effects. (*See* ACUPUNCTURE and ACUPRESSURE in PART 2 Treatment Section for additional information.)

Applied Kinesiology

Applied Kinesiology is excellent for reducing pain rapidly. The AK practitioner tests your muscles to determine the origin of your trigeminal neuralgia pain and then decides on the best course of action, choosing from a wide variety of therapeutic methods at her or his disposal. (*See* APPLIED KINESIOLOGY in PART 2 Treatment Section for additional information.)

Cupping

Cupping can ease the pain of trigeminal neuralgia. If the area is too painful to touch, cupping can be applied to the relevant acupuncture points. (*See* CUPPING in PART 2 Treatment Section for additional information.)

Exercise and Stretching

Exercise releases endorphins, your body's natural pain fighting chemicals. To avoid further damage, it must be carefully supervised in the beginning. (*See* EXERCISE, STRETCHING, and SPORTS in PART 2 Treatment Section for additional information.)

Guided Imagery and Visualization Techniques

These help to relieve stress and minimize pain. If your pain is a stabbing sensation, visualize a shield or barrier protecting the area. If you are having spasms, picture them as large waves and watch them grow smaller. (*See* GUIDED IMAGERY and VISUALIZATION in PART 2 Treatment Section for additional information.)

Osteopathic Manipulation

The goal of osteopathic manipulation in the treatment of trigeminal neuralgia is to decrease muscle tension and improve blood circulation. (*See* OSTEOPATHIC MANIPULATION in PART 2 Treatment Section for additional information.)

Reflexology

Reflexology massage therapy can be performed on the part of the foot or hand corresponding to the area that is in pain. The toes, and areas just beneath the toes, relate to facial structures. (*See* REFLEXOLOGY in PART 2 Treatment Section for additional information.)

Rolfing

Rolfing can be effective in the treatment of trigeminal neuralgia. It can have long-lasting effects. (*See* ROLFING in PART 2 Treatment Section for additional information.)

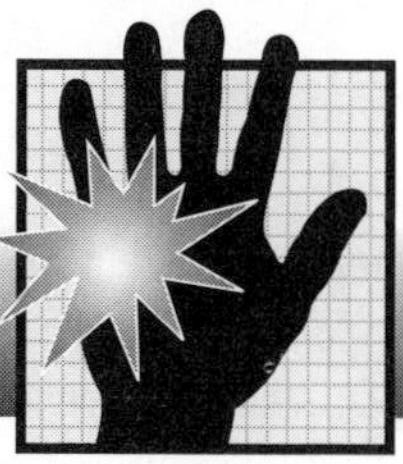

Trigger Finger

Trigger finger is an inflammation of the tendons in the palm of the hand (tendons are the fibrous cords of tissue that connect muscles to bones). Aging makes tendons more susceptible to injury, but anyone who performs repetitive motions or plays sports regularly can develop this form of tendonitis. The tendons in the palm are used for grasping and hand dexterity, and they work in a pulley system. If they become inflamed, a condition called tenosynovitis develops and a nodule forms. When you bend your finger, the nodule gets caught in the pulley system. Then when you try to extend your finger, it snaps (triggers) in its attempt to slide through the pulley.

Symptoms

A bump in the palm is a sign of this problem. There is pain when pressure is applied to the involved tendon, and the finger snaps when it is bent and straightened.

Common Causes

This problem can develop when there are occupations that require repetitive hand tasks. It can also result from direct pressure being applied to the hand in such sports as baseball, tennis, racquetball, or weightlifting.

Diagnosing the Problem

Diagnosis is determined by applying pressure to the area and observing whether pain occurs and the finger snaps when it is bent and straightened.

Conventional Treatments

- ❑ Avoiding the offending activities.
- ❑ Cortisone injections.
- ❑ Finger splinting to rest the tendon.
- ❑ Physical therapy.
- ❑ Surgery.

Problems with Some Conventional Treatments

- ❑ Injections can cause the condition to flare up. Corticosteroid injections can have serious side effects.
- ❑ Because of the number of nerves in the hand, if surgery is unavoidable, be sure to use a surgeon who specializes in hand surgery.

SELF-HELP ALTERNATIVE TREATMENTS

The following techniques can be done at home. Although they may not work as fast as drugs or surgery, natural alternatives help the body heal itself. All herbs, homeopathic remedies, packs, and supplements discussed here are available in health food stores and, increasingly, in large drug and grocery stores, as well as on the Internet.

Aromatherapy

Aromatherapy can help relieve the pain of trigger finger; particularly the essential oils of clove bud, marjoram, rosemary, and pine. Add a few drops to vegetable oil and massage into the affected area. Apply gently twice daily to the affected area. Do not use a vigorous massage over any swollen joint. Essential oils are available in health food stores and stores specializing in aromatherapy products, which you can find in the yellow pages. (*See* AROMATHERAPY in PART 2 Treatment Section for additional information.)

Castor Oil Packs

Dip a piece of white flannel into some warm castor oil. Wring it out and place it over the affected area. Cover with plastic and apply a heating pad for one hour. Do this twice daily. (*See* COMPRESSES, PACKS, and POULTICES in PART 2 Treatment Section for additional information.)

Diet

Trigger-finger tendonitis is inflammatory in nature so certain dietary modifications may be helpful.

Good Foods

All the foods listed below help to reduce inflammation.

- ❑ Foods that contain B vitamins, such as complex carbohydrates, fruits, nuts, seeds, vegetables, and whole grains.
- ❑ Fish, particularly wild salmon.
- ❑ Flaxseed meal.
- ❑ Fresh vegetables and fruits, preferably organically raised. Dark green vegetables contain antioxidants that help scavenge and neutralize the free radicals that are causing the inflammation.
- ❑ Garlic.

(*See* NUTRITIONAL THERAPY in PART 2 Treatment Section for additional information.)

Bad Foods

Avoid the following foods, which can all trigger an inflammatory reaction in your body.

- ❑ Alcohol.
- ❑ Processed foods and fast foods.
- ❑ Saturated fats, as found in meats and dairy products.
- ❑ Spicy foods.
- ❑ Sugary-type foods.
- ❑ White flour products, such as pasta and bread.

Exercise and Stretching

Hold the affected finger in the opposite hand and gently move it back—away from the palm—twenty times, four times a day or more. Be sure to stop at the point you feel any discomfort. (*See* EXERCISE, STRETCHING, and SPORTS in PART 2 Treatment Section for additional information.)

Heat Therapy/Cold Therapy

Applying cold to the painful area reduces swelling, and heat helps increase blood flow. (See HEAT THERAPY/COLD THERAPY in PART 2 Treatment Section for additional information.)

Herbal Remedies

- ❑ Black currant oil relieves pain and inflammation.
- ❑ Boswellia has anti-inflammatory properties and acts similarly to NSAIDs without the side effects of stomach irritation or ulceration.
- ❑ Cayenne ointment, applied topically, relieves pain.
- ❑ Coltsfoot and comfrey, used externally in soaks or poultices, reduce fluid retention. (Note: Comfrey taken internally has the potential to cause liver damage and should be used only under careful supervision.)
- ❑ Evening primrose oil relieves pain and inflammation.
- ❑ Ginger stimulates circulation.
- ❑ Hydrangea acts like cortisone.
- ❑ Watercress reduces fluid retention.
- ❑ White willow bark relieves inflammation and pain. Take 60–120 mg per day. Although its pain-relieving aspects are slower than aspirin, they last longer.
- ❑ Yucca is a precursor of synthetic cortisone. It enables your adrenal glands to produce and release their own cortisone into your system.

Take the above herbs as directed on label. They can also be used in teas and infusions. (*See* HERBAL REMEDIES in PART 2 Treatment Section for additional information.)

Homeopathic Remedies

You can self-treat with homeopathic remedies by selecting the one that most closely matches your symptoms. If you don't see improvement, try another, or a combination product. Follow the instructions on the label. If you do not have relief in a reasonable amount of time, consult a physician who specializes in homeopathic medicine.

- ❑ Arnica soothes inflammation. It is also available in cream and ointment form for external application.
- ❑ Calcarea phosphorica eases pain and stiffness.
- ❑ Hypericum eases nerve pain.
- ❑ Ruta graveolens helps ease stiffness and weakness.

Take the above remedies as indicated on label. Combination remedies sometimes work more effectively than single ones. (*See* HOMEOPATHY in PART 2 Treatment Section for additional information.)

Hydrotherapy

Running hot water over a painful area while in the shower or soaking in a hot tub can help diminish the pain. (*See* HYDROTHERAPY in PART 2 Treatment Section for additional information.)

Magnet Therapy

Magnet therapy relieves pain, accelerates healing, and reduces inflammation. (*See* MAGNET THERAPY in PART 2 Treatment Section for additional information.)

Supplements

- ❑ Bromelain is a digestive enzyme if taken with meals, but acts as an anti-inflammatory when taken on an empty stomach. Take 400 mg 3 times a day between meals.
- ❑ Flaxseed oil, 1–2 teaspoons daily.
- ❑ Magnesium citrate, 500 mg three times daily, acts as a muscle antispasmodic.
- ❑ Manganese, 25–100 mg twice a day during the acute phase. Then take 10–15 mg twice a day.
- ❑ Proteolytic enzymes taken between meals can reduce pain and swelling and help speed up the healing process. Take per instruction on label.
- ❑ Selenium, 100–200 mcg daily.

- ❑ Vitamin B_6 aids the normal function of nerve cells and helps reduce swelling because it has a natural ability to eliminate water retention. Dr. Edward M. Wagner, ND, recommends 200 mg three times a day. He says it is more effective to use the pyrodoxal #5 phosphate form of B_6, which has a higher assimilation rate than plain pyrodoxine.
- ❑ Vitamin B_{12}, sublingual, helps prevent nerve damage. Take 500 mcg twice daily. Note: For balance when taking individual Bs, be sure to supplement with a B-complex once daily, or a multivitamin containing Bs.
- ❑ Vitamin C (Ester-C), 1000 mg three times daily, is a general overall antioxidant.
- ❑ Vitamin E, 400 IU daily.

(*See* SUPPLEMENT THERAPY in PART 2 Treatment Section for additional information.)

ASSISTED ALTERNATIVE TREATMENTS

The following techniques may require specialized training or the aid of a healthcare professional.

Acupuncture and Acupressure

Acupuncture involves the insertion of extremely thin solid needles into specific points of your body to stimulate its own healing mechanism and improve blood flow to the affected areas. It also reduces inflammation, relieves pain, improves mobility, and there are rarely any risks or side effects. (*See* ACUPUNCTURE and ACUPRESSURE in PART 2 Treatment Section for additional information.)

Applied Kinesiology

Applied Kinesiology is excellent for reducing pain rapidly. The AK practitioner tests your muscles to determine the origin of your problem and then decides on the best course of action, choosing from a wide variety of therapeutic methods at his or her disposal. (*See* APPLIED KINESIOLOGY in PART 2 Treatment Section for additional information.)

Chiropractic

Chiropractic theory is based on the assumption that a properly aligned spine is essential for good health, and that any misalignment of the vertebrae in the spine causes pressure on the spinal nerves, leading to pain. The chiropractor makes spinal adjustments to move misaligned vertebrae to more normal positions, which helps the nervous system to function properly. (*See* CHIROPRACTIC in PART 2 Treatment Section for additional information.)

Guided Imagery

Guided imagery is a useful adjunct to help you manage your pain. In your mind, picture the affected area as an object and bring in the appropriate tools. (*See* GUIDED IMAGERY and VISUALIZATION in PART 2 Treatment Section for additional information.)

Massage

A massage helps bring blood to the affected area and relieve the pain. There are many kinds of massage therapies available and you can ask your practitioner to suggest the appropriate one for your problem. (*See* MASSAGE in PART 2 Treatment Section for additional information.)

Osteopathic Manipulation

The goal of osteopathic manipulation in the treatment of trigger finger is to increase range of motion, decrease muscle tension, and improve blood circulation. (*See* OSTEOPATHIC MANIPULATION in PART 2 Treatment Section for additional information.)

Physical Therapy

Physical therapy improves your body's natural healing mechanism. (*See* PHYSICAL THERAPY in PART 2 Treatment Section for additional information.)

Reflexology

Reflexology massage therapy can be performed on the part of the foot or hand corresponding to the area that is in pain. (*See* REFLEXOLOGY in PART 2 Treatment Section for additional information.)

Rolfing

Rolfing helps place your body in balance with gravity by releasing stress patterns that keep it out of alignment. It can have long-lasting effects in easing pain. (*See* ROLFING in PART 2 Treatment Section for additional information.)

PRACTICAL SUGGESTIONS

- ❑ Use as large a grip as possible on racquets, bats, and clubs.
- ❑ Be sure your hand is dry when gripping because more than a 50 percent grasp is needed to hold a racquet, bat, or club when your hand is wet.

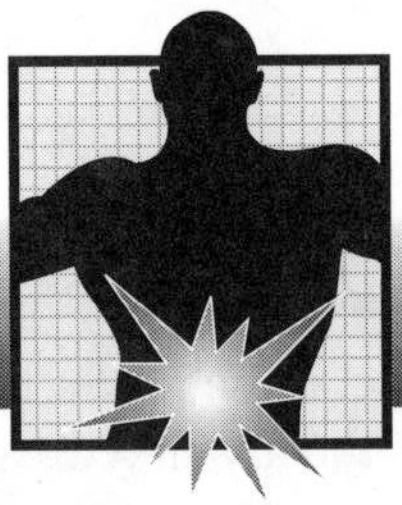

Ulcerative Colitis

Inflammatory bowel diseases (IBD) are disorders in which the bowel becomes inflamed, resulting in cramps and diarrhea. The IBD known as ulcerative colitis affects the mucous membranes lining the large intestine, causing it to become inflamed and ulcerated, and leading to bloody diarrhea, cramps, and fever. The bleeding can, in turn, lead to iron-deficient anemia. This inflammatory bowel disorder usually begins in the lower end of the large intestine (the rectum or sigmoid colon) and can, in time, spread throughout the entire large intestine (the condition does not affect the small intestine). It can come on at any age, but, as with another IBD, Crohn's disease, it usually starts between ages fifteen and thirty. And, as with Crohn's, flare-ups may be associated with inflammation of the joints, whites of the eyes, and skin problems.

Symptoms

Attacks may begin gradually, and symptoms can include:

- ❑ Abdominal pain;
- ❑ Blood and mucus in the stool;
- ❑ Cramps;
- ❑ Diarrhea;
- ❑ Fever;
- ❑ Hard, dry stools when the colitis is limited to the rectum and sigmoid colon;
- ❑ Loose bowel movements that occur frequently, as many as twenty times a day, accompanied by cramps and painful spasms if the colitis is higher up in the intestines;
- ❑ Weight loss.

Common Causes

The exact cause is unknown, but possibilities include an overactive immune response of the intestine, food allergies or sensitivities, heredity, or poor eating habits, such as eating too fast and not chewing food properly.

Diagnosing the Problem

Doctors suspect colitis when there is a history of watery loose stools accompanied by cramping. Blood tests can be done to see if the number of white blood cells has increased, if anemia is present, if albumin levels are low, and if the erythrocyte sedimentation rate is elevated. Stool analysis and sigmoidoscopy are also effective diagnostic tools.

Note: With ulcerative colitis, barium enema studies and a colonoscopy can also determine the extent of the colitis, but should not be performed when it is active because at those times there is an increased risk of perforating the colon.

Conventional Treatments

- ❑ Azathioprine and mercaptopurine help maintain remissions and decrease the need for corticosteroids.
- ❑ Codeine controls diarrhea.
- ❑ Corticosteroids control inflammation and can induce remission.
- ❑ Deodorized opium tincture controls diarrhea.
- ❑ Diphenoxylate also controls diarrhea.
- ❑ Mesalamine, olsalazine, and sulfasalazine all reduce inflammation and prevent symptoms from flaring up.
- ❑ Surgery to remove the large intestine and rectum can be a last resort.

Problems with Some Conventional Treatments

- ❑ Azathioprine and mercaptopurine take three to six months to be effective and can lead to allergic reactions.
- ❑ Corticosteroid therapy has side effects, such as fluid retention, a puffy face, bone loss, eye problems (glaucoma and cataracts), elevated blood pressure, and a lowered resistance to infections. Corticosteroids given to children for prolonged periods of time can suppress their growth.
- ❑ Sulfasalazine may cause allergic reactions, such as difficulty breathing, hives, rashes, and swelling of the tissues in the area around the eyes. Other side effects are hearing loss, insomnia and sun sensitivity. If you are taking this drug, you should have blood tests performed regularly for liver and bone marrow monitoring.
- ❑ Surgery. Although removal of the large intestine and rectum permanently cures ulcerative colitis, those who have undergone the operation have had to live with an opening in their abdominal wall and an ileostomy bag. There are newer procedures now that maintain continence, such as an ileo-anal anastomosis, in which a

small reservoir is created out of the small intestine and attached to the remaining portion of the rectum above the anus. However, complications such as inflammation of the reservoir may occur.

SELF-HELP ALTERNATIVE TREATMENTS

The following techniques can be done at home. Many medications for bowel problems have undesirable side effects so you may want to try alternative methods to promote wellness. All herbs, homeopathic remedies, packs, and supplements discussed here are available in health food stores and, increasingly, in large drug and grocery stores, as well as on the Internet.

Aromatherapy

Aromatherapy is particularly useful for relieving symptoms related to the digestive system. To relieve constipation, black pepper, cardamom, cinnamon leaf, citronella, ginger, and peppermint oils have a stimulating effect. Mix two or three drops of these oils with a carrier oil, such as sweet almond oil, and use to massage the abdomen in a clockwise direction. You can also add up to ten drops of these oils to your bath water, or soak a piece of flannel in hot water containing four or five drops of oil and apply it as a compress.

For control of diarrhea, chamomile, cinnamon, clove, geranium, ginger, lavender, nutmeg, tea tree oils, and thyme are beneficial. Use as above.

Do not ingest essential oils or use them full strength as they are very powerful compounds. They are available in health food stores and stores specializing in aromatherapy products which you can find in the yellow pages. (*See* AROMATHERAPY in PART 2 Treatment Section for additional information.)

Castor Oil Packs

Dip a piece of white flannel into some warm castor oil. Wring it out and place it over the affected area. Cover with plastic and apply a heating pad for one hour. Do this twice daily. (*See* COMPRESSES, PACKS, and POULTICES in PART 2 Treatment Section for additional information.) (*See also* AROMATHERAPY above in this entry.)

Diet

If you have any kind of bowel problem, you may have food intolerances. These are not true allergies caused by an immune system response, but are metabolic in nature and can best be evaluated by an elimination diet whereby suspected foods are avoided and then gradually reintroduced. This should be monitored by a qualified nutritionist.

NSAIDs AND PEPTIC ULCER DISEASE

Although our focus in this book is on long-term chronic pain, we are including a mention of peptic ulcer disease because roughly 4.5 million Americans experience the acute pain it can cause. After it was isolated, the *H. pylori* bacterium was thought to be, almost exclusively, the chief cause of peptic ulcer disease, but now NSAIDs (nonsteroidal anti-inflammatory drugs) are catching up as a primary cause. Use of these drugs is at an all-time high because people are living longer and are treating their arthritis with NSAIDS, which symptomatically lessen pain and decrease swelling. As palliative temporary drugs, the occasional use of NSAIDs for pain relief is considered acceptable, but it has been found that 25 percent of the people who use them chronically develop a peptic ulcer. And the many gastrointestinal complications that result from overuse of NSAIDs are known to cause more than 100,000 hospitalizations and 16,500 deaths annually in the United States. When relied on for chronic treatment, these insidious drugs can also cause excessive bleeding, fluid retention, kidney problems, and miscarriages, as well as microscopic damage to the stomach's mucosal layer.

To counter this, there is zinc-carnosine, a relatively new nutrient composed of zinc and L-carnosine that was developed in Japan in the late 1980s. Zinc-carnosine is considered a breakthrough treatment because of its two-way action to inhibit the *H. pylori* bacteria and to heal the sores of ulcer by stimulating the body's natural healing mechanism.

Dosage is 75 mg a day, preferably divided in two doses of 37.5 mg twice daily for eight weeks. Supplementation with zinc-carnosine is not a quick fix. Relief is gradual; some alleviation of the pain occurs after two weeks, but after eight weeks of supplementation, there is substantial long-term relief, with no harmful side effects.

You can read more about this breakthrough treatment in *Ulcer Free* by Georges Halpern, MD, PhD.

Good Foods

- ❑ Cabbage and carrot juices are nourishing and cleansing for colitis.
- ❑ During an acute attack, eat only steamed vegetables put through a food processor, or store-bought junior baby food.
- ❑ To keep stools soft and mobile, it is a good idea to add one tablespoon of oat bran or rice to your cereal or juice.

Bad Foods

The following foods may exacerbate your condition.

- ❑ Dairy products.
- ❑ Fried foods.
- ❑ Grains, except for brown rice.
- ❑ Nuts.
- ❑ Processed foods.
- ❑ Red meat.
- ❑ Seeds.
- ❑ Spicy foods.

Other Substances to Avoid

Anyone who has a bowel disorder has a problem with alcohol, caffeine, carbonated beverages, and tobacco because they are irritating to the gastrointestinal tract. Additionally, all artificial sweeteners, especially aspartame, minnitol, and sorbitol, can cause diarrhea.

Herbal Remedies

- ❑ Chamomile soothes the digestive system and relaxes the body.
- ❑ Dandelion helps relieve constipation.
- ❑ Feverfew helps relieve gas pains.
- ❑ Ginger relieves most digestive problems.
- ❑ Pau d'arco aids healing.
- ❑ Red clover is an anti-inflammatory and has antibacterial properties.
- ❑ Yarrow helps heal mucous membranes.

Take the above herbs as directed on label. They can also be used in teas and infusions. (*See* HERBAL REMEDIES in PART 2 Treatment Section for additional information.)

Homeopathic Remedies

You can self-treat with homeopathic remedies by selecting the one that most closely matches your symptoms. If you don't see improvement, try another, or a combination product. Follow the instructions on the label. If you do not have relief in a reasonable amount of time, consult a physician who specializes in homeopathic medicine.

The following homeopathic remedies are useful for *all* painful bowel problems, including ulcerative colitis.

- ❑ Argentum nitricum eases bloating, flatulence, and diarrhea that occurs after drinking water.
- ❑ Bismuth relieves diarrhea.
- ❑ Bryonia relieves constipation.
- ❑ Carbo veg controls diarrhea alternating with constipation.
- ❑ Chamomilla relieves diarrhea.
- ❑ Colocynthis eases abdominal pain and cramping that eases by bending over or applying pressure.
- ❑ Dulcamara helps control diarrhea containing mucous.
- ❑ Hydrastis relieves constipation.
- ❑ Iris ver also relieves constipation.
- ❑ Kali sulph relieves diarrhea containing mucous.
- ❑ Lycopodium helps control bloating, constipation, gas, heartburn, and pain.
- ❑ Mag phos is an antispasmodic.
- ❑ Nat mur aids digestion.
- ❑ Nux vomica helps relieve gas, cramps, and muscular soreness in the abdomen.
- ❑ Podophyllum helps control diarrhea that alternates with constipation and is accompanied by weakness.
- ❑ Sulphur is useful for anyone with morning diarrhea and excessive gas.

Combination remedies sometimes work more effectively than single ones. (*See* HOMEOPATHY in PART 2 Treatment Section for additional information.)

Meditation

Meditation can help if the ulcerative colitis is stress-related. (*See* MEDITATION in PART 2 Treatment Section for additional information.)

Supplements

The following help your body function better and make it more resistant to ulcerative colitis.

- ❑ Acidophilus twice a day between meals helps normalize intestinal bacteria.
- ❑ Alfalfa, per label, supplies chlorophyll and vitamin K

to aid healing of tissues (a deficiency of vitamin K has been linked to intestinal disorders).

- ❑ Folic acid supplements, per label, are important because intestinal absorption of this nutrient is impaired.
- ❑ Garlic capsules, per label, help heal the colon.
- ❑ Iron supplements, per label, help to treat anemia resulting from bleeding.
- ❑ Mineral supplements that contain calcium, chromium, magnesium, and zinc, per label, because people with ulcerative colitis have problems absorbing them.
- ❑ Proteolytic enzymes, per label, reduce inflammation and aid digestion.
- ❑ Vitamin A, 25,000 IU daily, for tissue repair.
- ❑ Vitamin B-complex, 50–100 mg daily, for normal function of all body cells and to help maintain muscle tone in the digestive tract.
- ❑ Vitamin C with bioflavanoids, per label, aids healing.

(*See* SUPPLEMENT THERAPY in PART 2 Treatment Section for additional information.

ASSISTED ALTERNATIVE TREATMENTS

The following techniques may require specialized training or the aid of a healthcare professional.

Acupuncture and Acupressure

Acupuncture involves the insertion of extremely thin solid needles into specific points of your body to stimulate its own healing mechanism and improve blood flow to the affected areas. It also reduces inflammation, relieves pain, improves mobility, and there are rarely any risks or side effects. (*See* ACUPUNCTURE and ACUPRESSURE in PART 2 Treatment Section for additional information.)

Applied Kinesiology

Applied Kinesiology is a non-invasive, non-toxic method that can correct imbalances in the body. It is excellent for reducing pain rapidly, including abdominal pain. (*See* APPLIED KINESIOLOGY in PART 2 Treatment Section for additional information.)

Biofeedback

Biofeedback is useful for reducing stress in anyone with painful bowel problems. (*See* BIOFEEDBACK in PART 2 Treatment Section for additional information.)

Chiropractic

Chiropractic theory is based on the assumption that a properly aligned spine is essential for good health, and that any misalignment of the vertebrae in the spine causes pressure on the spinal nerves, leading to pain. The chiropractor makes spinal adjustments to move misaligned vertebrae to more normal positions, which helps the nervous system to function properly. (*See* CHIROPRACTIC in PART 2 Treatment Section for additional information.)

Craniosacral Therapy

Craniosacral therapy is a form of energy healing that can help balance your system. It has been shown to be effective for soothing bowel problems. (*See* CRANIOSACRAL THERAPY in PART 2 Treatment Section for additional information.)

Cupping

Cupping helps to promote energy flow and reduce pain. (*See* CUPPING in PART 2 Treatment Section for additional information.)

Exercise and Stretching

Stretching exercises help improve digestion. To avoid damage, they must be carefully supervised at the beginning. (*See* EXERCISE, STRETCHING, and SPORTS in PART 2 Treatment Section for additional information.)

Guided Imagery

Guided Imagery helps relieve stress and manage pain. Visualizing your abdominal area as soft and relaxed can be useful to help relieve the stress associated with pain. (*See* GUIDED IMAGERY and VISUALIZATION in PART 2 Treatment Section for additional information.)

Hypnosis

Hypnosis is useful for reducing stress in those with an IBD. (*See* HYPNOSIS in PART 2 Treatment Section for additional information.)

Massage

A massage helps bring blood to the affected area to relieve the pain. There are many kinds of massage therapies available and you can ask your practitioner to suggest the appropriate one for your problem. (*See* MASSAGE in PART 2 Treatment Section for additional information.) (*See also* AROMATHERAPY above in this entry.)

Oxygen Therapy

Oxygen therapy helps enhance your body's ability to heal itself. Inflammatory bowel diseases respond well to ultraviolet irradiation of blood (UVIB). (*See* OXYGEN THERAPIES in PART 2 Treatment Section for additional information.)

Reflexology

Reflexology massage therapy can be performed on the part of the foot or hand corresponding to the abdominal area that is in pain. (*See* REFLEXOLOGY in PART 2 Treatment Section for additional information.)

Tai Chi, Qigong, and Yoga

These therapies help your body to enter a relaxed state and also increase production of endorphins, which are natural painkillers. (*See* TAI CHI, QIGONG, and YOGA in PART 2 Treatment Section for additional information.)

PRACTICAL SUGGESTIONS

Do not wear tight clothing around your waist.

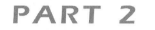

PART 2

Treatments

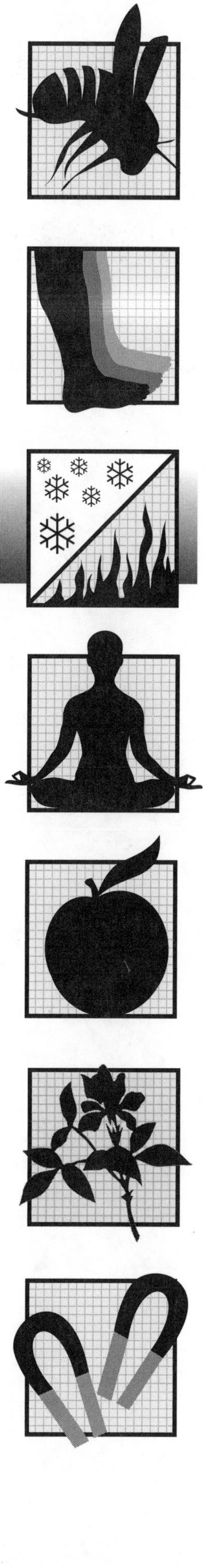

Acupuncture and Acupressure

Acupuncture and acupressure are methods used to create a smooth flow of vital energy, or chi, throughout the body. The aim of both methods is to heal the body by balancing its energy flow. Considered alternative/complementary treatments in the United States, they have been standard treatment in China for many millenia. Needles are used for acupuncture, and fingertips for acupressure. In the United States, those who practice acupuncture are either licensed practitioners or physicians. Acupressure is used by some chiropractors and massage therapists, and can even be used for self-treatment. It has been referred to as acupuncture without needles.

THE HISTORY OF ACUPUNCTURE

Except for Chinese neighborhoods, acupuncture was virtually unknown in the United States until 1971 when James Reston, a *New York Times* foreign correspondent, had an emergency appendectomy while he was on an assignment in China. Following the surgery, Reston was treated with acupuncture, which he reported effectively blocked his pain. Nowadays, both physicians and nonphysicians practice acupuncture. In the United States, 4,000 of the 10,000 licensed acupuncturists are physicians, but the majority are practitioners of traditional Chinese medicine (TCM).

HOW ACUPUNCTURE WORKS

Practitioners of TCM believe that your body is electrical in nature and has positive and negative poles that should be in balance. According to this belief, sickness occurs when there is a disruption in the balance of the electromagnetic fields in your body and brain, and it often disappears when that balance is restored. A basic component of this belief system is that the life forces in your body, called yin and yang, should be in balance in order for energy to flow smoothly along your body's thirty-two interconnected primary meridians. (It should be noted that the number of meridians, as well as the number of acupuncture points, varies widely from practitioner to practitioner.)

These meridians, located on each side of your body, are close to the surface at 671 different points, and each meridian services one or more of your body's areas or organs. To correct imbalances between yin and yang, acupuncturists stimulate the appropriate meridian by inserting tiny steel needles into the specific point(s) related to the particular illness or symptom. This helps your energy to become evenly dispersed instead of remaining blocked, thereby restoring balance so your body can heal itself. An acupuncturist in New York, Anuthep Benja-Athon, MD, PC, believes that the body is 50 percent chemical makeup and 50 percent electrical, and that acupuncture works on the 50 percent that is electrical.

Acupuncture is just one of the modalities used in TCM, which also includes herbs, nutrition, physical therapy, and special exercises, such as tai chi and qigong. The goal of all TCM methods and procedures is to correct small imbalances in the body's energy before they lead to major health problems.

The thought of having needles inserted into your body can be a frightening one, but acupuncture is not a painful experience. The needles are so fine that most people are not aware they have been inserted and often ask the practitioner when the needle insertion is going to start.

Jacques Depardieu, MS, LAc, is a licensed acupuncturist and a certified Chinese herbalist who practices TCM at The Center for Integrative Chinese Medicine in Darien, Connecticut. He says, "Sometimes one treatment may be all that is necessary, although it usually takes four to six treatments for acupuncture to be effective. If there are no positive results after four to six treatments, the person should talk with the practitioner." Depardieu gives seasonal treatments that he refers to as tune-ups, important because energy travels through the organs differently at different times of year and the meridians in the body change with the seasons. He says Chinese medicine is exceedingly specific, and even though there are many methods, they all work because they all encourage the body's own natural tendency toward health. He treats the pain, and addresses its underlying cause with herbs, nutrition, and exercise. "My goal is to empower the patient, says Depardieu. "I do not want people to be dependent on me, or any practitioner. The idea is to get people back in balance and out the door as soon as possible."

Treatments are generally performed weekly in the West, more frequently if the pain has reached an acute stage. Depending on the condition, an arthritic joint for instance, your acupuncturist may want to complete a course of treatment, then treat you again in three or four months. One positive aspect of acupuncture is that subsequent treatments are just as effective as the initial treatment.

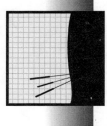

The Western approach is to treat the patient when there are symptoms present. Conversely, practitioners of traditional Chinese medicine believe in keeping their patients in a healthy state, before they display any symptoms, and may suggest treating chronic conditions more often. Eastern and Western philosophies differ. Most Westerners believe that acupuncture is an alternative treatment for pain, while the Chinese have a more holistic approach. They want to treat the entire body as an integrated system and, in support of this view, many people report that, after receiving acupuncture for what ails them, they find their other problems have also been resolved.

PAINFUL CONDITIONS THAT RESPOND WELL TO TREATMENT

Although acupuncture is used in China for all kinds of diseases, in the West it is used for treating pain. The World Health Organization lists more than 100 conditions that may benefit from treatment with acupuncture, including gastrointestinal disorders, neurologic disorders, sciatica, and various rheumatoid and osteoarthritis conditions.

Almost all of the painful conditions addressed in this book can be helped by acupuncture. (*See* Quick Help Chart for synopsis of suggested treatments for all conditions covered in this book.)

ADVANTAGES OF ACUPUNCTURE AND ACUPRESSURE

- ❑ They are non-toxic methods of healing the body.
- ❑ While treating for pain, other conditions often improve.
- ❑ They can eliminate or reduce your dependence on pain medications.

HOW ACUPUNCTURE AND ACUPRESSURE ARE USED

Acupuncture is not a self-help treatment since it involves the insertion of needles into specific body points, but since acupressure is applied to acupuncture points with the fingertips, it *is* a technique you can learn and use on yourself. You can use your fingertip or the eraser end (not the point) of a pencil. Here are a few quick fixes you might want to try.

Back Pain

Press the central area between your nose and upper lip. Maintain deep pressure for several seconds and then release. Repeat from five to ten times.

Apply pressure between your inside ankle bone and Achilles tendon for several seconds. Then release. Repeat five to ten times.

Headaches

Apply pressure to the center of the webbing in your hand, between your thumb and index finger. Maintain pressure for at least two minutes while taking slow deep breaths. Then repeat this on your other hand.

Leg or Foot Cramps

Pinch your upper lip for a minute or two. This is especially useful if your foot cramps while swimming or snorkeling with fins.

Neck or Shoulder Tightness

Pinch the skin above each eyebrow in three places, the middle, the left end, and the right end of the brow.

ACUPUNCTURE RESOLVES ORIGINAL PROBLEM TWO YEARS LATER

Alice M, a seventy-year-old woman, went to see acupuncturist Jacques Depardieu at the center in Darien, CT because she had been in great pain with unexplained nausea for the previous two years. In her attempt to relieve this problem, she had gone to a highly regarded clinic attached to a top university where she had been given anti-convulsant medicine, an anti-emetic, and a G.I. stimulant. The side effects from one of the medications had given her Parkinson-like symptoms, which stayed with her even after the pills were stopped, becoming an ongoing addition to her original problem. She was subjected to MRI's and CAT Scans, and they even removed her gallbladder, only to discover, oops, that was not the problem. Her nausea, meantime, was unrelieved, and Alice went into a deep downward spiral, eventually ending up with Depardieu. He diagnosed her in TCM terms as having "live invading stomach," and in just one acupuncture treatment (after two years of misery), he was able to relieve 90 percent of her cascading problems. Two months and six treatments later, the nausea, all her painful stomach problems, and all the side effects of the medications, including the Parkinson's symptoms—clenched jaw and shoulders, deviated (twisted) tongue, and tremors—were a thing of the past. Although no one could ever give Alice back her gallbladder, she was fine on her last visit to the center a year ago, and fine, too, on the most recent sighting of her—in a restaurant where she was eating away and fully enjoying herself, her painful years behind her.

Animal Injuries

If your pet has been injured and is in shock, press its upper lip just below the nose for several seconds at a time. This can be a lifesaving maneuver while on your way to emergency veterinary care.

CAUTIONS

Acupuncture has its strengths and weaknesses, just as Western medicine does, but it is safe and effective when it is performed by a practitioner who is properly trained and licensed. Your acupuncture practitioner should be aware of his or her limitations, and if you have an acute or life-threatening condition, you should seek treatment by Western medical doctors.

An accurate diagnosis is also essential. Marshall H. Sager, DO, Diplomat American Board of Medical Acupuncturists (DABMA), Fellow of American Academy of Medical Acupuncturists (FAAMA), and President of the American Academy of Medical Acupuncture, tells of a patient who came to him complaining of fatigue and a lack of energy. After treating him twice with acupuncture, Dr. Sager saw some improvement, but said, "I was not happy with his response and I sent him for more testing." It turned out the man had leukemia, but fortunately it was caught early enough that he was able to have a positive response to treatment (early detection is crucial in cases like these).

CLINICAL STUDIES

Doctors trained in orthodox Western medicine have a difficult time accepting acupuncture because it has not been subjected to what they consider scientific studies. Practitioners of TCM think it is non-productive to waste time and money trying to convince Western doctors of something that has been successfully used for thousands of years. Some skeptical Western doctors believe that acupuncture works best in suggestible individuals who would likely have similar results with hypnosis, or they merely chalk it up to a distraction factor. Those who believe in acupuncture point to the fact that animals respond well to acupuncture and animals are not suggestible.

The following figures are based on the clinical experience of acupuncture practitioners.

Most acupuncturists believe about 70 percent of people with painful musculoskeletal conditions do get significant relief from acupuncture treatments.

About 65 to 95 percent of people with headaches are helped. The headaches either disappear completely or occur with markedly less frequency and intensity.

Up to 70 percent, more than two-thirds, of those with trigeminal neuralgia gain some improvement with acupuncture.

About 40 percent of those with post-herpetic neuralgia can be helped. It is interesting to note that this condition is rare in China because they treat all cases of shingles with acupuncture before the neuralgia develops.

The following recent studies are three among thousands that have shown the efficacy of acupuncture for pain relief.

Carlsson, CP, Sjolund, BH. "Acupuncture for chronic low back pain: a randomized placebo-controlled study with long-term follow-up." *Clinical Journal of Pain.* December 2001; 17(4):296–305.

The authors of this six-month Swedish study of thirty-six people concluded that there was a long-term pain-relieving effect of needle acupuncture compared with true placebo in people with chronic low back pain.

Molsberger, A, Hille, E. "The analgesic effect of acupuncture in chronic tennis elbow." *British Journal of Rheumatology.* December 1994; 33(12):1162–1165.

The results of this single-blind, placebo-controlled German study of forty-eight people showed that true acupuncture following Chinese acupuncture rules has an intrinsic pain-relieving effect in the treatment of tennis elbow which exceeds that of placebo acupuncture (no penetration of the skin with the needle).

Sun, KO, Chan, KC, Lo, SL, et al. "Acupuncture for frozen shoulder." *Hong Kong Medical Journal.* December 2001; 7(4):381–391.

This randomized, controlled trial of thirty-five people showed that the combination of acupuncture and shoulder exercise was a more effective treatment for frozen shoulder than exercise alone.

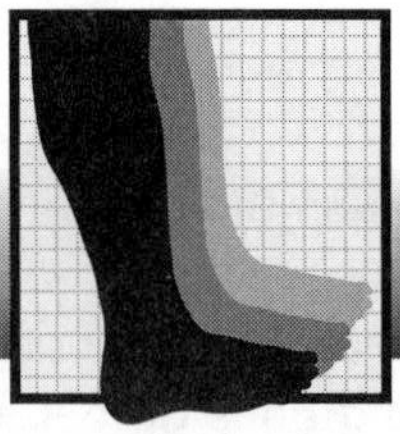

Applied Kinesiology

Applied kinesiology (AK) is a diagnostic system that involves the use of manual muscle testing to detect structural, electromagnetic, and biochemical imbalances in the body. It is a whole-body approach which recognizes that, in order to be healthy, there has to be balance between all the body's different parts. According to Dr. Robert Porzio, DC, a Board Certified Diplomate of the International Board of Applied Kinesiology, "the thing that differentiates applied kinesiology from almost anything else in the natural healthcare arena is that we have the means of evaluating the treatment of a weak muscle immediately in terms of observing any changes relative to the normal strength of a muscle. The ongoing research shows that a muscle can be strengthened or weakened, and can, therefore, be stimulated to improve its functioning."

His colleague, Dr. Avery H. Ferentz, also a Board Certified Diplomate, said, "Applied kinesiology has proven to me that it is a very efficient, predictable set of techniques. One technique is 'therapy localization' which first pinpoints where the pain is, then directs where the therapy is to be applied for relief of the pain, not necessarily the same place. This reliable diagnostic method leads to a whole array of different, effective therapeutic measures that can correct the imbalance and relieve the pain or discomfort. And, by correcting that imbalance and restoring the muscles to their normal state, many times we find that the misalignments end up correcting themselves."

Although usually practiced by chiropractors in the United States, applied kinesiology uses muscles instead of joints to monitor a change in the nervous system. In comparing AK to traditional chiropractic care which uses an examination with the hands, or x-rays, and then manipulates joints in a short dynamic thrust, both doctors quoted here said that the AK methods of detecting imbalances are an addition to chiropractic and are, therefore, more accurate, more efficient, and more inclusive.

Once the AK muscle testing has isolated the problem, the therapeutic approach then overlaps with many other healthcare systems, allowing the corrections to take many forms: osteopathic and chiropractic manipulations, subtle craniosacral therapy, heavy-handed rolfing, acupressure, exercise, homeopathic remedies, nutritional therapy, and a few manipulative procedures that are currently unique to applied kinesiology. Chronic pain requiring longer care can also include lifestyle modifications. Whichever methods are used, however, all are intended to restore balance and maintain well-being throughout life.

Seventy-five percent of AK patients arrive seeking relief from some kind of joint pain, usually in the back or neck. On average, you need between four and fifteen visits to alleviate the problem, and probably more if the problem is chronic.

According to Dr. Ferentz, applied kinesiology is an excellent method for achieving *rapid pain reduction.* In fact, one recurring problem in his over twenty years in practice was with the many patients whose pain went away so fast they forgot how significant their injury was. "They may have been bedridden or disabled for two weeks," he said, "but when they come in for treatment and get eighty percent better in twenty minutes or half an hour, they say, 'Oh, it couldn't have been too bad in the first place, look how fast it feels better,' and then become active again much too soon, promptly reinjuring themselves, of course."

Applied kinesiology has been used since 1964 on many world class and professional athletes worldwide, including marathon winner Greta Weitz, baseball's star pitcher, Tom Seaver, top triathlete Mark Allen, and race-car driver, Michael Andretti.

THE HISTORY OF APPLIED KINESIOLOGY

Practicing as a chiropractor in the 1960s, Dr. George J. Goodheart made the discovery that specific muscle functions are related to certain body systems and can be used to diagnose a wide range of disorders. He observed that postural distortion is usually associated with muscles that test weak and found that applying the appropriate therapy would make the muscle test strong and would change the postural distortion.

In 1964, Dr. John Thie met Dr. Goodheart and learned from him that the body's muscle functioning and strength could change just by the simple act of rubbing reflex points on the body. Amazed by this technique, he promptly spread the word among his colleagues, and in 1976 he and a group of like-minded doctors founded the *International College of Applied Kinesiology* (ICAK), which now certifies health professionals to become licensed AK practitioners. Dr. Thie became its first chairman and Dr. Goodheart became the first research chairman, a position he still holds. Dr. Goodheart was also a member of the United States Olympic Sports Medicine Committee at the 1980 winter games in Lake Placid New York, the first non-medical practitioner to hold such a position.

Today, applied kinesiology is used by approximately 37 percent (18,600) of the chiropractic profession in the

United States. In many countries throughout the world, there are thousands of doctors practicing AK and they come from all professions—dentistry, medicine, osteopathy, and podiatry, just to name a few. In addition to its many chapters in the United States, ICAK has chapters in Australasia, Canada, and Europe, with hundreds of seminars being taught by certified teachers, and new chapters being added each year.

HOW APPLIED KINESIOLOGY WORKS

Dr. Goodheart developed a now universally accepted equilateral triangle as a logo for applied kinesiology: the base represents structure which consists of the body's physical parts and their various relationships; one of its sides represents chemistry which includes nutrition and the effects of drugs and other substances; and the other side is mental, including emotions, moods, and attitudes. For optimum health, you need to have a balance between all three of these equally important sides. Using the manual muscle test, it is found that, for some, an emotional issue is causing the muscle to be out of balance, and for others it's a biochemical or structural issue, but for most people it's a little bit of all three. So, by monitoring the body's response to different stimuli and using a muscle test to measure that response, the doctor is able to discern where the imbalance is and what the appropriate therapy may be.

Manual muscle testing is both a science and an art and the examiner must be trained in the anatomy, physiology, and neurology of muscle function in order to be an effective therapist. AK practitioners are constantly subjecting their patients to different stimuli—touch, pressure, rubbing, etc.—and then seeing how each affects the muscle test. The general rule is that the body should react to stimuli by being strong all the time. Everything should be efficient and the muscles should be strong, so if the doctor takes your joint and pushes it and that triggers a muscle weakness, then he or she knows something is wrong with the joint that was pushed. If the muscle that is touched does *not* get weak, then the doctor knows that's not the problem area, and doing this routinely is how the exact spot of weakness is ferreted out.

Similarly, if you touch the joint in your own body that is misaligned, that will cause the corresponding muscle to weaken. The key thing is that, if the pain is due to tissue irritation that is secondary to a muscular imbalance, AK provides a mechanism for detecting the muscle imbalance. And, once detected, there are a variety of therapeutic measures that could potentially be brought in to correct your muscular imbalance.

The unique contribution of AK is that it is a hands-on diagnostic method that uses your own muscles and nerves to determine an over, under, or normally stimulated muscular function. Using manual muscle testing as a tool, the practitioner is able to evaluate a whole host of therapies to see which ones make the difference, and start the healing process for you.

PAINFUL CONDITIONS THAT RESPOND WELL TO APPLIED KINESIOLOGY

- ❑ Achilles tendonitis.
- ❑ Back pain, including herniated discs, neck pain.
- ❑ Bursitis.
- ❑ Carpal tunnel syndrome.
- ❑ Cluster headaches.
- ❑ Crohn's disease.
- ❑ Dental pain.
- ❑ Diverticulitis.
- ❑ Endometriosis
- ❑ Frozen shoulder.
- ❑ Irritable bowel syndrome.
- ❑ Migraine headaches.
- ❑ Osteoarthritis.
- ❑ Pelvic floor tension myalgia.
- ❑ Peripheral neuropathy.
- ❑ Post-polio syndrome.
- ❑ Premenstrual syndrome.
- ❑ Reflex sympathetic dystrophy syndrome (RSDS).
- ❑ Rheumatoid arthritis.
- ❑ Rotator cuff tendonitis.
- ❑ Sciatica.
- ❑ Tarsal tunnel syndrome.
- ❑ Temporomandibular joint (TMJ) syndrome.
- ❑ Tennis elbow.
- ❑ Tension headaches.
- ❑ Trigeminal neuralgia.
- ❑ Trigger finger.
- ❑ Ulcerative colitis.

In addition to these painful conditions, applied kinesiology is also effective with allergies, anxiety and stress, dyslexia and related learning disabilities, general malaise, postmenopausal hormonal imbalances in women, and tinnitus.

ADVANTAGES OF APPLIED KINESIOLOGY

- ❑ It is non-invasive and non-toxic.
- ❑ It is an umbrella diagnostic tool for detecting muscle imbalance that causes pain.
- ❑ It has proven to be a very efficient, reliable set of techniques for pain relief, chronic and acute.
- ❑ It is an excellent method for achieving *rapid pain reduction.*
- ❑ It is a full-body, full-psychology, full-biochemistry approach that helps restore balance between all the different parts of the body.
- ❑ It helps the body reach a threshold where it is healthier than it is sick; it allows the body to balance itself and proceed in its natural tendency toward optimum good health.
- ❑ It alone, among the other natural healing approaches, is able to deal effectively with vague, general malaise.
- ❑ It can detect a problem before it manifests obvious symptoms, thereby allowing preventive therapeutic measures to ward off the problem before it becomes acute.
- ❑ It can help to strengthen muscles weakened by aging or misaligned joints.
- ❑ It can reduce dependence on pain medication.

HOW APPLIED KINESIOLOGY IS USED

If you come in with pain, the doctor might first do a postural examination that involves looking at your body's symmetries. Is one shoulder higher than another? One arm rotated more, one hip higher? These are all clues as to what might be out of balance. After that, the doctor could feel for little nodules that develop along the temporosphenoidal line on the side of your head. These help to guide her or him in determining which acupuncture and muscle circuits are out of balance.

Muscle testing then helps to pinpoint the exact location of your problem. The doctor might ask you to raise your right arm above your head and tell you to resist while downward pressure is applied to it. The doctor may then bend your arms or legs at different angles, again asking you to resist as he/she applies counterpressure. Your ability to withstand, or not, these and similar tests is what provides the clues that help zero in on your body's trouble spots.

Testing the muscles is only part of the story, however, because the most important part of any pain treatment is to correctly diagnose the cause. Muscle testing is not intended to stand on its own for this, but rather to act as part of a full diagnostic workup which involves laboratory testing, x-rays if needed, orthopedic tests, and neurologic tests, with everything corroborating. AK practitioners can do all your tests themselves, one-stop-shopping style, or they can gather your additional diagnostic information from other sources.

Along with several other pain-reducing modalities in this book, AK is not technically a self-help treatment, but if you have tried established medical procedures and treatments and have yet to find relief, it is perhaps time to consider applied kinesiology.

CAUTIONS

As with any doctor, it is important to check the credentials of the therapist using the applied kinesiology techniques to make sure that this person has valid training. Look for a board-certified practitioner with a broad diagnostic scope that enables her or him to apply any one of a number of different therapies to your problem and and see what makes a difference.

(*See also* ACUPUNCTURE and ACUPRESSURE, CHIROPRACTIC, CRANIOSACRAL THERAPY, and ROLFING in PART 2 Treatment Section.)

CLINICAL STUDIES

Since the organization of ICAK, there have been over 2,000 clinical research papers published by, and for, its membership. In addition, clinicians in the fields of biochemistry, dentistry, neurology, nutrition, and psychology, among other component aspects of the AK approach, have also conducted electrophysiological research relating to applied kinesiology because AK practitioners integrate a variety of assessment and therapeutic methods into their comprehensive system of healing.

The following three studies are among the many that directly support applied kinesiology methods.

Leisman, G, Shambaugh, P, Ferentz, A. "Somatosensory evoked potential changes during muscle testing procedures." *The International Journal of Neuroscience.* 1989; 45:143–151.

This study shows that changes take place in the brain during muscle testing.

Leisman, G, et al. "Electromyographic effects of fatigue and task repetition on the validity of estimates of strong and weak muscles in applied kinesiology muscle testing procedures." *Perceptual and Motor Skills.* 1995; 80:963–977.

This paper describes the results of six studies which all demonstrated that weak and strong muscles are in fundamentally different states, that weak muscles differ from fatigued muscles, that AK muscle-testing procedures can be objectively evaluated, and that the cause and effect of AK treatment can be plotted over time.

Perot, C, Meldener, R, Gouble, F. "Objective measurement of proprioceptive technique consequences on muscular maximal voluntary contraction during manual muscle testing." *Aggressologie.* 1991; 32(10):471–474.

This French study established that there was a significant difference in electrical activity in the muscles that corresponded with the perceived strong-versus-weak outcomes in tests perfomed by AK practitioners.

There are additional ongoing studies at universities, clinics, and the nonprofit *Foundation of Allied Conservative Therapies Research* founded by ICAK to promote quality research in applied kinesiology.

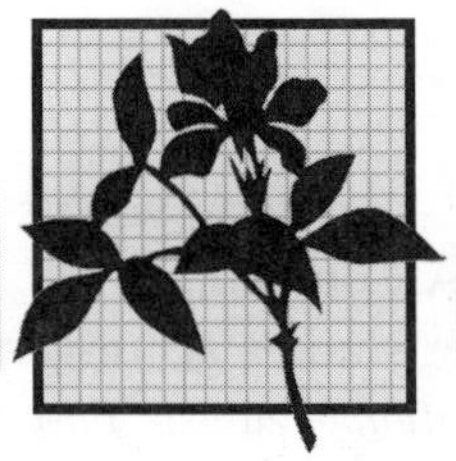

Aromatherapy

Aromatherapy is the use of essential oils from plants to treat a wide variety of conditions. It may be considered a subspecialty of herbal therapy. The essential oils used in aromatherapy are condensed from those parts of the plant that give them their fragrance, protect them from predators, and attract insects for pollination. These essential oils carry the plant's vital energy which, in turn, raises the vital energy of the person who uses them. They help balance the body's functioning and alleviate some medical conditions. Essential oils can stimulate the immune system to develop natural antibodies.

There are three main ways that essential oils are used:

- ❑ Direct inhalation;
- ❑ Steam inhalation;
- ❑ Application to the skin for absorption.

THE HISTORY OF AROMATHERAPY

Aromatherapy is based on one of the ancient medical systems that, along with other alternative/complementary therapies, represent a return to nature. Although seen by some as a new-age modality, it was widely used in Ancient Egypt and Greece, and is a much older form of treatment than Western orthodox medicine.

Its first use in the West came about seventy-five years ago when a French fragrance chemist, René-Maurice Gattefosse, burned his arm at work and immediately plunged it into the closest thing at hand, a container of lavender oil. To his surprise, his pain eased immediately, his burn healed quickly, and he had no scarring. Gattefosse attributed all these positive results to lavender oil's antiseptic and anti-inflammatory properties, as well as its potent scent. He was so deeply impressed by his experience that he spent the rest of his life studying essential oils, while continuing his career as a perfume maker.

By the 1970s, the use of aromatherapy had grown widely in Europe and Japan. In France, medical students are now taught how to prescribe essential oils, and prescriptions for aromatherapy are covered by insurance there and in many other European countries.

The use of essential oils suffered a setback about fifty years ago when antibiotics and other "wonder drugs" first arrived on the scene. Essential oils, as well as herbs, came to be viewed as archaic and outmoded and were even banned in some places. Now the scientific world is changing its stance on natural remedies and is beating a path back to them since synthetic drugs have been shown to have so many harmful side effects.

HOW AROMATHERAPY WORKS

Aromatherapy works in two ways, by inhalation and by absorption.

Inhalation

With inhalation, the essential oils release a gaseous vapor into the air, and when you inhale that vapor your bloodstream absorbs it through your lungs and your olfactory nerve, which is connected to your sense of smell.

Aromatherapy treats your mind and body together. The oil has a chemical effect on your body while the scent affects your emotions. Your sense of smell is one of your most acute senses. When odor molecules strike nerves in your nasal passages, they are transformed into nerve impulses. These impulses travel to the olfactory (smell) bulbs in your brain, which are connected to the limbic system (primitive brain), the portion that controls memory and emotion. Information is then passed on to the hypothalamus which controls the pituitary gland, and which then releases hormones that are essential for most basic body functions.

Some essential oils are known as adaptogens because they have a regulating effect. Lavender, for example, can act as a sedative or a stimulant, depending on what your body needs at the time.

Absorption

If you use essential oils in your bath, or add them to massage oils, they are absorbed through your skin into your bloodstream and are carried to your joints, muscles, organs, and tissues. This is similar to the nicotine or nitroglycerin patches that are used to deliver medicines to the body. When you have an essential oil massage, there is a synergistic effect on your body due to the interaction of touch and smell.

PAINFUL CONDITIONS THAT RESPOND WELL TO AROMATHERAPY

- ❑ Achilles tendonitis.
- ❑ Back pain.
- ❑ Bursitis.
- ❑ Cluster headaches.

- ❑ Crohn's disease.
- ❑ Dental pain.
- ❑ Diverticulitis.
- ❑ Endometriosis.
- ❑ Fibromyalgia.
- ❑ Gout.
- ❑ Irritable bowel syndrome.
- ❑ Migraine headaches.
- ❑ Neuroma.
- ❑ Osteoarthritis.
- ❑ Pelvic floor tension myalgia.
- ❑ Peripheral neuropathy.
- ❑ Postherpetic neuralgia.
- ❑ Post-polio syndrome.
- ❑ Premenstrual syndrome
- ❑ Reflex sympathetic dystrophy syndrome (RSDS).
- ❑ Rheumatoid arthritis.
- ❑ Rotator cuff tendonitis.
- ❑ Sciatica.
- ❑ Temporomandibular joint (TMJ) pain.
- ❑ Tennis elbow.
- ❑ Tension headaches.
- ❑ Trigeminal neuralgia.
- ❑ Trigger finger.
- ❑ Ulcerative colitis.

ADVANTAGES OF AROMATHERAPY

Aromatherapy is a holistic approach to health. In an aromatherapy massage, the oils produce both physiological and psychological benefits. Some of those using aromatherapy report they can decrease the amount of anti-inflammatory drugs they had been taking.

HOW TO USE ESSENTIAL OILS

Absorption Method—Baths

Put three to six drops of the selected essential oil in a tub half full of comfortably hot water. Soak in the treated bath for at least fifteen minutes.

Absorption Method—Compresses

Use two to four drops of oil for each cup of warm water. Soak a clean cloth in the water and place it over the affected part. Cover the compress with a towel or bandage and leave it on for half an hour.

Absorption Method—Massages

Add two to four drops of essential oils to two teaspoons of a carrier oil, such as sweet almond or apricot kernel oil. Whatever carrier oil you choose, be sure it is unrefined and cold-pressed. Store it in a lightproof container in the refrigerator. Other carrier oils you can use include avocado, canola, hazelnut, and olive oil. After you dilute the essential oil with one of these carrier oils, place a small amount in your palm, rub your hands together to warm it, and then massage it over the area you want to treat. The best time for an aromatherapy massage would be after a bath or shower, but if you do apply the oil beforehand, wait at least two hours to take a bath or shower in order to give the oil a chance to soak in.

Inhalation Methods

Put five drops of oil into a saucer of warm water and place it on a radiator. The aroma of the warmed oil will radiate out into the room.

Put two drops of oil onto a tissue and seal it in a plastic bag to be opened and inhaled when needed.

Put five to ten drops of oil into a basin of hot water, cover your head with a towel, and inhale.

CAUTIONS

- ❑ Do not use essential oils full strength because they are highly concentrated and can cause irritation. Diluting them in a carrier oil does not alter their therapeutic effects.
- ❑ Use essential oils only in their pure form. A synthetic

ESSENTIAL OILS REDUCE NSAID INTAKE

Geraldine DePaula, MD is the founder of a company that makes blends of essential oils for specific purposes. Dr. DePaula tells of a woman she treated, who had acute arthritis in the knees. The amount of NSAIDs this woman was taking to control her pain and inflammation caused her to have severe stomach problems. And then, in an all-too-familiar case of one medication necessitating another, she was prescribed medication for the stomach problems, and that made her dizzy and lightheaded. But two weeks after using a blend of Dr. DePaula's essential oils for arthritis, the woman was able to cut her dose of NSAIDs in half, and she was able to be more active, which was beneficial to the health of her cartilage because it is a living tissue that gets its nourishment during movement of the joints.

fragrance may smell the same, but it does not have the same therapeutic effect.

- ❑ Since essential oils are quite powerful, even diluted in a carrier oil, it is a good idea to test them on a small area before applying them.
- ❑ Two essential oils *can* be used full strength. Lavender oil, which helps your skin heal, can be applied directly to burns, cuts, insect bites, and rashes. And tea tree oil, which has anti-infectious, anti-inflammatory, antiseptic, antiviral, and antifungal properties, is a remarkably useful oil. It has been referred to as a first-aid kit in a bottle.
- ❑ Avoid using essential oils that are derived from plants to which you are allergic.
- ❑ Keep essential oils away from your eyes.
- ❑ Do not use sweet fennel oil if you have epilepsy.
- ❑ If you have high blood pressure, do not use rosemary oil, sage oil, or thyme oil.
- ❑ Do not use clary sage oil for several hours before or after consuming alcohol because it can cause nausea and can exaggerate the effects of the alcohol.

CLINICAL STUDIES

Although aromatherapy has been used worldwide to help reduce pain and stress, and positive results have been noted, double-blind studies have not been performed because smell and touch cannot be hidden from those participating in studies.

Bee Venom Therapy

Bee venom therapy, also referred to as Apitherapy or BVT, involves the use of a superior type of live honeybee, apis mellifera, or injections of bee venom into painful areas, such as the spine, joints, or extremities. The therapists are either beekeepers who work from their homes and use live honeybees to sting their clients, or doctors who give injections of bee venom in their offices. People who have been helped by the treatment tell stories of dramatic relief from their arthritis pain, or the enormous improvement they see in their MS symptoms. Although most conventional practitioners do not trust the therapy, some are beginning to use it.

THE HISTORY OF BEE VENOM THERAPY

Bee venom has been used for over 2,000 years to treat inflammation in both the East and the West. It is believed that, in ancient China, stings were the first acupuncture needles, and bee venom is mentioned in the Koran and the Bible. Hippocrates, the fifth century BC Greek physician, who is considered "the Father of Medicine," was aware of its anti-inflammatory properties and referred to it as "a strange and mysterious medicine." Galen, the second century AD Roman physician, wrote of bee venom treatment, and Charlemagene (742–814 AD) is said to have had himself treated with bee stings for his stiff joints.

The real progress with apiculture and the scientific study of bees came with the Austrian physician, Philip Terc, who advocated the intentional use of bee stings in his 1888 work, "Report about a Peculiar Connection Between the Beestings and Rheumatism." And in 1928, Dr. Franz Kretschy, another Austrian, developed a subcutaneous injectable venom, which was less painful than the stinging process.

The history of bee venom therapy in the United States dates back over a hundred years and includes Dr. Bodog Beck whose classic 1935 book, *Bee Venom Therapy,* was based on his work in the late 1920s. His student, Charles Mraz, the late beekeeper of Middlebury, Vermont, is credited with popularizing bee venom therapy in the United States. After a severe attack of rheumatic fever, Mraz decided to listen to the old wives' tales about the therapy, and woke up pain-free for the first time in months after using it. From that point on, he considered it reasonable to try bee venom therapy in any situation where nothing else worked, and used bee stings to treat people with arthritis (and later multiple sclerosis) until his death in 1999. Today thousands of medical practitioners and lay professionals use bee venom therapy worldwide.

HOW BEE VENOM THERAPY WORKS

The theory is that bee venom helps to stimulate the immune system. The venom contains at least eighteen active substances, the most prevalent of which, melittin, has bacteriocidal properties and is one of the strongest anti-inflammatory agents known—it is said to be 100 times more powerful than hydrocortisone. After the venom is absorbed by the blood, it stimulates the pituitary gland to release ACTH, a hormone which, in turn, stimulates the adrenals to make cortisol, the body's own natural form of cortisone. It also improves blood circulation and oxygen flow to the affected areas. Part of its action is to cause temporary redness and heat, which helps the healing. In fact, heat, swelling, and itching are all signs that BVT is working effectively. Overall, it can be said that bee venom produces a unique reaction that helps the body to heal itself.

PAINFUL CONDITIONS THAT RESPOND WELL TO BEE VENOM THERAPY

❑ Bursitis.

❑ Endometriosis.

❑ Fibromyalgia.

❑ Migraine headaches.

❑ Osteoarthritis.

AN UNEXPECTED BENEFIT OF BEE VENOM THERAPY

Charles Mraz thought his bee venom treatments had successfully rid a woman of her arthritis, but when her symptoms returned after a five-year hiatus, her doctor told her she didn't have arthritis, she had multiple sclerosis, and probably had for the past ten years. She returned to Mraz to tell him he had accidentally—and successfully—treated her for MS, and from that point on he began also treating people for this degenerative nerve disease, work that has since been carried forward by his students and other licensed health practitioners.

- ❏ Postherpetic neuralgia.
- ❏ Premenstrual syndrome (PMS).
- ❏ Rheumatoid arthritis.
- ❏ Tennis elbow.

Additionally, research by the American Apitherapy Society into the therapy's effectiveness for symptoms of muscle strains and multiple sclerosis and other conditions has been ongoing for several years, and the studies show promise.

Other conditions that have responded favorably to BVT include asthma, facial twinges, infections, and skin conditions.

ADVANTAGES OF BEE VENOM THERAPY

Its anti-inflammatory properties help it to reduce pain, it increases the immune response, and it may lead to increased mental alertness and improved concentration. Many swear that the venom from honeybees can provide pain relief for inflammatory and degenerative diseases within minutes.

HOW BEE VENOM THERAPY IS USED

You may be stung by live honeybees, where the practitioner uses long tweezers to place the bees, one by one, close to the areas that need treatment, or the venom may be injected with a hypodermic needle. When live bees are used, some therapists hold an ice pack over the area to help numb it and reduce the sensitivity before you are stung. The number, sites, and frequency of the stings or injections depend on the person and the condition to be remedied. A simple problem like tendonitis might take only two to three stings/injections a session for two to three sessions, whereas something more complex, like arthritis, might take two to three stings/injections a session, two to three sessions a week, for one to three months. Most practitioners believe it is better to sting or inject directly at the source of the pain, but they sometimes go by acupuncture points.

SHUTTING OUT SHINGLES

Dr. Andrew Kochan has done groundbreaking work on the efficacy of BVT for postherpetic neuralgia, the pain that can persist for four months (or even years, in the worst cases) following the onset of an outbreak of herpes zoster (shingles). His studies have shown that treatment with the European honeybee, apis mellifera, has reduced the pain 70–100 percent in just four treatments.

Regarding costs for BVT, the American Apitherapy Society says that many apitherapists do not charge; they ask for a donation to AAS for treatments. If you go to an acupuncturist, naturopath, or green-medicine (natural plant-and-herb medicine) doctor, they ask their customary fees. Some doctors who specialize in pain, and do not necessarily practice green medicine, also do apitherapy by injection or bee venom (two such doctors are listed in Resources in this entry). M. Simics of Apitronic Services says that most doctors use injections because it is difficult for them to keep bees in their offices. You can find apitherapy practitioners by contacting the American Academy of Neural Therapy or the American Apitherapy Society.

CAUTIONS

Bee venom therapy could be harmful, even fatal, if you have an allergic reaction to bee venom, so if this is the case, you should be very careful and have professional supervision when using this therapy. Fortunately however, many allergies that are attributed to honeybee venom are in fact to yellow jacket or wasp venom. If you ever had a bad reaction to stepping on bees, for example, chances are you were stung by yellow jackets because honeybees do not live on the ground. And since the honeybee venom accounts for only 5 percent of all adverse stinging-insect reactions, and is not closely related to wasp or yellow jacket venom, an allergy to the latter does not necessarily negate your chances of being able to benefit from bee venom therapy. But supervision and careful pretesting are important here.

Additionally, bee venom should not be used on anyone who has diabetes, gonorrhea, heart disease, hypoglycemia, kidney disease, or tuberculosis.

(*See also* ACUPUNCTURE and ACUPRESSURE.)

CLINICAL STUDIES

One difficulty with controlled double-blind studies of bee venom is that it is impossible to create a proper placebo—if you're stung by a bee, you know it. Also, there is no safe substance that provokes a skin reaction similar to that provoked by bee venom. But randomized clinical studies do exist.

Kwon, YB, Kim, JH, Yoon, JH, et al. "The analgesic efficacy of bee venom acupuncture for knee arthritis: a comparative study with needle acupuncture." *American Journal of Chinese Medicine.* 2001; 29(2):187–199.

This four-week, randomized clinical study conducted at the Seoul National University in South Korea compared two groups, one receiving BV acupuncture, the other receiving traditional needle acupuncture. It was observed that more of those receiving bee venom therapy in traditional acupuncture sites reported substantial pain relief than those receiving only traditional needle acupuncture therapy in the same sites.

Kwon, YB, Lee, JD, Lee, HJ. "Bee venom injection into an acupuncture point reduces arthritis associated edema and nociceptive responses." *Pain.* February 15, 2001; 90(3):271–280.

Another South Korean study conducted on animals at the same university found that BV acupuncture may be a promising alternative medicine therapy for the long-term treatment of rheumatoid arthritis.

Won, Choong-Hee, Hong, Seong-Sun, Kim, Christopher. "Efficacy of Apitox (Bee Venom) for Osteoarthritis: A Randomized Active-Controlled Trial." *Journal of the American Apitherapy Society.* 2000; 7(3):11–15; 7(4):10–12; 8(1):11–18.

The International Pain Institute, USA, sponsored this six-week study of 101 participants with knee or lumbosacral osteoarthritis, with follow-up four weeks after the last treatment. There were three groups on different dosage levels of the bee venom, and a control group on an NSAID. The overall efficacy of the bee venom was shown to be greater in the minimum-dose group and significantly greater in the two groups receiving medium and maximum doses of apitox (bee venom) than in the control group given the NSAID.

A Beekeeper's Remedy

More than twenty-five years ago, Charles, a beekeeper in Yarmouth, Maine got tired of taking 100 aspirins a week for his rheumatoid arthritis, so he put his bees to work to help rid him of the painful spasms that would twist him up so severely he wasn't able to run or play with his children, and the stiffness that would cause him to get out of bed in the morning by sliding to the floor. Charles's problems ameliorated soon after he began stinging himself, up to three times a week, depending on the severity of his symptoms, and he has now had decades of pain relief, thanks to his bees. And, since they say beekeepers tend to live longer than the rest of the population, Charles will probably continue to get relief for some time to come.

There is also much anecdotal evidence reported by people who have either arthritis or MS and feel greatly improved after bee sting therapy.

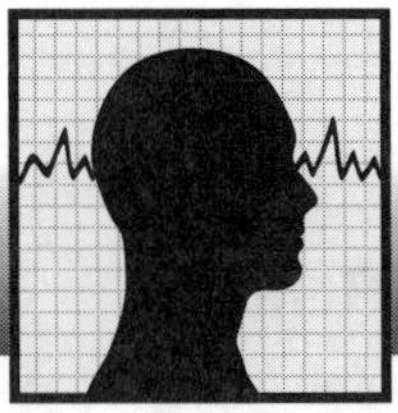

Biofeedback

Biofeedback teaches you how to consciously regulate your involuntary bodily functions, which include blood pressure, brain waves, heart rate, muscle tension, and even your body temperature. These processes are monitored by specialized equipment that feeds back information about your body. For instance, with a biofeedback machine you might see flashing lights or hear a beep whenever your muscles tense. Depending on which body part they are targeting, the machines can vary. They might be blood pressure devices, modified cardiac monitors, electroencephalograph machines (for brain waves), flowmeters (for breathing), motility sensors for gastrointestinal problems, or electrodermal machines for measuring skin temperature. At first the machines help you monitor your responses. When you can see graphically how your body reacts, you can train yourself, with the help of a therapist, to alter the lights or beeps, slowing them down by relaxing your muscles. Eventually you can alter your physiological responses without the machine or the therapist.

THE HISTORY OF BIOFEEDBACK

In the late 1960s, researchers designed laboratory procedures for training research subjects to control their bodies by altering their blood pressure, brain activity, heart rate, temperature, and other body processes that were not voluntarily controlled. While some of their high hopes, for instance doing away with medications, were not met, the research demonstrated for almost the first time that people do have more control over their involuntary functions than was previously thought possible. According to the Association for Applied Psychophysiology and Biofeedback, there are currently about 4,000 biofeedback practitioners in the United States.

HOW BIOFEEDBACK WORKS

Biofeedback works by reducing stress and the physical responses associated with it. When you are under stress, your sympathetic nervous system responds to the strong emotions aroused by producing physical responses. This system is known to prepare you for emergencies, and elicits what is commonly called the fight or flight response. Even though we do not face as many physical threats nowadays, your body reacts to stress as though it were under attack by a wild animal. Your heart pounds, your blood pressure rises, and the blood vessels under your skin contract to help control bleeding. At the same time, the blood vessels in your brain and muscles dilate to increase their oxygen supply, and your digestive system slows down. If these programmed responses occur too frequently and remain overactive, they can eventually cause damage to your body's tissues. This is where biofeedback comes in. If you learn this skill and practice it, biofeedback can help you change how you react to stress.

PAINFUL CONDITIONS THAT RESPOND WELL TO BIOFEEDBACK

Studies have shown that biofeedback techniques can be used to treat many conditions, including any conditions aggravated by stress.

- ❑ Angina.
- ❑ Back pain (spinal injuries).
- ❑ Cluster headaches.
- ❑ Diverticulitis.
- ❑ Endometriosis.
- ❑ Fibromyalgia.
- ❑ Irritable bowel syndrome.
- ❑ Migraine headaches.
- ❑ Pelvic floor tension myalgia
- ❑ Phantom pain.
- ❑ Postherpetic neuralgia.
- ❑ Premenstrual syndrome.
- ❑ Reflex sympathetic dystrophy syndrome (RSDS).
- ❑ Temporomandibular joint (TMJ) pain.
- ❑ Tension headaches.
- ❑ Ulcerative colitis.

In addition to its use for painful conditions addressed in this book, biofeedback is also being used to help control an abnormal heartbeat, alcoholism, asthma, drug addiction, epilepsy, high blood pressure, movement disorders, Raynaud's disease (a circulatory problem that causes abnormally cold extremities), and Tourette's syndrome.

ADVANTAGES OF BIOFEEDBACK

These procedures are safe, effective, and non-invasive. By examining your daily life, you can learn to change particular behaviors that add to stress, and it is a well-known fact that lowered stress is crucial to good health. Some who practice biofeedback are able to cut down on, or eventually stop taking medication. People who are partially paralyzed due to strokes have been known to regain the use of their limbs through biofeedback techniques. The monitor shows them there is some activity in the affected area and they can see the changes that occur when they perform their therapy.

Note: Do not reduce or stop any medication without first consulting your healthcare practitioner.

HOW BIOFEEDBACK IS USED

Psychologists are the primary health professionals to train you in the use of biofeedback, but the list also includes dentists, nurses, physical therapists, and physicians. Your therapist attaches sensors to your body to monitor your physiological responses—an electrode placed on your chest will measure your heart rate, or an electrode on your head will measure your brainwave activity. You watch a computer screen to check the readings. If your heart rate is rapid, your therapist teaches you special techniques, such as deep breathing or visualization, to slow down the readings. You check the screen to see how well you are doing, and eventually you can alter your responses without the machine. It does take practice, however, and you must commit yourself to practice the techniques taught to you.

The cost of treatment varies from $70 to $200 a session, depending on whom you see. A psychologist will likely charge more than a clinician in an educational facility. You will probably need from ten to thirty sessions until you are able to control your responses without the specialized equipment, but you should begin to see improvement after ten sessions. You can find a practitioner by contacting your state biofeedback society or the psychology department at a university.

CAUTIONS

Be sure your therapist is qualified and has been trained to use biofeedback, and be aware that reputable practitioners will not treat you until you have had a thorough physical examination to rule out any conditions that could require conventional medical treatment. Also, be aware that, while biofeedback may help, it is not a substitute for conventional treatment for such serious conditions as diabetes, heart disease, or high blood pressure. It is not recommended for fractures or slipped discs, and if you have a pacemaker, tell your therapist and check with your doctor before using biofeedback.

Except for the possibility of a minor skin irritation in the area where the electrodes are attached, there are no side effects.

CLINICAL STUDIES

The National Institutes of Health has endorsed biofeedback for helping to alleviate insomnia and tension headaches, and a number of studies have been done to date.

Brucker, BS, Bulaeva, NV. "Biofeedback effect on electromyography responses in patients with spinal cord injury. *Archives of Physical Medicine and Rehabilitation*. February 1996; 77(2):133–137.

This study of one hundred people showed that biofeedback was able to increase voluntary electromyography (EMG) responses in people who had cervical spinal cord injuries of more than one year. All participants had less than normal strength and recordable EMG activity from the triceps, and had reached a plateau in return of function, but after only one biofeedback treatment session, there was a significant increase in muscle strength. Further significant increases occurred in subsequent treatments.

Nadler, RB. "Bladder training biofeedback and pelvic floor myalgia." *Urology*. December 2002; 60(6 Suppl): 42–43; discussion 44.

This study at Northwestern University Medical School in Chicago used biofeedback and pelvic floor re-education in the treatment of chronic pelvic pain syndrome (CPPS) instead of the traditionally administered drugs. Pelvic floor tension myalgia is considered a contributing factor in CPPS, and a preliminary study showed that eight out of eleven people had an improvement in their level of pain with biofeedback, leading to a recommendation for further evaluation of this method for pain relief.

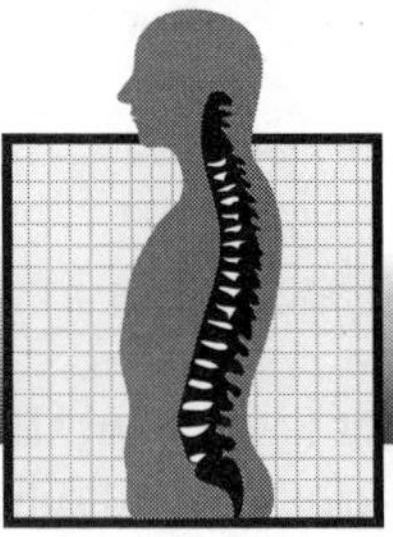

Chiropractic

Chiropractic is a means of treating physical problems including, but not limited to, back and neck pain, and headaches. Chiropractors manually manipulate (adjust) vertebrae that have become misaligned, because they believe that any misalignment of bones, particularly in the spine, is the basis for a wide variety of ailments, and that when the spinal column is readjusted to restore the normal relationship of one vertebra to another, the energy blocks in the body are eliminated. Chiropractic is believed by many to be the treatment of choice for a variety of lower back problems, and chiropractors are, in fact, the second largest group (after MDs) of primary-care health providers in the United States—a 1998 study in JAMA (*Journal of the American Medical Association*) reported that chiropractors treated more than 11 million adults a year.

Although the more than 60,000 chiropractors in practice concentrate mainly on neurological and musculoskeletal diagnosis and treatment, many people often find that a variety of other conditions also respond to chiropractic care.

Before students are accepted at chiropractic school, they are required have a minimum of two years in college. Training at a chiropractic school consists of courses in anatomy, physiology, neurology, and x-ray interpretation. Before they can practice, graduates have to pass four national board examinations and a state chiropractic board examination. Chiropractors are trained to recognize when spinal manipulation is contraindicated, and most of them work in cooperation with other healthcare practitioners.

THE HISTORY OF CHIROPRACTIC

Spinal manipulation has been performed since ancient times. As early as 2700 BC, civilizations in Babylonia, China, and Tibet used one form or another. In 460 BC, Hippocrates used manipulation to cure a wide variety of ailments, and in the second century AD, Galen, a Roman physician who had been born in Greece, used spinal manipulation. One of his success stories was manipulating the seventh cervical (neck) vertebra to resolve a patient's hand weakness and numbness. From the dark ages to the beginning of modern times, manipulative therapy techniques were passed from generation to generation and became well-known in folk medicine.

Daniel David Palmer, a self-educated healer who referred to himself as "old dad chiro," founded chiropractic on the premise that vertebral subluxations (misalignments in the spine) caused *all* diseases and that chiropractic adjustments could cure them. Palmer believed that when nerves were pinched, the body's health was impaired. He developed the theory of chiropractic, which suggested that when spinal bones were misplaced, they impinged on nerves and caused disease.

Since conventional medicine in the United States uses drugs as the primary healing modality, the medical profession regarded chiropractic as an economic competitor because of its premise to heal without drugs. They staged continuing assaults on chiropractors, arranging for many to be sent to jail for practicing medicine without a license. In 1906, Dr. Palmer was among those so charged; he spent twenty-three days in jail and also paid a $350 fine.

In 1976, five chiropractors set out to right the wrongs done to their profession for too many years by filing an anti-trust suit against the American Medical Association. They lost their suit, but later won it on appeal, and in 1991 the Supreme Court affirmed the ruling of Appeals Court Judge, Susan Getchendanner, which declared that the American Medical Association et al. was guilty of anti-trust violations that were part of an ongoing conspiracy to "contain and eliminate" the chiropractic profession.

HOW CHIROPRACTIC WORKS

The theory of chiropractic is that when the bones of the spine are improperly positioned, they pinch nerves. These misalignments in the spine, referred to as subluxations, can lead to pressure, causing symptoms in the back and other parts of the body. Chiropractic treatment attempts to realign the vertebrae in order for the nervous system to function properly when the joints are adjusted and the subluxations removed. Larry S. Segal, DC, a practitioner in Philadelphia, PA, says that, "The chiropractor's primary goal is to fix the joint. Without joint movement, the muscular system will not function adequately. The

REALIGNED SPINE RESTORES HEARING

In 1895, D.D. Palmer restored the hearing of Harvey Lillard, a janitor of his acquaintance who had been deaf for seventeen years, by pushing a vertebra in his spine back into its proper position. This restoration was permanent and Mr. Lillard went to his grave a hearing man.

body will adapt to the decrease in motion, causing the muscle to contract and, in turn, cause chronic pain. Chiropractic can reverse that."

PAINFUL CONDITIONS THAT RESPOND WELL TO CHIROPRACTIC

These are the conditions most commonly treated with chiropractic.

- ❏ Achilles tendonitis.
- ❏ Back pain, including neck pain.
- ❏ Carpal tunnel syndrome.
- ❏ Cluster headaches.
- ❏ Crohn's disease.
- ❏ Dental pain.
- ❏ Diverticulitis.
- ❏ Endometriosis.
- ❏ Frozen shoulder.
- ❏ Irritable bowel syndrome.
- ❏ Migraine headaches.
- ❏ Osteoarthritis.
- ❏ Pelvic floor tension myalgia.
- ❏ Peripheral neuropathy.
- ❏ Phantom pain.
- ❏ Post-polio syndrome.
- ❏ Premenstrual syndrome.
- ❏ Reflex sympathetic dystrophy syndrome (RSDS).
- ❏ Rheumatoid arthritis.
- ❏ Rotator cuff tendonitis.
- ❏ Sciatica.
- ❏ Tarsal tunnel syndrome.
- ❏ Temporomandibular joint (TMJ) pain.
- ❏ Tension headaches.
- ❏ Trigger finger.
- ❏ Ulcerative colitis.

Since the body functions at its optimum level when the nervous system is working properly, chiropractic is useful for all the painful conditions addressed in this book. Additional ailments that respond well to chiropractic include the common cold, high blood pressure, menstrual difficulties, and respiratory and gastrointestinal disorders.

ADVANTAGES OF CHIROPRACTIC

- ❏ Chiropractic can strengthen your immune system.
- ❏ Your general health will benefit because adjusting the spine improves the nerve flow to your organs.
- ❏ When your body functions at its optimum level, it is able to heal itself.

HOW CHIROPRACTIC IS USED

When you first see a chiropractor, she/he will take a detailed case history and perform a chiropractic examination, which includes checking your spine and nervous system, analyzing your posture and, if necessary, ordering x-rays. Then the appropriate spinal adjustments are performed, with direct pressure being applied to your spine and joints. In order to readjust your spinal column, the chiropractor may twist or squeeze your torso, pull or twist your arms or legs, or manipulate your head or back. This readjusts your spinal column, and with the energy blocks eliminated, your vertebrae can have normal relationships to each other.

CAUTIONS

Chiropractors are trained to recognize if a problem is beyond their scope of expertise. Be sure that whomever you see has a working relationship with other conventional practitioners.

CLINICAL STUDIES

Chiropractic has been repeatedly attacked as unscientific because only anecdotal evidence has been presented. This, however, is a hypocritical bias on the part of conventional medicine because, of all the highly touted orthodox medical interventions, only about 15 percent have been validated by rigorous scientific research. The other 85 percent, including that indispensable staple of establishment medicine, aspirin, have not.

Every year, there are more and more studies published in medical and chiropractic journals that expand the range of conditions where chiropractic should be considered the treatment of choice.

Cassidy, JR, Kirkaldy-Willis, WH. *Canadian Family Physician* reported a 1985 Canadian study done by this chiropractor and renowned orthopedic surgeon which showed excellent results following two to three weeks of daily chiropractic adjustments for severe and chronic lower back pain.

Meade, TW, et al. "Low Back Pain of Mechanical Origin: Randomized Comparison of Chiropractic and Hospital Outpatient Treatment." *British Medical Journal* June 1990; 300 (6737):1431–1437.

This British study performed by Dr. Thomas Meade demonstrated long-term chiropractic benefits for his patients with low back pain.

Shekelle, Paul, et al. "The Appropriateness of Spinal Manipulation for Low Back Pain: Indications and Ratings by a Multidisciplinary Expert Panel." Los Angeles, CA: Rand Corporation Study, 1991.

The study at this healthcare think tank recognized spinal manipulation as an appropriate treatment for some patients with low back pain.

Studies in Australia and the Netherlands have also shown that chiropractic manipulation was a benefit to people with back and neck pain.

A study done in Florida showed that, compared to conventional medical care for similar conditions, those receiving chiropractic care had half the amount of disabilities, hospitalizations, and bills.

In another study, spinal manipulation was shown to be more effective than medication for headache relief.

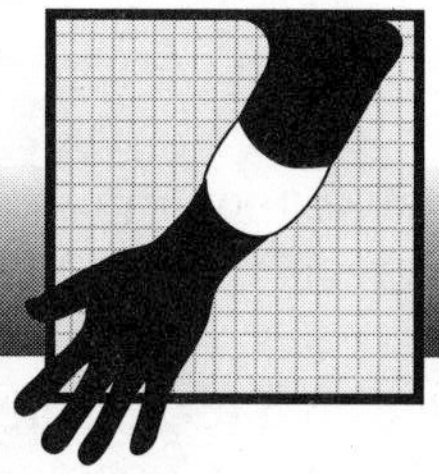

Compresses, Packs, and Poultices

Compresses, packs, and poultices are useful forms of externally applied therapy for reducing pain and inflammation. Although they seem similar, the preparation varies for each.

Compresses are prepared using cotton material (gauze, washcloths, towels) soaked in water or herbal mixtures. Depending on the condition being treated, these compresses may be applied either hot or cold.

Packs are prepared by saturating cloth, usually flannel, with mineral oil or castor oil, or spreading the cloth with a mixture of mustard, flour, and water (the mustard plasters of bygone days).

Poultices are paste-like mixtures that variously consist of herbs, clays, or powders. Dr. Emily Kane, ND, says that, "a poultice is the therapeutic application of a soft moist mass to the skin (usually fresh herbs, sometimes minerals or food pulp) for the purpose of drawing out toxins, encouraging local circulation, and relieving pain," adding that "Traditional Chinese medicine provides many combination herbal poultices for a wide variety of applications."

THE HISTORY OF COMPRESSES, PACKS, AND POULTICES

Before contemporary medicine, and far back in history, these were the treatment of choice for relieving pain and congestion in the body.

HOW COMPRESSES, PACKS, AND POULTICES WORK

Some draw impurities out through the skin, others are absorbed into the tissues, some do both. Warm compresses draw out impurities. They help bring blood to the area, and the oxygen helps nourish the tissues. Cold compresses can reduce swelling. The substance in the packs gets absorbed into tissues (the oil in a castor oil pack, for example, is taken in by the skin).

Dr. Kane says a poultice can work two ways in the body: It can draw waste products (dead white blood cells, nitrogen, saturated oils, viral residues) out through the skin, or it can transfer therapeutic nutrients into the body. Poultices can be particularly useful when, for example, someone is very debilitated and cannot eat or assimilate nutrients. This is because, although the skin is not as absorptive as the mucous membrane of the small intestine, in a pinch it can help transfer herbs and minerals into the bloodstream.

PAINFUL CONDITIONS THAT RESPOND WELL TO THERAPY

- ❑ Achilles tendonitis.
- ❑ Back pain.
- ❑ Bursitis.
- ❑ Carpal tunnel syndrome.
- ❑ Cluster headaches.
- ❑ Crohn's disease.
- ❑ Dental pain.
- ❑ Diverticulitis.
- ❑ Endometriosis.
- ❑ Frozen shoulder.
- ❑ Gout.
- ❑ Irritable bowel syndrome.
- ❑ Migraine headaches.
- ❑ Neuroma.
- ❑ Osteoarthritis.
- ❑ Pelvic floor tension myalgia.
- ❑ Phantom pain.
- ❑ Post-polio syndrome.
- ❑ Premenstrual syndrome.
- ❑ Rheumatoid arthritis.
- ❑ Rotator cuff tendonitis.
- ❑ Sciatica.
- ❑ Tarsal tunnel syndrome.
- ❑ Temporomandibular joint (TMJ).
- ❑ Tennis elbow.
- ❑ Tension headaches.
- ❑ Trigeminal neuralgia.
- ❑ Trigger finger.
- ❑ Ulcerative colitis.

All three types of therapy work well with inflammatory conditions. In addition, they are helpful with abscesses, fevers, injuries and bruises, insomnia, and painful perineum following childbirth (the perineum is the area between the vagina and anus that is either torn, cut, or stretched during childbirth.)

ADVANTAGES OF COMPRESSES, PACKS, AND POULTICES

They stimulate circulation when the blood flow is compromised or the lymphatic system is not adequately draining an area. They also help draw out impurities and are non-invasive.

HOW TO USE COMPRESSES, PACKS, AND POULTICES

Compresses

Soak a cloth or towel in hot water (up to 180° F), cold water, warm herbal tea, or the appropriate aromatherapy oils (diluted). Apply the soaked cloth to the affected area, cover with a towel to retain the heat or the cold and leave in place for twenty to thirty minutes. Use cold compresses for headaches, fever, inflammation, swelling, and new injuries. Hot compresses are useful for congestion, aching muscles, and increasing the circulation.

Packs

Also referred to as plasters, packs are made two ways. One is to saturate a flannel cloth with mineral oil or castor oil, apply it to the affected area, cover it with plastic and a heating pad, and leave in place for an hour at a time. The other way is to make a paste out of *hot* herbs, such as cayenne or mustard mixed with flour and water in approximately a ten to one proportion, and spread it between layers of cloth so the preparation does not come in direct contact with the skin. Mustard packs work wonders for bronchitis, and mustard plasters (applications of mustard through a thin cloth over the lungs, front and back, and covered with heat) were used to break up pneumonia before antibiotics were discovered, says Dr. Kane, who often teaches patients with weak lungs to apply these packs at the first hint of respiratory trouble.

Like compresses and poultices, simple castor oil packs have been used for centuries to produce wonderful results, including relief of pain and reduction of inflammation when applied directly over the affected area and covered in plastic, with a hot water bottle or heating pad placed on top of it. Dr. Kane says that putting castor oil packs over a painful abdominal area can also bring relief from constipation. While a pack is on, usually about twenty to forty-five minutes several times a week, you can meditate, do deep-breathing exercises, or just relax and let your mind wander. The same pack is good for weeks or months; just add one tablespoon of castor oil every four to five uses, and store it in a cool place between uses.

According to Cathy Rogers, ND, mud (peat) baths are also used extensively. Dr. Kane adds that the mud can be ordinary garden variety in a pinch, but that other types are considered more therapeutic. Usually applied in baths or compresses, mud is anti-inflammatory and is a very effective way to get heat into the body to stimulate the perspiration that helps draw toxins out. For example, a cloth pack soaked in peat (mud), then applied to joints sore from arthritis and held in place with plastic wrap and blankets for about thirty minutes, can go a long way toward easing the pain in those joints. There are also the cosmetic muds, green clay, which is widely used in salons or for home facial treatments, or the famous Moor mud, formed by the decomposition of medicinal plants over hundreds of years.

POULTICES

Poultices of herbs, mashed vegetables, or similar organic substances are spread onto cheesecloth or flannel, covered with a second layer of cloth, then packed or tied loosely onto the part of the body that is aching, and left there for up to an hour while you relax and rest. Dr. Kane cites the benefits of specific poultices for specific conditions: carrot poultices for mastitis; comfrey for broken bones; and oatmeal for the nervous system (putting this poultice in the warm bath with you smooths your skin as it is soothing your nerves). And she adds that some kind of mentholated poultice would work very well for most pain syndromes. Others say that a poultice made of the herb goldenseal can be used to treat all kinds of painful inflammations, as can a combination of the herbs fenugreek, flaxseed, and slippery elm.

The materials for all of these applied therapies are reasonably priced and can be obtained in health food or grocery stores.

CAUTIONS

Take care not to burn the skin with hot compresses and remember that cold applications also have to be used with caution. Do not apply ice directly to the skin or use a cold application for more than twenty minutes at a time. Some *hot* herbs, such as mustard and cayenne, can burn the skin if they come in direct contact with it. Keep checking the area and remove if any redness occurs.

Castor oil stains clothing and bedding, so be sure to carefully cover the wrap with plastic, and do not use a pack during heavy menses.

Dr. Kane cautions that, if you are experiencing pain in

such places as the abdomen or the pelvis, you should be careful to first rule out more serious conditions before applying any of these therapies.

(*See also* AROMATHERAPY, HEAT THERAPY/COLD THERAPY, HYDROTHERAPY, and HERBAL REMEDIES in PART 2 Treatment Section.)

CLINICAL STUDIES

Although scientific research has not been conducted on the efficacy of compresses, packs, and poultices, they have been used in many cultures since ancient times, and holistic practitioners often recommend them because they are so effective.

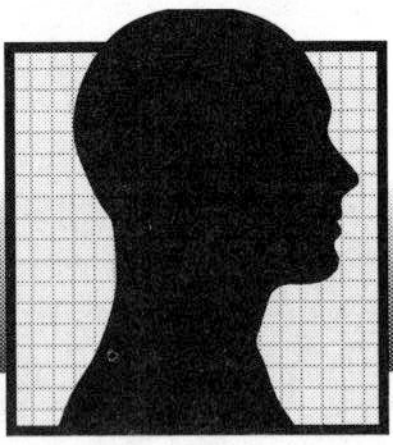

Craniosacral Therapy

The craniosacral system includes the bones of your skull, face, and mouth, which make up the cranium, and extends down to the sacrum at the bottom of your spine. It consists of a sac filled with cerebrospinal fluid that moves via hydraulic pressure stemming from pulsating ventricles in the brain, and surrounds, nourishes, and protects the brain and spinal cord. Just as your cardiovascular system has a rhythm that medical practitioners can feel or listen to throughout your body, so can practitioners of craniosacral therapy monitor the craniosacral rhythm. Using expert palpation, primarily of the eight bones that make up the skull which are constantly moving, they can locate the source of an obstruction or stress. Since your bones are in constant motion (although you are not conscious of it), as this cerebrospinal fluid gets pumped through your body, a practitioner can detect any minute variations in the bones' movement and can perform techniques to free up the flow of the fluid if any blockage restricting the craniosacral rhythm is found.

THE HISTORY OF CRANIOSACRAL THERAPY

In the early part of the twentieth century, Dr. William Sutherland, an osteopathic physician, discovered that the skull bones were designed to move, a finding that put him at odds with most of the medical community because *Gray's Anatomy,* the bible of anatomical reference books (as well as other anatomy texts) held that skull bones were immobile. Another osteopathic physician and surgeon, Dr. John Upledger, a professor of biomechanics at Michigan State University from 1975 to 1983, led a team of twenty-seven research scientists in a project to study and evaluate the craniosacral system, and found that "it had a pretty good scientific basis." Out of this research and Dr. Upledger's subsequent clinical application of the theories he found to be valid, craniosacral therapy was developed.

HOW CRANIOSACRAL THERAPY WORKS

The theory is that physical injuries and emotional traumas are stored or frozen in the body until they are released, and trained practitioners can feel out, through expert, gentle manipulation (primarily of the skull), those areas where normal tissue function is restricted, usually due to these physical or emotional traumas. They can ferret out these craniosacral rhythms because they are transmitted by your muscular, nervous, and fascial systems, and can be monitored. The fascia is the connective tissue that runs from the top of your head to the bottom of your feet. It is made up of layers, between which are pockets that contain your organs, muscles, and bones. Being elastic, the fascia can glide about a millimeter, and noting how well it glides is one method the practitioner has for determining what areas may be restricted and not moving as easily as others.

PAINFUL CONDITIONS THAT RESPOND WELL TO THERAPY

- ❑ Back pain.
- ❑ Cluster headaches.
- ❑ Crohn's disease.
- ❑ Dental pain.
- ❑ Diverticulitis.
- ❑ Endometriosis.
- ❑ Irritable bowel syndrome.
- ❑ Migraine headaches.
- ❑ Osteoarthritis.
- ❑ Pelvic floor tension myalgia.
- ❑ Postherpetic neuralgia.
- ❑ Premenstrual syndrome.
- ❑ Rheumatoid arthritis.
- ❑ Sciatica.
- ❑ Temporomandibular joint (TMJ) pain.
- ❑ Tension headaches.
- ❑ Ulcerative colitis.

According to practitioners at The Center for Human Integration in Fox Chase, PA, craniosacral therapy is good for all painful conditions, especially those with an emotional component, which could cause stress leading to chronic pain.

In addition to its help with painful conditions, craniosacral therapy is also good for allergies, autism, brain and spinal cord injuries, blood pressure normalization, depression, injuries and bruises, MS, strokes, post-operative complications, posttraumatic stress disorder, sinusitis, tinnitus, and vertigo. It can also shorten labor.

ADVANTAGES OF CRANIOSACRAL THERAPY

Since craniosacral therapy is such a gentle form of treatment, it can even be performed on newborn babies and very young children. Correcting problems early on in this system may help avoid problems in the digestive and respiratory tracts, and even prevent such conditions as hyperactivity, scoliosis, and seizure disorders later in life. Although CST originated as an adjunctive medical modality, it can be incorporated with various theories involving energy healing. Practitioners can be chiropracters, massage professionals, MDs, osteopaths, or physical therapists. They do not have to be medical professionals.

HOW CRANIOSACRAL THERAPY IS USED

Your therapist will place his or her hands on specific areas of your body, primarily your head, but also your neck, lower back, and ankles, to assess the state of your craniosacral system. Then she or he applies very light force, possibly lifting your arms and legs and moving them gently to allow your tissues to unwind themselves. While receiving CST you may experience a variety of feelings, ranging from deep relaxation to insights into problems in your life and memories of prior physical sensations.

CAUTIONS

Craniosacral therapy is safe and has no adverse side effects.

CLINICAL STUDIES

Research into the craniosacral system is ongoing at the Colorado Cranial Institute, the Society of Ortho-Bionomy, and the Upledger Institute.

In 1999, the Upledger Foundation sponsored a study using intensive craniosacral therapy on veterans with posttraumatic stress disorder (PTSD). Independent reports noted a more than 95-percent correlation between the impressive reduction of the PTSD symptoms and the treatment program.

CST Brings Relief to Bill's Bell's Palsy

When Bill woke up one morning, his facial muscles felt twisted, his neck felt out of alignment, and he was sure he'd had a stroke. A doctor, however, diagnosed his condition as Bell's Palsy, a sudden, unexplained facial paralysis which distorts the face. The steroids prescribed only made things worse for Bill, so he went to see a local craniosacral therapist. As soon as she touched his face with opposing forces against the muscles, Bill began to feel dramatically better, and after two weeks of therapy, his condition was almost completely relieved. Most people with Bell's Palsy are never told about craniosacral therapy, but in Bill's opinion, it's the first treatment they should look for in order to avoid having the problem drag on for months and months, maybe even forever.

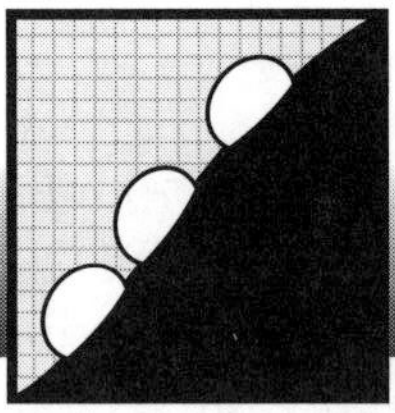

Cupping

Cupping is an ancient method of treatment in which a cup of some type is heated and applied to the skin. This creates suction, which draws the skin and underlying muscle area into the cup. Many types of cups can be used for this process, including ones made of bamboo, glass, plastic, rubber, or even the hollowed-out animal horns that the Chinese used. A partial vacuum is created in cups placed on the skin when heat (fire) or suction is used. Another, newer type of cup creates suction by using a pump. The cups come in various sizes depending on the area to be treated.

THE HISTORY OF CUPPING

Cupping has been used for millenia by Asian, Arabian, and Indian cultures, as well as the indigenous peoples of the Americas and Africa. The Ethiopians have always used cupping to treat chest pain, and traditional Chinese medicine (TCM) has always considered cupping an important tool in its storehouse of methods, often linking it to acupuncture and the meridians of the body. The earliest recorded use of cupping was *A Handbook of Prescriptions for Emergencies,* written by Ge Hong, a famous Taoist alchemist and herbalist who lived from 281 to 341 AD. Since animal horns were used then, the process was known as the Horn Technique. Later, cups were often made of metal or pottery but with these materials the person doing the cupping couldn't see the skin inside the cup. Transparent drinking glasses were better for that purpose and came to be used more often. Then, toward the end of the twentieth century, the suction type, described below, was developed.

HOW CUPPING WORKS

Pain can be due to a lack of oxygen in the cells. Cupping increases circulation, bringing blood and oxygen to the cells. It can reach up to four inches into the tissues, causing them to release toxins, activate the lymphatic system, and activate and clear the veins, arteries, and capillaries, among other benefits. Cupping can reduce swelling and pain, and is considered probably the best deep-tissue massage available, as well as the best way to open the meridians of the back to promote energy flow through every part of the body.

PAINFUL CONDITIONS THAT RESPOND WELL TO CUPPING

- ❑ Back pain (arm and shoulder pain).
- ❑ Cluster headaches.
- ❑ Crohn's disease.
- ❑ Diverticulitis.
- ❑ Irritable bowel syndrome.
- ❑ Migraine headaches.
- ❑ Postherpetic neuralgia.
- ❑ Sciatica.
- ❑ Temporomandibular joint (TMJ) pain.
- ❑ Tension headaches.
- ❑ Trigeminal neuralgia.
- ❑ Ulcerative colitis.

Other conditions that respond well to cupping include asthma, bronchitis, a chronic cough, the common cold, and insomnia.

ADVANTAGES OF CUPPING

Cupping is a non-invasive, non-pharmaceutical method of pain control. It is considered safe, free from side effects, and can be easily learned and incorporated into a health regimen.

HOW CUPPING IS USED

Cupping techniques can vary, but they all depend on either heat or suction. With suction, the area to be treated is covered with a slippery substance, such as petroleum jelly, and the edges of the cups (transparent in order to easily observe the skin changes within the cup) are also lubricated to form a tight seal. This lubrication allows for ease of movement around the affected area and easy removal when the treatment is over.

The older cupping method uses fire to create suction. Cotton soaked in alcohol and held with forceps is ignited, placed briefly in the cup, then removed, and the cup is immediately placed on the skin.

With the pump type of cupping, the cup has a nipple on its top. When the cup is placed over the area to be treated, the pump gets attached to the nipple and goes to work sucking out the air.

Following treatment, the cupping area develops a color ranging from pink to red to purple that generally disappears in about twenty-four hours. Pain relief is usually immediate and it continues to improve. Some practitioners believe the treated area is vulnerable and should be kept warm and covered for twenty-four hours to avoid catching a cold.

Cupping is usually performed by acupuncturists or massage therapists. In addition to applying the cups directly to the painful areas, they may be applied to acupuncture points that relate to the painful areas. Wet cupping might be performed before the cup is applied. This is when the practitioner does bloodletting—pricking the area with a needle to express a few drops of blood. Some practitioners believe this increases the effects of cupping and that it is particularly useful to relieve swelling.

To find a practitioner, check with an acupuncturist, a holistic healthcare center, or a hospital with an Integrative Medicine Department.

CAUTIONS

The fire method can cause burns on the skin. Use of the pump type is much safer. Do not use cupping therapy if you are taking blood thinners because there can be excessive bleeding.

(*See also* ACUPUNCTURE and ACUPRESSURE in PART 2 Treatment Section.)

CLINICAL STUDIES

Kemper, KJ, Sarah, R, Silver-Highfield, E, et al. "On pins and needles? Pediatric pain patients' experience acupuncture." *Pediatrics.* April 2000; 105(4):941–947.

Data for this unusual study of pediatric patients treated with acupuncture, magnets, and cupping showed that the young subjects found all the treatments pleasant and useful. Further studies were recommended.

Sherman, KJ, Cherkin, DC, Hogeboom, CJ. "The diagnosis and treatment of patients with chronic low-back pain by traditional Chinese medical acupuncturists. *The Journal of Alternative Complementary Medicine.* December 2001; 7(6):641–650.

This analysis of the acupuncture treatments of 150 people with low back pain also included adjunctive treatments, such as cupping. Although there was improvement shown, it was recommended that researchers develop a treatment with less variability that contained broad features characteristic of patterns in clinical practice.

Zhilong, Zhang. "Observation on therapeutic effects of bloodletting puncture with cupping in acute trigeminal neuralgia." *Journal of Traditional Chinese Medicine.* 1997; 17(4):272–274.

This study of forty-five people with trigeminal neuralgia showed that bloodletting puncture with cupping was an effective therapy for the condition.

MIGRAINE BE GONE

Tim, a forty-four-year-old man, had lived in pain from recurring migraine headaches for about twenty years. After a decade of excruciating pain, he had changed his diet completely, becoming a vegetarian, but it didn't help, so he knew his problem wasn't diet-related. He had also tried chiropractic and other alternative therapies, again with no improvement. His pain was so unbearable, he said, that he took pain medication two to three times a day. A shower hitting the meridians on the top of his head helped, but one half-hour afterwards, the pain started up again.

Dr. Maria Elena Boekemeyer, a naturopath and bioresonance practitioner at the New Hope Clinic in California, relates that Tim was desperate for relief when he came to them for a cupping session. To assess the cause of his condition, the doctors first placed cups along his spine and, based on the color of his skin after suction was applied, they were able to determine which organ was affected (in his case, the gallbladder). The second round of therapy was wet cupping (where a small prick releases blood) and they were able to further assess and confirm the cause of his problem based on the gasses that were released. Thanks to the use of the cupping techniques, combined with a very advanced bioresonance machine, the diagnosis had been confirmed in just two visits, and he was put on a gallbladder flush consisting of garlic, olive oil, and lemon.

After two weeks, Tim reported that he hardly had any migraines anymore, and the severity of those he did have was greatly diminished. After a month of undergoing cupping therapy at the clinic, he was completely migraine-free. Dr. Boekemeyer says he calls in every three months, and each time is happy to report that he is still free of the disabling pain that had plagued him for twenty years, and immeasurably grateful to the clinic that made this happen.

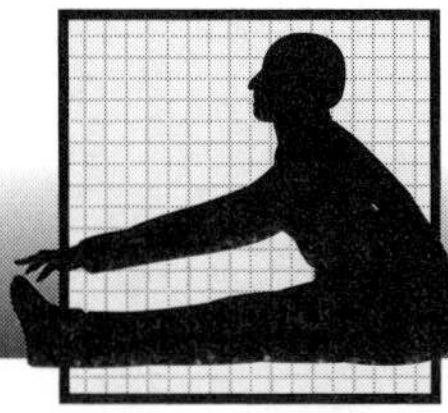

Exercise, Stretching, and Sports

Exercise, stretching, and sports keep your body strong and flexible and protect your cardiovascular system. When muscles are properly warmed up and stretched they work better. Although many with chronic pain conditions fear exercise will stress their bodies and make their conditions worse, the reverse is true. Immobility, not exercise, is the factor leading to more deterioration and pain.

For good health, it is important to keep active. A great percentage of back problems are caused by a lack of exercise. Those who play racquet sports or golf tend to use one side of their body more than the other, and it is important for them to also engage in exercise that uses both sides of the body.

THE HISTORY OF EXERCISE, STRETCHING, AND SPORTS

People have always moved, there's never been a time when they didn't, and sports have been around for millenia. In ancient times, they were a form of competition between tribes, which evolved over the centuries into modern day sports, particularly spectator sports. Now, in addition to watching sports, many people participate in them as a form of enjoyable exercise.

The more structured forms of participatory exercise are really a twentieth-century phenomenon, starting with such workouts as calisthenics in the military and the gym classes that most kids hated. Prompted in large measure by doctors who considered lack of exercise a health risk, exercise routines increased in popularity, and with the advent of health clubs and their ever-widening memberships, working out is now an ingrained aspect of contemporary life, so much so that it's hard to imagine there was ever a time when people considered non-sporting physical exercise beneath them.

HOW EXERCISE, STRETCHING, AND SPORTS WORK

Exercising, stretching, and participating in sports release endorphins, your body's natural painkillers and mood lifters. Strengthening the muscles that support your joints helps to increase their stability.

PAINFUL CONDITIONS THAT RESPOND WELL TO THERAPIES

All painful musculoskeletal conditions respond favorably to proper exercising, stretching, and sporting activities. (*See* Quick Help Chart for synopsis of suggested treatments for all conditions covered in this book.)

ADVANTAGES OF EXERCISE, STRETCHING, AND SPORTS

You can do some form of exercising anywhere. Resistance training and weightlifting:

- ❑ Help build stronger bones;
- ❑ Build physical strength;
- ❑ Help turn fat into muscle.

Besides being good for your cardiovascular system, the type of aerobic exercise that increases your heart rate, also:

Functional Fitness

Unlike most fitness programs, which isolate individual parts of the body for cosmetic toning purposes, the goal of this transformative new school of thought is to prepare your entire body to do daily activities—bending, climbing stairs, lifting, walking—without pain, injury, or discomfort. Balancing on yoga blocks, racing up and down stairs, and using oversized rubber balls in pursuit of balance, coordination, flexibility, and strength, this whole-body regimen borrows from many disciplines—dance, physical therapy, Pilates, and yoga among them—to achieve its aims.

According to Michael A. Clark, President of the National Academy of Sports Medicine in Calabasas, CA, functional fitness is "very much the direction of the fitness industry." The method teaches all those with injuries how to use multiple muscle groups in an integrated way to alleviate their back pain, their knee pain, or other painful problems. The workouts are all about head-to-toe fitness and they "challenge the body collectively, as a whole, firing up the muscles in a sequential way," says advocate Jarrod Jordan, a fitness trainer in the Sports Center at Chelsea Piers in New York. Done properly, and accompanied by a change in the way you move on a daily basis, this approach could help keep you fit and free of pain for a lifetime.

- ❑ Helps keep your joints loose;
- ❑ Helps your body absorb nutrients more efficiently and helps you get rid of waste products;
- ❑ Improves blood flow, which helps deliver oxygen and nutrients to the area;
- ❑ Increases blood flow to your muscles and connective tissues, which helps make them more elastic.

Stretching is useful to:

- ❑ Help improve posture;
- ❑ Help keep you from feeling sore after you exercise;
- ❑ Help reduce stiffness;
- ❑ Help relieve back pain, joint pain, and muscle pain;
- ❑ Help you perform your daily activities more easily;
- ❑ Improve your athletic performance because it makes you more flexible;
- ❑ Increase your range of motion;
- ❑ Prevent injuries;
- ❑ Strengthen your ligaments and tendons.

Since exercising and stretching are inherent parts of any sporting activities, their advantages apply equally to sports.

HOW TO USE EXERCISE, STRETCHING, AND SPORTS

Choose activities that you enjoy and try to vary them so you use different parts of your body. It is important to warm up with some type of moderate activity, such as walking or running slowly in place. This will allow more blood to reach your muscles and tendons before you stretch them so you are not stressing cold muscles. Then you should stretch, do your workout, and stretch again.

One of the best stretching methods is to hold your stretch as you exhale and try stretching a bit farther as you do so.

Walking in water (the shallow end of a pool), or performing water aerobics are excellent non-impact and non-weight-bearing ways of exercising without stressing your joints. The water also provides resistance, which improves muscle tone and flexibility.

For specific stretches, consult an exercise physiologist, a trainer at a gym, a physical therapist, or a chiropractor. This will help insure that you are doing them properly.

Other activities can include:

- ❑ Aerobics classes;
- ❑ Biking;
- ❑ Dance classes;
- ❑ Gardening;

FOR INTERMITTENT CLAUDICATION, TRY EXERCISING

Intermittent claudication, a peripheral artery disease that causes pain in the lower legs, particularly when walking, is a systemic condition comparable to angina pain in the arteries that feed the heart. It is caused by a narrowing of the arteries in the lower legs that prevents an adequate supply of oxygenated blood from reaching the muscles. In addition to pain, the legs and feet may become discolored, swollen, numb, or cold, and may be accompanied by a tingling sensation. The risk factors for this painful condition include smoking, diabetes, high cholesterol, high blood pressure, obesity, and aging. A supervised exercise program that includes the use of a treadmill to extend the distance a person can walk without pain can help improve circulation and be a good alternative to drug therapy.

- ❑ Golf;
- ❑ Jogging;
- ❑ Pilates classes;
- ❑ Rowing machines;
- ❑ Stepping machines;
- ❑ Swimming;
- ❑ Tennis and other racquet sports;
- ❑ Walking;
- ❑ Water aerobics;
- ❑ Weightlifting.

CAUTIONS

Always be sure to warm up before you stretch. Do not bounce while stretching, and do not stretch too far. If you feel pain while exercising or stretching, stop, because you are most likely doing something wrong. Consult an athletic trainer or physical therapist if you feel you are not doing the exercises or stretches properly. If you participate in a sport where you are performing repetitive motions on one side of your body only, make sure to balance them out with exercises for the other side.

CLINICAL STUDIES

Rogind, H, Bibow-Nielsen, B, Jensen, B, et al. "The effects of a physical training program on patients with osteoarthritis of the knees." *Archives of Physical Medicine and Rehabilitation.* November 1998; 79:1421–1427.

Pilates Techniques

Developed in the 1920s, Pilates (pron: puh-LAH-teez) is an exercise and body- conditioning program that is useful for preventing back and postural problems, increasing flexibility and strength, and preventing injuries.

Joseph Hubertus Pilates was a frail child who dedicated himself to becoming stronger, and grew up to become a boxer, circus performer, and self-defense trainer who studied yoga and meditation. He developed his unique techniques while interned as an enemy alien in England during WWI. Using springs from old-fashioned hospital beds, he devised special machines that provided progressive resistance to heal and strengthen muscles.

His method, especially popular with dancers, is a series of controlled movements performed on these machines, or on mats, under the supervision of highly trained teachers. Its benefits include: learning how to maintain better posture, which contributes to the overall health of the body; long, flexible muscles; increased joint range of motion; a flat, lean stomach; improved circulation and stamina; better coordination; and all this without the pain and soreness often caused by conventional forms of exercise, an especially important benefit for anyone already experiencing a painful condition.

A three-month study of twenty-five people with osteoarthritis of the knees focused on general fitness, balance, coordination, stretching, and lower-extremity muscle strength, and included a daily home-exercise program. At the end of the three months, there was sufficient improvement in the pain experienced by the study's participants to consider general physical training beneficial for anyone with osteoarthritis of the knees.

Sexton-Radek, K, Ator, R, Keenum, M, et al. "Conjunctive measurement of aquatic exercise in an office setting." *Psychological Report*. October 2001; 89(2):237–242.

In this unusual in-office study of twenty-four people, a Hydrotrack, a treadmill immersed in a water bath, was used for rehabilitation treatment, and results of the study confirmed the usefulness of the aquatic device.

Shrier, I. "Does stretching improve performance? A systematic and critical review of the literature." *The Clinical Journal of Sports Medicine*. September–October 2004; 14(4).

Dr. Ian Shrier of the SMBD-Jewish General Hospital in Montreal, Canada reviewed 23 studies on the effects of "acute" stretching immediately prior to sport or exercise and determined that this hindered, even reduced, sport performance. Dr. Shrier reports that regular stretching performed "after exercise, or at a time not related to exercise" was found to be more beneficial, probably because it increases muscle strength.

Dr. Shrier does not see a case for stretching just prior to exercising and cites many studies in this article to back up his findings that pre-exercise stretches are not effective in reducing injury.

Shrier, I. "Does stretching improve performance?: a systematic and critical review of the literature." *Clinical Journal of Sport Medicine*. September 2004; 14(5):267–273.

Dr. Ian Shrier of the SMBD-Jewish General Hospital in Montreal, Canada reviewed 23 studies on the effects of "acute" stretching immediately prior to sport or exercise and determined that this hindered, even reduced, sport performance. Dr. Shrier reports that regular stretching performed "after exercise, or at a time not related to exercise" was found to be more beneficial, probably because it increases muscle strength.Strauss-Blasche, G, Ekmekcioglu, C, Vacariu, G, et al. "Contribution of individual spa therapies in the treatment of chronic pain." *Clinical Journal of Pain*. September-October 2002; 18(5):302–309.

This three-week study of 153 people with chronic back pain used various methods of spa treatments, including exercise, which were found to be beneficial for relieving pain on both a short-term and a long-term basis.

Stretching for Conditioning, Stiffness, and Pain

Dr. Ian Shrier, MD, PhD, Assistant Professor at McGill University in Montreal, Canada, and past president of the Canadian Academy of Sport Medicine, questions the value of stretching immediately before exercising, saying that it does not prevent injury. He adds that stretching at other times "may or may not prevent injury, there is very little research in this area." From his clinical experience, he believes that stretching is beneficial for people with morning stiffness. For people with painful injuries, he believes that strengthening is more important than stretching, but says there are exceptions, and some believe that people with the stiffness of frozen shoulder must stretch in order to increase range of motion. Dr. Shrier also says that a little-known benefit of stretching comes with what he calls "stretch tolerance, in which the stretching acts like an analgesic. Initially a stretch is painful," he says, "but when repeated, one is not aware of the pain."

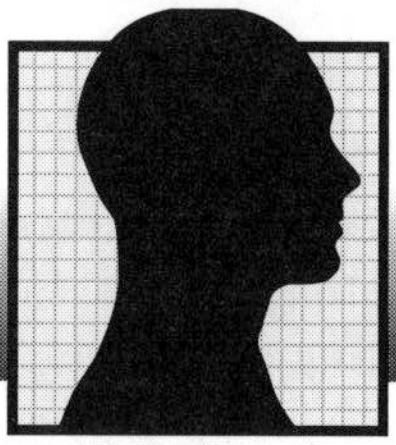

Guided Imagery and Visualization

Guided imagery and visualization, or creative visualization, are techniques that use the power of your mind to elicit a physical response. With guided imagery, images come either from a therapist or a tape, and can be auditory, aural, tactile, or visual. With visualization, or creative visualization, the visual images are self-induced. Whether you are working alone or with a therapist, the techniques are the same. They can all be used to relieve stress and manage pain, and are all based on the theory that your mind can influence your body. A typical example of the power of visual imaging is that, when you think of something you really like to eat, a juicy orange for example, you are likely to start salivating. If you think of something that frightens you, such as falling from a great height or being stuck in an elevator, your heart will start to pound and your blood pressure will rise. Although it is not a cure-all, imagery can be miraculous for some, and a high percentage of those who have tried imaging and/or visualization find the techniques a helpful adjunct for pain relief.

Guided imaging and visualization have wide applications and can be very effective for improving athletic performance, preparing yourself for public speaking, or rehearsing music, but here we are concentrating on their usefulness for pain management.

THE HISTORY OF GUIDED IMAGERY AND VISUALIZATION

Since ancient times, imagery and visualization have been used by people in many different cultures, including Egyptian, Greek, Hebrew mystic, and Native American. After disappearing for centuries, the techniques again became popular in the early 70s to help athletes and musicians perform better. Studies have shown that basketball players who visualize their shots do just as well as those who actually practice them. Beyond improving performance, imagery and visualization are increasingly winning acceptance as ways of controlling chronic pain.

HOW GUIDED IMAGERY AND VISUALIZATION WORK

If you have ever worried (and who hasn't), you have practiced imagery. According to David Bresler, PhD, co-director of the Academy for Guided Imagery in Mill Valley, California, "If you are good at worrying, you're good at using imagery."

Your body cannot differentiate between having a physical experience and imagining one. Have you ever noticed at a scary movie, how your heart pounds just watching the onscreen action? Your flight-or-fight response has been activated and it reacts just the same as if you were actually having the experience.

The mind is so powerful that if a shaman curses a believing tribesman, he will likely die. Guided imagery and visualization work by helping you relax and by triggering the release of endorphins (hormones that help you feel good).

PAINFUL CONDITIONS THAT RESPOND WELL TO THERAPIES

All the painful conditions discussed in this book respond to imagery and visualization. (*See* Quick Help Chart for synopsis of suggested treatments for all conditions covered in this book.)

ADVANTAGES OF GUIDED IMAGERY AND VISUALIZATION

- ❑ Since imagery relaxes your body and reduces stress, it is especially useful for conditions that are stress-related, such as back pain, headaches, digestive, and menstrual problems.
- ❑ Both can be done with a therapist or alone, and are techniques you can practice yourself at little or no cost. There are many excellent tapes and CDs you might want to try, all available in bookstores or at Internet booksellers online.
- ❑ These techniques are less expensive than most methods of pain control and have no side effects. William L. Mundy, MD, of Shawnee Mission, KS, who uses imagery principally for allergy control, but also sings its praises for pain relief, likens visualization techniques to chicken soup, saying, "If it doesn't help, it won't hurt."

HOW GUIDED IMAGERY AND VISUALIZATION ARE USED

When working with a practitioner, a session starts by helping you achieve a relaxed state. The therapist may guide you through deep-breathing exercises, have you picture yourself in a tranquil place, such as a beach at twilight, or lead you through progressive relaxation by having you tense and then relax various muscle groups. Some practitioners have you imagine you are on a down escalator or on descending stairs, and feeling more and more relaxed as you are going down.

You might learn how to meet an imaginary guide and ask what he is doing to cause your pain and how you can get him to stop. For example, if you have a splitting headache and the guide is wielding an axe, you can ask what you have to do to make him put it down. Or, if you have a vise-like pain in your head, you can ask what you can do to loosen the vise. You might gain insight into what lifestyle changes of yours need modification.

Self-Treatment Techniques

Although it is best to have some sessions with a professional to get you started visualizing, here are some techniques you can try yourself.

First, loosen any tight clothing, find a comfortable position, and get into a relaxed state by one of the above methods. Then:

- ❑ Visualize the painful area being injected with a numbing substance.
- ❑ Use glove anesthesia. Concentrate on one of your hands becoming extremely cold. You can do this by picturing that you are holding a snowball in your bare hand or soaking your hand in a bucket of ice until it becomes numb. Then place your cold hand over the painful area, allowing its numbness to ease your pain.
- ❑ Give the pain a symbol that represents it, such as a bright light bulb or a dial with numbers. Gradually dim the light or dial the numbers lower, lessening their intensity.
- ❑ Form a picture of your pain. For example, if it is a burning sensation, picture it as a fire and then think of ways to extinguish the fire, such as using a fire extinguisher, or a stream of water. If the pain feels like pressure, picture a vise and what will loosen it. If you have joint pain due to lack of lubrication, picture taking an oilcan and injecting the lubricating oil into the joint.
- ❑ Change your pain into an object. Visualize how large it is and what shape it has. Give it a color. See what it smells and tastes like.
- ❑ As with any skill, it is important to practice imaging. The more you practice, the better you can visualize.

To review, first create an image of your pain and then find an image to counteract it. As you keep practicing, you may find that all you have to do is think of the image that counteracts the pain. The important thing is to find those images that help you visualize the outcome you desire.

CAUTIONS

- ❑ Anyone with psychoses, who cannot tell the difference between reality and suggested images, should not use guided imagery and visualization.
- ❑ Anyone with a serious condition should not use guided imagery and visualization as a substitute for conventional medical care. For instance, if you or your child has a high fever, or a sudden onset of chest or abdominal pain, you should seek medical attention.
- ❑ Be sure you have been properly evaluated by a medical professional to determine what is causing your pain.
- ❑ Do not listen to guided imagery tapes or practice imagery while driving a car.

(*See also* BIOFEEDBACK, HYPNOSIS, and MEDITATION in PART 2 Treatment Section.)

PEACE FOR THE PEACE CORPS VOLUNTEER

Andy was a Peace Corps volunteer in Senegal and he suffered from such severe headaches that he had to spend hours lying in the shade. Painkillers were not particularly effective, and most of his fellow workers were not sympathetic—they thought he was slacking off to keep out of the heat. His friend, Lisa, who had had very good results using visualization techniques for severe menstrual cramps, offered to work on Andy. Although skeptical, he was willing to try anything because he really wanted to stay in the Peace Corps.

Lisa led him through progressive relaxation techniques and then had him concentrate on his breathing to induce a relaxed state. His pain was like having his head in a vise, he told Lisa, so she got him to mentally loosen this vise while he was in the relaxed state. To his amazement, when he did this, the pain began to lessen and he was able to function. From then on, whenever Andy felt the first stirrings of a headache, all he had to do was visualize the vise loosening and the pain would go away, giving him peace *and* keeping him in the Peace Corps, right where he wanted to be.

CLINICAL STUDIES

Studies at hospitals and universities are examining the effectiveness of imaging and visualization on patients with AIDS, asthma, cancer, cardiac, and pulmonary problems. The Office of Alternative Medicine at the National Institutes of Health is funding some of these studies. Unfortunately, however, most funding for medical research comes from drug companies who have little to gain financially from drug-free or alternative methods, so major sources of funding for alternative methods are difficult to find. (Even Dr. Dean Ornish, very well known for his work using diet and relaxation techniques to reverse heart disease, was not able to get grants from the government or the American Heart Association.)

Studies have shown that patients who practiced imagery and visualization while undergoing minor surgery recovered faster, and with less pain.

Below are several studies on guided imagery for chronic pain conditions.

Fors, EA, Sexton, H, Gotestam, KG. "The effect of guided imagery and amitriptyline on daily fibromyalgia pain: a prospective, randomized, controlled trial." *Journal of Psychiatric Research.* May-June 2002; 36(3):179–187.

This twenty-eight day Norwegian trial of fifty-five women studied the effects of pleasant, attention-distracting guided imagery compared to an attention-focusing imagery and the drug amitriptyline. The pleasant imagery was more effective in reducing the pain of fibromyalgia than either the attention-focusing imagery or the drug, which showed no significant advantage over the placebo.

Mannix, LK, Chandurkar, RS, Rybicki, LA, et al. "Effect of guided imagery on quality of life for patients with chronic tension-type headache." *Headache.* May 1999; 39(5):326–334.

In this study at the Headaches Wellness Center in Greensboro, North Carolina, the people who received therapy and listened to a guided-imagery tape for a month showed significantly more improvement than the control group who had only therapy. The conclusion drawn was that guided imagery is an effective adjunct therapy for chronic tension-type headaches.

Heat Therapy/Cold Therapy

Heat therapy/cold therapy, also known as thermotherapy, is the therapeutic application of heat or cold to provide relief from many forms of pain, and it is one of the first tools that therapists turn to for this purpose. Heat therapy causes the blood vessels to dilate, while cold therapy causes them to constrict. Applying heat makes blood rush to the area, nourishing and cleansing it. Applying cold does just the opposite; it decreases blood flow to the area, which helps reduce inflammation.

THE HISTORY OF HEAT/COLD THERAPY

These treatments have been used since ancient times to help relieve pain. The use of cold therapy can be traced back to the time of Hippocrates, known as "the Father of Medicine," who noted that snow and ice produced beneficial results following soft-tissue injury. Heated water treatments (baths) were regular therapy for the Greek physician Galen, and water's healing effects have been attributed to its value as a medium for heat and cold.

HOW HEAT/COLD THERAPY WORKS

Temperature change works the same, whether it's in your body or everywhere else: cold constricts and heat expands. Heat therapy works by increasing blood flow to the painful area, and making muscles relax, and cold therapy keeps blood flow away from the area, which reduces swelling and inflammation.

PAINFUL CONDITIONS THAT RESPOND WELL TO HEAT/COLD THERAPY

- ❑ Achilles tendonitis
- ❑ Back problems.
- ❑ Bursitis.
- ❑ Carpal tunnel syndrome.
- ❑ Cluster headaches.
- ❑ Dental pain.
- ❑ Endometriosis.
- ❑ Fibromyalgia.
- ❑ Frozen shoulder.
- ❑ Gout.
- ❑ Migraine headaches.
- ❑ Neuroma.
- ❑ Osteoarthritis.
- ❑ Pelvic floor tension myalgia.
- ❑ Peripheral neuropathy.
- ❑ Phantom pain.
- ❑ Plantar Fasciitis.
- ❑ Postherpetic neuralgia.
- ❑ Plantar fasciitis.
- ❑ Postherpetic neuralgia.
- ❑ Post-polio syndrome.
- ❑ Reflex sympathetic dystrophy syndrome.
- ❑ Rheumatoid arthritis.
- ❑ Rotator cuff tendonitis.
- ❑ Tarsal tunnel syndrome.
- ❑ Temporomandibular joint (TMJ) pain.
- ❑ Tennis elbow.
- ❑ Tension headaches.
- ❑ Trigeminal neuralgia.
- ❑ Trigger finger.

ADVANTAGES OF HEAT/COLD THERAPY

These forms of therapy are inexpensive and easy to do. They are non-invasive, and they are a drug-free form of pain relief.

HOW TO USE HEAT/COLD THERAPY

Heat Therapy

Heat therapy treatments are used in different forms: moist heat, dry heat, paraffin, Jacuzzis, or whirlpool baths. Moist heat penetrates more deeply than dry heat and can be applied by using special hot packs that retain heat. Known as hydrocollator packs, these canvas bags are filled with gel or silicon dioxide, which absorbs many times its own weight when exposed to moisture. The packs are kept in hot water (140–160° F) and then applied to the area over layers of towels to prevent burning the skin. Electric hydrocollators that deliver moist heat are also available. They have a safety switch you have to hold down to keep the heat on, so if you fall asleep while using one, the heat will go off.

Dry heat is applied by using the old familiar heating pads. Some of these can be applied over a damp towel to get the effect of moist heat.

Generally, moist heat is better to use than dry heat because it penetrates deeper. Dry heat is easier to apply and feels good, but it pulls moisture out of the area and may dehydrate your skin.

Paraffin is a combination of wax and mineral oil that has a temperature between 120 and 130° Fahrenheit. It is usually used to treat arthritis of the hands and feet. The hand or foot is dipped into the warm paraffin several times until a thick coating forms. Then a towel is wrapped around the hand or foot to retain the heat.

Whirlpools or Jacuzzis are tubs with jets that agitate water kept between 100 and 104° Fahrenheit. The agitation of the jets helps the water move around the body to improve circulation.

If you are camping or in an area without electricity, you can carry an old-fashioned hot-water bottle and fill it with water heated over a fire.

Cold Therapy

Cold therapy (aka cryotherapy) is used to decrease swelling and pain. It can be applied by using cold packs, ice, snow, sprays, or coldwater baths. A simple way to do cold therapy is to put crushed ice into a paper or Styrofoam cup and rub the cup over the affected area for up to twenty minutes. You can also put ice in a ziplock bag and apply it over a damp cloth placed against the painful part of the body you are treating. Or you can buy gel packs to keep in the freezer. Packs of frozen vegetables, such as peas or corn, can also be used, but as with all cold packs, there should be a layer of material, such as a thin towel, between the pack and the skin to minimize the risk for frostbite. Apply cold for up to thirty minutes every three hours, and when using cold therapy alone for that length of time, be sure to wait at least two hours between treatments to allow for rewarming of the skin (cooled tissue returns to normal temperature more slowly than heated tissue). Since cold increases the stiffness of collagen, which results in decreased flexibility, therapeutic cold should be applied only after physical therapy sessions or any athletic participation.

Heat/Cold Therapy—Which to Use and When

If you are not sure whether to use heat or cold, the general rule is to use cold for swelling or injuries, and after activities that cause pain or discomfort. Use heat to relieve stiffness and muscle spasms, but wait until any swelling goes down before using it because the increased blood flow to the painful area can increase the swelling. Unlike cold therapy, which decreases flexibility, applying heat before physical therapy sessions or athletic participation can help you loosen up and can diminish your chances of injury or reinjury.

ALTERNATING HEAT/COLD THERAPIES

Some therapists recommend alternating heat and cold applications, which produces a pump-like effect that can break up painful muscle spasms. This therapy, originally derived from the contrast baths that naturopaths recommend, can be especially helpful for anyone with rheumatoid arthritis or reflex sympathetic dystrophy. It involves dipping the affected body region into a warm bath (105–110° F) for five minutes, then into a cold bath (50–60° F) for one to two minutes, and repeating the cycle for thirty minutes, ending with the cold application to minimize chances of soft-tissue swelling. If there is any initial swelling, once this has gone down, you can take a hot shower or soak the affected area in hot water, and then apply cold water for up to ten minutes.

CAUTIONS

- ❑ Don't stay in Jacuzzis more than twenty minutes at a time because you might get lightheaded or dizzy.
- ❑ Do not consume alcohol in Jacuzzis.
- ❑ Do not use heating pads for more than thirty minutes at a time. If they feel uncomfortably hot, put more towels between the pad and your skin.
- ❑ Heat is relaxing, so to avoid burning yourself, be careful not to fall asleep while using a hot pad.
- ❑ While heat can cause burns, cold may also be dangerous because it can cause frostbite. Do not apply ice directly to the skin.
- ❑ Do not use heat on acute injuries because it can increase swelling.
- ❑ Do not use heat if you have dermatitis or a skin irritation.

(*See also* HYDROTHERAPY in PART 2 Treatment Section.)

CLINICAL STUDIES

Nadler, SF, Steiner, DJ, Erasala, GN, et al. "Continuous low-level heat wrap therapy provides more efficacy than ibuprofen and acetaminophen for acute low back pain." *Spine.* 2002; 27:1012–1017.

As the title suggests, of the 371 people in this study, those using the heat wraps for lower back pain had significantly greater pain relief than those taking either of the two drugs.

Schlesinger, N, Detry, MA, Holland, BK, et al. "Local ice

therapy during bouts of acute gouty arthritis." *Journal of Rheumatology.* February 2002; 29(2):331–334.

This study of nineteen people at the University of Medicine and Dentistry of New Jersey showed that the group treated with ice had significantly greater reduction in pain compared to the control group. It was concluded that cold applications can be useful in the treatment of gouty arthritis.

Stitik, TP, Nadler, SF. "Sports Injuries: When and How to Use Cold Most Effectively." *Consultant.* December 1998, 2881–2890. (*See* insert:"Doctors' Perspective on Heat and Cold Therapy.")

Stitik, TP, Nadler, SF. " Sports Injuries: When and How to Apply the Heat." *Consultant.* January 1999, 144–157. (Ibid.)

Doctors' Perspective on Heat and Cold Therapy

The December 1998 and January 1999 issues of *Consultant* contain two articles discussing the uses of thermotherapy that were researched and written by Todd P. Stitik, MD, and Scott F. Nadler, DO. Both doctors are physiatrists and assistant professors in their respective specialties at the University of Medicine and Dentistry of New Jersey, in Newark.

"Part 1: When—and How—to Use Cold Most Effectively" listed different modalities, and compared the advantages and disadvantages of each in reducing inflammation and pain. Citing JD Loeser in a *Health Communications* publication, they list three ways that cold diminishes pain: first by slowing or blocking sensory nerve impulses on their way to the central nervous system (CNS); second by lessening muscle spasms which diminishes the pain; third by transmitting signals to the spinal cord that override pain impulses. This can be understood, they say, in terms of the gate theory of pain modulation (discussed in the introduction of this book). Drs. Stitik and Nadler say, in addition to its use for musculoskeletal injuries, cold acts as a direct analgesic for chronic pain conditions, perhaps by some of the mechanisms discussed above.

"Part 2: When—and How—to Apply the Heat" also listed the advantages and disadvantages of various heat modalities. They prefer moist heat over dry heat since they believe the moisture helps heat penetrate more deeply into muscle tissue. They postulate that heat relieves muscle spasms by several (still-unknown) mechanisms which activate pain-inhibiting systems: it overrides pain signals entering the spinal cord, and it acts to decrease pain perception in the brain. Their list of the benefits of heat includes an analgesic (painkilling) effect, decreased muscle spasms, and an enhanced metabolic rate. They caution against the prolonged use of heat, which can cause skin mottling and swelling, or the overuse of heating pads, which can lead to burns.

Drs. Stitik and Nadler believe in the importance of heat and cold modalities as effective methods of combating and controlling painful conditions, and this is what they impart to their patients.

Herbal Remedies

Herbalism is the use of berries, flowers, leaves, stems, and roots of plants to perform healing functions in the body. The botanical definition of an herb is a seed-producing annual, biennial, or perennial plant that does not develop woody tissue and dies down at the end of the growing season. There are more than 260,000 herbs classified as higher plants (those capable of photosynthesis) that have the potential to offer medical benefits, although only about 10 percent of these have been studied to date.

Many of today's familiar medications are isolated from herbal sources. Salicyclic acid, a precursor of aspirin, was derived from white willow bark, cinchona tree bark is the source of quinine, and digitalis, used for heart conditions, comes from the foxglove plant, for example.

THE HISTORY OF HERBAL REMEDIES

Herbal remedies have been used throughout history. In ancient China, doctors created manuals depicting the plants that were used for medicinal purposes, and a Chinese text from 2700 BC lists thirteen herbal prescriptions. The *Papyrus Ebers,* written in ancient Egypt in 1500 BC, contains references to more than 700 herbal remedies. In ancient Greece, Hippocrates, considered "the Father of Medicine," often used diet and herbs as the basis of his treatments, and later, Pedanius Dioscorides, also a Greek physician and pharmacologist, living in the latter part of the first century AD, compiled *De Materia Medica.* This herbal treatise described approximately 1000 drugs and remedies, and for the next 1500 years was considered the foremost authority in the West on botany and pharmacology. Herbs were also extensively used in the Roman Empire.

In 1649, Nicholas Culpepper wrote *A Physical Directory,* and a few years later he wrote *The English Physician,* an herbal pharmacopeia suitable for the lay-person to use. To this day, his manual is still referred to and widely quoted.

Herbal remedies were used for centuries, up to World War II and the advent of the new wonder drugs. After some decades of decline while drugs reigned supreme, herbal medicine is now regaining popularity because herbs are considered a safe, effective alternative to drugs with their potentially harmful side effects. Before antibiotics, the herb echinacea, in particular, was the treatment of choice for infections, and it is again coming to the fore as an impressive infection fighter without the undesirable side effects of antibiotics. Echinacea, which comes from the purple coneflower, is also an immune-system booster, aiding your immune system by stimulating production of the white blood cells necessary to fight disease.

HOW HERBAL REMEDIES WORK

While preventive herbal remedies do not provide the quick fix of most pharmaceutical medications, unlike drugs they *do* address the underlying conditions that cause problems. They work gently to help your body return to its natural state of well-being by strengthening its systems and organs. Garlic, for example, a popular culinary herb, has been used throughout the ages to effectively treat all kinds of infections, as well as respiratory ailments and high blood pressure.

Herbalism does not rely on one particular ingredient extracted from the plant. There is a synergistic interaction among all its ingredients. Although many pharmaceutical preparations have been developed from botanicals by isolating and synthesizing those parts of the plants thought to contain the medicinal properties, this differs from, and is considered by many not as effective as, using the herb in its whole form. The reasoning here is that the remaining unused active ingredients in an herb may be the very ones which give the plant its healing properties, or act as natural safeguards, working in harmony with its more powerful components and enabling the body to utilize the herb's natural balance of pharmacologically active compounds.

PAINFUL CONDITIONS THAT RESPOND WELL TO HERBAL REMEDIES

Herbal remedies are useful for both acute and chronic conditions. In this book, we are focusing on chronic conditions, all of which can be helped by herbal remedies. Refer to individual entries in Conditions Section for specific herbal treatments. (*See also* Quick Help Chart for synopsis of suggested treatments for all chronic pain conditions covered in this book.)

ADVANTAGES OF HERBAL REMEDIES

- ❑ Herbs have a cleansing effect.
- ❑ Herbs help normalize body functions.
- ❑ In some cases, herbs are actually more effective than conventional medication. For example, ginger has been shown to work better than dimenhydrinate (Dramamine) in preventing motion sickness, and saw palmetto is proven to be every bit as useful as many pharmaceuticals in treating enlarged prostate glands.

- ❑ Herbs help nourish your body and raise its energy level.
- ❑ Herbs strengthen your immune system, and encourage your body's natural healing mechanisms.
- ❑ Herbal remedies are gentle, effective, and inexpensive alternatives to conventional medications.
- ❑ Herbs can often be used in conjunction with conventional medication. (*See* Cautions below.)
- ❑ Herbs are safer than drugs, have fewer side effects, and are also less expensive than conventional medications.
- ❑ Herbal remedies work to eliminate the causes of symptoms, not just suppress them.

HOW TO USE HERBAL REMEDIES

You can buy the remedies in health food stores, some pharmacies, or on the Internet. Herbs are available in many forms: as the fresh or dried plants themselves; as tinctures and extracts in liquid form; as lozenges; as components of ointments and salves; and in capsules, tablets, and teas. Or you can make any of the following herbal remedies yourself.

- ❑ A cold extract. Add one to two ounces of the plant's parts to a pint of cold water and let the mixture stand for twelve hours.
- ❑ A decoction. Simmer half an ounce of plant parts in one cup of water for twenty to thirty minutes.
- ❑ An infusion (similar to tea). Pour one pint of boiling water over one-half to one ounce of plant parts and let it steep for ten minutes.
- ❑ A tea. For each cup of tea, steep a tablespoon or two of plant parts in one cup of boiling water.
- ❑ A tincture. Combine four ounces of a finely cut or powdered herb with one pint of brandy, gin, or vodka, cover the mixture tightly, and shake it several times a day for two weeks, then strain the liquid before you use it.

It is important to mention here that the whole herb plant is to be used for each of these methods above, as it is for all herbs discussed in the Conditions entries.

CAUTIONS

Some herbs have an anticoagulant effect and can keep your blood from clotting. While this may be beneficial for stroke or heart-attack prevention, if you are going to have surgery you should tell your doctor, who will likely tell you to stop taking the herbs for a week or two prior to the procedure. The doctor might question you about taking aspirin, NSAIDs, or Vitamin E, but be sure to also inform him or her if you are taking any anticoagulant herbs, such as feverfew, garlic, ginger, or ginkgo.

EPHEDRA—THE WHOLE PLANT

An herbal remedy that has been much in the news the past few years is a prime example of why it is important to use the whole herb plant rather than isolated individual elements taken from it. For centuries, ephedra, one of the best bronchodilators in the plant kingdom, has been extremely valuable for use with painful asthma and allergy conditions. And its thermogenic (heat-producing) qualities have also made it effective for weight loss.

Ephedra, the plant, is vastly safer than the two drugs isolated from it, ephedrine and pseudoephedrine, which can have negative cardiovascular effects (rapid heartbeat, palpitations, or worse), and their entry into the marketplace has caused unfair accusations against this beneficial whole herb plant, ephedra—that it is dangerous, which it is not—and it has now been taken off the market, which leaves people with nothing to alleviate their symptoms but drugs.

The confusion over what causes the harmful side effects exists because the manufacturers who isolate ephedrine have boosted it to dangerously high amounts, notably for their weight loss products. In the whole herb plant, ephedrine accounts for approximately 1 percent of the plant's substances, and each plant may contain up to 50 mg of ephedra, which yields .5 mg of ephedrine. By contrast, the manufactured herbal drug pills may each contain up to 20 mg of this isolated ephedrine, a vastly increased amount. At this level, it's small wonder that problems crop up, but they are with the *isolated herbal drug ephedrine*, not the whole herb plant ephedra, and this is a crucial difference to note.

It's also important to remember that all whole herb plants are foods and, as such, are taken into the body through its enzyme activity, whereas drugs, even herbal drugs, are not. And remember, too, that whole plants have built-in protective, balancing qualities, whereas drugs, even herbal drugs, do not.

If you are taking diuretic medications (for high blood pressure) along with herbs, particularly the stimulant herbal laxatives aloe, cascara sagrada, or senna, you may be depleting your body of potassium, which can lead to confusion, muscular weakness, and an irregular heartbeat.

You may be consuming herbs without realizing it, as many of them—cayenne, garlic, and ginger, for example—are also popular foods.

If you are allergic to ragweed, do not use chamomile tea because it is from the same family of plants.

Prolonged use of licorice can increase blood pressure.

Keep in mind that just because something is natural, it is not necessarily safe. Case in point—poison ivy.

CLINICAL STUDIES

In the United States, a lack of research funds delays FDA approval of herbal remedies. This underfunding is due to the fact that, since these remedies can't be patented, the drug companies have no financial incentive to invest large amounts of money into studying something that can easily be imitated by others. If, therefore, an herb has not made FDA approval, that does not mean it isn't safe or effective. Unfortunately, because the drug companies in the United States are not interested in spending money or time in botanical research, most current studies are only being done overseas, particularly in China, Germany, Russia, and Taiwan; and in a perverse Catch-22 situation, the FDA does not accept any findings from foreign studies.

Chrubasik, S, Eisenberg, E, Balan, E, et al. "Treatment of low back pain exacerbations with willow bark extract: A randomized double-blind study." *American Journal of Medicine*. 2000; 109:9–14.

In Germany, clinical trials were performed on willow bark extract to see how effective it was in treating low back pain. Results showed that both high (240 mg/day) and low (120 mg/day) doses gave significantly more relief than a placebo. Participants taking the higher dose noted significant pain relief after only one week.

Loch, E-G, Selle, H, Boblitz, N. "Treatment of premenstrual syndrome with a phytopharmaceutical formulation containing Vitex agnus castus." *Journal of Women's Health and Gender-Based Medicine*. 2000; 9(3):315–320.

In another German study, 93 percent of the female participants reported that their PMS symptoms either disappeared or decreased following treatment with vitex over the course of three menstrual cycles.

Piscoya, J, Rodriquez, Z, Bustamante, SA, et al. "Efficacy and safety of freeze-dried cat's claw in osteoarthritis of the knee: mechanisms of action of the species *Uncaria guianensis*." *Inflammation Research*. 2001; 50:442–448.

Cat's claw has long been a highly regarded treatment for chronic inflammation in South America. This four-week, placebo-controlled, double-blind Peruvian study, funded by grants from the National Institutes for Health, Bethesda, MD, clearly showed that cat's claw is an effective treatment for osteoarthritis of the knee, with the major benefits found in alleviating exercise-related pain.

Randall, C, Randall, H, Dobbs, F, et al. Randomized controlled trial of nettle sting for treatment of base of thumb pain. *Journal of the Royal Society of Medicine*. 2000; 93:305–309.

A small placebo-controlled study in Britain showed that daily application of fresh stinging nettle leaf (*urtica dioica*) was significantly more effective than a placebo in relieving osteoarthritis at the base of the thumb.

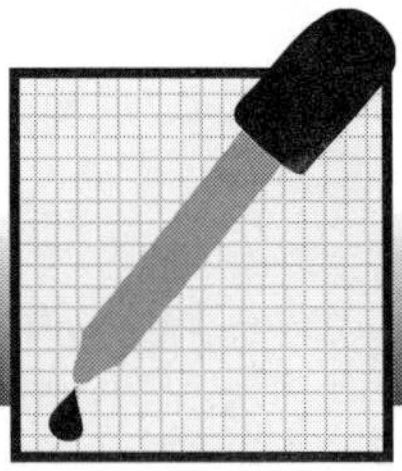

Homeopathy

The principle of homeopathy is to work with your symptoms, rather than suppress them, because symptoms are looked upon as your body's efforts to restore itself to health. The homeopathic approach, completely opposite to mainstream medicine, which treats most conditions with substances designed to suppress symptoms, is to treat by stimulating your body's own disease-fighting mechanisms. It does this by using extremely small doses of a substance that will trigger these mechanisms in order to allow them to do the healing. The word *homeopathy* comes from the Greek words *homoios,* which means *like,* and *pathos,* which means *suffering.*

THE HISTORY OF HOMEOPATHY

Unlike most natural therapies, homeopathy is a relative newcomer to the realm of naturopathic remedies. It began in the latter part of the eighteenth century when Dr. Samuel Hahnemann, a German physician, became frustrated with the medical practices then in vogue. Such methods as blistering, bloodletting, and purging were so horrifying to him that he left a successful medical practice to seek what he believed were safer ways to treat his patients.

One of Dr. Hahnemann's initial investigations focused on malaria treatment. He dosed himself with quinine, a drug used to treat malaria (quinine is still being used today) and noticed that he experienced the same malaria symptoms, chills and fever, that the drug was supposed to cure. In addition to testing his remedies on himself, Dr. Hahnemann also used his seven children as guinea pigs.

Since he believed in minimal intervention, he wanted to determine how small an amount of medication could be given to promote healing, so he began diluting his remedies. From these experiments, he formulated the basis for the two tenets of homeopathy—the Law of Similars and the Law of Infinitesimals, which are described fully in the following section.

Several doctors who had studied in Europe brought homeopathy to the United States in 1825, and for the rest of the nineteenth century, homeopathy was very popular in the United States. By the early part of the twentieth century, 40 percent of the doctors in the United States were homeopathic physicians, and there were more than a hundred homeopathic hospitals. Then, with the advent of antibiotics, regarded as wonder drugs, interest in homeopathy waned, especially in the United States. Another reason for its decline was the growing power of the American Medical Association, the AMA. Homeopathic facilities could not receive accreditation from the AMA and were forced to close. But, since many of the remedies were already being used before the AMA insisted on rigorous drug testing, they were grandfathered into their regulations. Interestingly, and probably because of their pre-AMA use, even though the FDA does regulate the manufacture of homeopathic *drug* remedies, they are available without a prescription.

In the middle 1980s, when the so-called wonder drugs began to demonstrate harmful side effects and overall flaws in their effectiveness, the circle came round again to an interest in natural remedies, and mainstream medical journals began publishing studies supporting homeopathy. In the three-year period from 1988 to 1991, sales of homeopathic remedies grew from $11 million to $150 million, and by 1996, sales had reached $227 million and were increasing by 12 percent a year. In 1970, there were 200 homeopathic practitioners in the United States, and 3,000 by 1996. Many conventional physicians also practice homeopathy, but a homeopathic practitioner does not have to be a medical doctor.

HOW HOMEOPATHY WORKS

Homeopathy works with your symptoms to cure your condition. Its fundamental principle is that symptoms are your body's efforts to heal disease. The use of extremely diluted amounts of a substance that, in a more concentrated form would make you sick, encourages your body to bring its own defenses to the rescue.

Immunizations and allergy shots are two types of conventional treatments that are similar to homeopathy, and both are given in small amounts to stimulate your body's immune response. Immunizations help protect your body from a disease that would result from exposure to a large amount of the offending substance. Allergy shots supply small amounts of an allergy-triggering substance to encourage your body to develop tolerance to larger amounts of the allergen.

The Law of Similars states that like cures like. If a substance produces debilitating symptoms in a healthy person, then a small dose of that substance could be used to treat the same symptoms in a person who is ill.

The Law of Infinitesimals states that the more a remedy is diluted, the stronger it will be. This concept is very difficult for most lay people and researchers to understand because it goes against most laws of physics and chemistry. Homeopathic remedies are prepared by diluting the active ingredient in water or alcohol, shaking it, diluting it again and shaking it again. This process is done repeatedly. Opponents of homeopathy say there is not enough of the original remedy left to do any good, while those who are believers say the shaking process triggers the effects of the original substance, creating an electrochemical pattern that remains in the diluted solution, and when the remedy is ingested, it gets circulated throughout the system via the water in the body.

PAINFUL CONDITIONS THAT RESPOND WELL TO HOMEOPATHY

Homeopathy is useful for all the conditions discussed in this book. Refer to individual entries for suggested remedies. (*See also* Quick Help Chart for synopsis of suggested treatments for all chronic pain conditions covered in this book.)

ADVANTAGES OF HOMEOPATHY

- ❑ The remedies have no side effects.
- ❑ They activate the immune system without causing any negative reactions.
- ❑ They are easy to use.
- ❑ They are available without a prescription.
- ❑ They work well for all kinds of ailments.
- ❑ They are very inexpensive. The average cost for a remedy is about $6.
- ❑ Your body will use only the amount of medicine it actually needs.

HOW TO USE HOMEOPATHY

You can visit a homeopathic practitioner who will design a program specifically for you, or you can self-treat. The remedies are available by mail order, through the Internet, at health food stores, and over the counter at many pharmacies. If you visit a practitioner, she or he will tell you how to take the suggested remedies. If you elect to self-treat, just read the label, which will tell you what it contains, the type of condition it helps, and how to use it. Most of the time the remedies are placed under your tongue, and you should take them at least ten minutes before or after eating or brushing your teeth. The preparations are available in various strengths (X, C, or M, which are the Roman numerals for 10, 100 and 1000). Those with lower numbers and the letter X indicate lower dosages. It helps to read the label, which tells you what the remedy contains, the types of conditions it is useful for, and directions as to its proper use.

MIGRAINE-FREE AT LAST

Following three years of unsuccessful conventional treatment, David M, a fifty-five-year-old man, was referred to Glasgow Homeopathic Hospital for his severe migraines that would start with nausea and be followed by vomiting every hour for twelve hours, during which time he also experienced a relentless throbbing pain on the left side of his head. A homeopathic physician at the hospital, who also had extensive experience in the diagnosis and treatment of headache disorders, consulted with David and prescribed a single homeopathic remedy, *bronia,* which completely and immediately reduced his pain and nausea. In a follow-up visit two months later, David reported that he had taken the *bronia* for three weeks (ie. twelve doses), was still headache-free, and had lost no further time from work. Thanks to homeopathy, he has remained attack-free for three years and counting, and now leads a migraine-free life.

CAUTIONS

Although homeopathic remedies have a high safety factor and work *with,* rather than against, your body, they are not a substitute for conventional medical treatment when in a life-threatening situation.

CLINICAL STUDIES

Even though homeopathy challenges orthodox medical thinking, of all the natural remedies, it is the one that can best be tested by controlled studies.

Fisher, P, Greenwood, A, Huskisson, EC. "Effect of Homoeopathic Treatment on Fibrositis." *British Medical Journal*. August 5, 1989; 299:365–366.

This double-blind British study comparing rhus toxicodendron to a placebo showed tender spots were reduced by 25 percent when test subjects were given the homeopathic medicine, as compared to those given the placebo.

Kleijnen, J, Knipschild, P, ter Riet, G. et al. "Clinical Trials of Homeopathy." *British Medical Journal*. February 9, 1991; 302:316–323.

Another British study reviewing more than 100 studies of homeopathic medicine showed positive effects in 77 percent of them. The researchers concluded that the evidence presented in the review would probably be sufficient for establishing homeopathy as a regular treatment for certain indications.

Linde, K, Clausius, N, Ramirez, G, et al. "Are the Clinical Effects of Homeopathy Placebo Effects? A Meta-analysis of Placebo-Controlled Trials." *The Lancet.* September 20, 1997; 350:834–843.

An article in the prestigious British medical showed that people taking homeopathic medicines were 2.45 times more likely to experience a positive therapeutic effect than those taking a placebo.

Shealy, CN, Thomlinson, RP, Borgmeyer, V. "Osteoarthritic Pain: A Comparison of Homeopathy and Acetaminophen." *American Journal of Pain Management.* 1998; 8:89–91.

A double-blind American study comparing homeopathic remedies with acetaminophen in the treatment of osteoarthritis concluded that homeopathic treatments were safe and at least as effective as acetaminophen, without its potential side effects of possible liver or kidney damage.

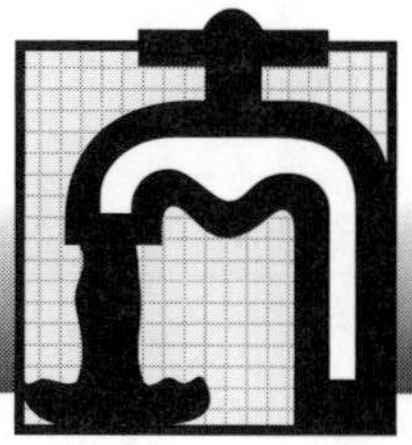

Hydrotherapy

Hydrotherapy is the use of all three forms of water (liquid, steam, and ice) to treat what ails you. Its name is derived from *Hydro,* the Greek word for water and there are two main therapeutic water methods. Hydrotherapy refers to the passive method, and aquatic therapy is the active method. Passive therapy involves relaxing in a warm or hot bath or shower, a Jacuzzi, or alternating hot and cold, a method known as contrast hydrotherapy, while in active therapy, exercises are performed in water, often under the supervision of a physical therapist. (Discussed separately in PHYSICAL THERAPY entry in PART 2 Treatment Section.) Both methods can be effective for the same condition.

THE HISTORY OF HYDROTHERAPY

Water-based treatments are as old as humans but, ironically, these effective natural therapies, which have been used since before recorded history, have to be rediscovered in each era. One of the first written mentions of water as medicine came in Greece, well before Hippocrates. In his time, the "Father of Medicine," stressed its importance as a therapeutic tool to treat illnesses and injuries, and in the second century, the physician Galen advocated specific baths as an integral part of his remedies. In ancient Rome, cold baths reputedly cured the Emperor Augustus of a mysterious disease that had not responded to any other remedies, and after that, cold baths, and water therapy in general, became a part of Roman social life.

In the early nineteenth century, an Austrian farmer, Vincent Priessnitz, rediscovered hydrotherapy for his time after several severe injuries of his had been successfully treated with cold compresses. He learned about the power of water healing firsthand, understood its power, and laid the foundation of today's water therapy by developing an entire therapeutic system of treatment. He eventually incorporated his therapies into the spa he opened in his village of Grafenberg, now a part of the Czech Republic.

Father Sebastian Kneipp of Bavaria, a priest who had benefited greatly from water therapy, believed in Pressnitz's treatments, and wherever natural spring water was available in Europe, spas were built where he developed innovative procedures. Under his aegis, water therapy became truly international, and now, spas incorporating hydrotherapy methods have spread out from Europe and are becoming increasingly popular all over the world. In Europe and the United States (where spas have gone from being vacation spots in the late nineteenth/early twentieth century, to luxury resorts today), hydrotherapy treatments are covered by most insurance companies.

"Taking the waters," as it used to be known, is still a popular activity in such places as Saratoga Springs in upstate New York, or the many natural hot springs (thermal spas) in California, Colorado, and other parts of the Western United States. Franklin D. Roosevelt used hot springs to ease the effects of his polio, and a number of people have reported miraculous healings after soaking in the Dead Sea in Israel. Hydrotherapy equipment is now everywhere—in health clubs, schools, gyms, offices of physical therapists and mental health specialists, and rehabilitation facilities—and spa staples, such as hot tubs, saunas, and whirlpool baths, are routinely installed in private homes.

HOW HYDROTHERAPY WORKS

Hydrotherapy works by conducting heat into or out of the body. The goal of the therapy is to improve the circulation and quality of blood so that healing nutrients can be effectively delivered, and toxins, which cause tissue and organ degeneration, can be removed. Hydrotherapy is regularly and successfully used, among other things, to alleviate muscular tension and the pain and swelling of injuries, eliminate fever, improve the function of the immune system, and reduce stress. Alternating hot and cold applications of water, a method known as constitutional, or contrast, hydrotherapy, first expands the blood vessels, allowing more blood to flow in, and then constricts them, forcing the blood to move on to other parts of the body, in the process improving circulation.

When water is applied to one part of the body, its other parts are similarly stimulated due to a reflex action. For example, if one foot is broken and in a cast, the other foot can have the alternating hot and cold therapy and the incapacitated foot will reap the benefits of the treatment, a method that, applied to the feet, also works for the sinuses or the throat, according to Dr. Cathy Rogers, ND, whose specialty as a naturopath is hydrotherapy.

PAINFUL CONDITIONS THAT RESPOND WELL TO HYDROTHERAPY

❑ Achilles tendonitis.

❑ Back pain.

Whirlpool Success

Dana, a sixteen-year-old high school student, sprained her ankle playing basketball. Fortunately, her school's new athletic center had a stainless whirlpool tub in the training room, and the trainer had her do hydrotherapy in it until the swelling went down. For ten minutes at a time, several times a week, Dana sat on the metal seat of the short tub, with her right ankle positioned under the high-pressure faucet as icy jets of water were applied to it. Although the therapy was very numbing, the pain did subside, and it became easier for Dana to walk on that ankle. She still feels a twinge when playing basketball, but says it is minor, she can play through it, and is just grateful that the proper treatment with water kept her acute problem from becoming acute chronic.

- ❑ Bursitis.
- ❑ Carpal tunnel syndrome.
- ❑ Fibromyalgia.
- ❑ Frozen shoulder.
- ❑ Gout.
- ❑ Neuroma.
- ❑ Osteoarthritis.
- ❑ Peripheral neuropathy.
- ❑ Phantom pain.
- ❑ Plantar fasciitis.
- ❑ Postherpetic neuralgia.
- ❑ Post-polio syndrome.
- ❑ Reflex sympathetic dystrophy syndrome (RSDS).
- ❑ Rheumatoid arthritis.
- ❑ Rotator cuff tendonitis.
- ❑ Sciatica.
- ❑ Tarsal tunnel syndrome.
- ❑ Tennis elbow.
- ❑ Trigger finger.

Other conditions that respond well to hydrotherapy include: severe burns (burn victims should soak in 93° water for long periods of time to remove dead skin and help prevent loss of body heat), cerebral palsy, and fever.

ADVANTAGES OF HYDROTHERAPY

- ❑ It is readily available, inexpensive, easy to learn and perform, and can be done at home.
- ❑ It is painless, with no harmful side effects.
- ❑ It is almost always a pleasurable experience, and often improves emotional and psychological well-being.
- ❑ It helps to support body weight by reducing the effect of gravity, thereby taking pressure off your joints and putting less stress on the body in general.
- ❑ It increases the range of motion.
- ❑ It increases circulation, and allows more oxygen to reach the muscles.
- ❑ The resistance of the water helps strengthen muscles.
- ❑ The water's hydrostatic pressure helps reduce swelling.
- ❑ It is also a useful tool for treating animals with musculoskeletal problems.

HOW TO USE HYDROTHERAPY

Hydrotherapy can be used in pools, spas, and natural mineral springs. Or you can soak in a Jacuzzi, a hot tub, or a bathtub filled with diluted aromatherapy oils or herbs. A hot bath or shower increases blood flow to the surface of the skin, and can also relax you, lower stress, and draw out toxins. A cold bath or shower reduces blood flow to an injured area, which can help reduce inflammation and pain there, and can also energize and stimulate you. A coldwater rinse can boost your immune system and improve blood flow. Immersing your feet and ankles in hot water for ten to thirty minutes can draw blood from inflamed areas of your body, and sitz baths covering your body from the waist down can powerfully affect your abdominal and pelvic organs.

If you visit a naturopath, he or she may recommend constitutional (contrast) hydrotherapy, which increases the immune system's functioning and promotes health in general. This treatment, consisting of a sequence of hot, then cold towels applied to your chest and back, is slightly more complicated than other hydrotherapy methods, but it is considered highly effective for most conditions, including arthritis, and painful digestive and pelvic problems.

According to Dr. Rogers, spas in Europe have MDs who receive an additional three years of training in balneology (bathing) and rehabilitation. These physicians prescribe specific waters for bathing (high calcium, high sulphur, etc.) and tell which to use for which condition. The waters in Europe are generally high in carbon dioxide, she says, and the mineral-water baths are applied at a neutral temperature to assure that the CO_2 remains in contact with the body. For pain conditions, such as fibromyalgia, arthritis, or psoriatic arthritis, brine baths (salt or seawater) are used, again at neutral temperature. Additionally, for painful conditions, such as arthritis, they use carbon dioxide gas baths, and subcutaneous injections of CO_2 as well, the idea here being to stimulate oxygenation. Peat baths are also used extensively. The peat (mud) is anti-inflammatory and is usually applied in baths or compresses. Combinations of these treatments are used daily over a four-week period of time and are typically paid for by government insurance.

Dr. Rogers continues that, "From a naturopathic perspective, toxicity is a major contributor to congestion and inflammation—and therefore pain." In her month-long cleanse class at her Chico Water Cure Spa on Puget Sound, she regularly sees a reduction of joint pain, back pain, and headaches from using techniques that include contrast showers, brine baths at neutral temperatures, and other water therapies.

CAUTIONS

- ❑ Be sure the water is neither too hot nor too cold.
- ❑ Do not consume alcohol.
- ❑ If you have peripheral vascular disease or diabetes, you should avoid sitz baths. There can be a loss of peripheral sensation or even unconsciousness.
- ❑ If you have an acute bladder infection, it is best to avoid constitutional hydrotherapy treatments.
- ❑ If you have hypertension, you should be cautious about using hot tubs, saunas, and steam baths, which can raise blood pressure.
- ❑ Hot tubs should be well maintained to guard against harmful microorganisms, mold, and yeast.

(*See also* AROMATHERAPY, HEAT THERAPY/COLD THERAPY, HERBAL REMEDIES, and Water Aerobics in EXERCISE, STRETCHING, and SPORTS, in PART 2 Treatment Section.)

CLINICAL STUDIES

Hashkes, PJ. "Beneficial effect of climatic therapy on inflammatory arthritis at Tiberias Hot Springs." *Scandinavian Journal of Rheumatology.* 2002; 31(3):172–177.

One hundred thirty-six Swedish men and women with inflammatory arthritis underwent four weeks of therapy at the Tiberias Hot Springs in Israel and, when examined at the conclusion of the study, most showed significant benefit from the therapy. Long-term follow-up was recommended.

Konrad, K, Tatrai, T, Hunka, A, et al. "Controlled trial of balneotherapy in treatment of low back pain." *Annals of Rheumatic Disease.* June 1992;51(6):820–822.

The National Institute of Rheumatology and Physiotherapy in Budapest, Hungary conducted a four-week study on 158 people to determine the effectiveness of this type of hydrotherapy. Balneotherapy, underwater traction bath, and underwater massage all equally improved the non-specific lumbar pain, it was found, and all test subjects undergoing these therapies were less reliant on analgesics (painkillers) at four weeks. After one year, the analgesic consumption of this group was significantly lower than for the control group, which had not undergone the three forms of hydrotherapy.

Kristof, O, Gatzen, M, Hellenbrecht, D, et al. "Analgesic effect of the serial application of a sulfurated mud bath at home." *Forsch Komplementarmed Klass Naturheilkd.* October 2000; 7(5):233–236.

This randomized, controlled Swiss study of twenty-five people with back pain was divided into two groups. In a two-week period, thirteen people took six sulfurated mud baths, and twelve people took six tap-water baths. After the final bath, the group taking the mud baths had a greater reduction in pain intensity than the control group, suggesting a significantly stronger anal-

SHOWER THERAPY

Andrea's hip replacement—the end result of a running injury mistreated, first, by a podiatrist, then by a chiropractor who actually dislocated the hip with a too-forceful outward rotation—was very successful and gave her no trouble at all, but an unexpected side effect left her with chronically stiff, sore muscles in her upper right leg, and an accompanying pain that traveled down to her right ankle. Determined to stop favoring that side, Andrea began stretching and flexing her seized-up leg and her ankle under hot running shower water every day. Because the muscles were so out of use, the stretching was extremely painful at first, but she persevered, and eventually the daily therapy with the hot water succeeded in loosening the stiffness. For the first time in years, Andrea was able to go through her day with a flexible, pain-free gait, no longer listing to the right as she walked.

In light of recent findings that doing yoga stretches in excessive heat can be counterproductive, this moderate exposure to hot water can provide exactly the right balance for relaxing and stretching the muscles.

gesic (painkilling) effect from taking the sulfurated mud baths than from taking the plain tap-water baths.

Mannerkorpi, K, Ahlmen, M, Ekdahl, C. "Six-and 24-month follow-up of pool exercise therapy and education for patients with fibromyalgia." *Scandinavian Journal of Rheumatology.* 2002; 31(5):306–310.

This Swedish study followed twenty-six people with fibromyalgia at six- and twenty-four month intervals after they had completed a program of pool exercise therapy and education based on their health problems. The study found that, two years later, all twenty-six still showed improvements in the severity of their symptoms, and in their physical and social functioning.

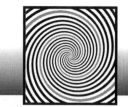

Hypnosis

The term hypnosis is derived from the Greek word *hypnos*, which means sleep. It refers to a trance-like state resembling, but not the same as, sleep, and it can either be self-induced or induced by a hypnotherapist. Hypnosis is an altered state of awareness in which you are susceptible to suggestions (some consider both guided meditation and guided imagery and visualization to be forms of hypnosis). In 1958, the American Medical Association accepted clinical hypnosis as an adjunct to standard medical care in the United States.

THE HISTORY OF HYPNOSIS

From ancient times right up through the middle ages, it was believed that evil spirits were the cause of disease. In order to expel these spirits, healers would use prayers and rituals to put people into trance-like states, and then give them something to eat or drink and suggest this would help the problem. Mind over matter being what it is, it did help in many cases.

In the late eighteenth century, Franz Anton Mesmer, a German physician who believed that human bodies contained a magnetic fluid affected by the planets, developed a theory about the magnetic influence of the planets on health. He tied groups of people together in tubs filled with iron filings and, touching them with a glass rod, "magnetized" them, after which many exhibited hysterical behaviors that he interpreted as spirit possession. While in this possessed state, Mesmer gave them suggestions that were often curative, an effect he named mesmerism, and claimed that these cures were transferred from him through his rod. He was eventually declared a fraud and it was determined that his *cures* came from the imaginations of the people he touched with a glass rod, not magnetism. To this day the term mesmerism is associated with hypnotism.

After Mesmer was discredited, many doctors using hypnosis were called quacks; some even lost their licenses and were considered blasphemous. But hypnotism was still used after that in many parts of the world, notably as a form of anesthesia. In a prison hospital in India in the mid-nineteenth century, where 3,000 surgical procedures were performed using hypnotism, the mortality rate dropped from almost 50 percent to 5 percent. This phenomenon—that when hypnosis is used for anesthesia, the subconscious mind helps the body fight infection—is still being studied today.

In the latter part of the nineteenth century, hypnosis was studied by prominent neurologists, among them Sigmund Freud, and was well on its way to becoming a legitimate medical practice. In the twentieth century, following World Wars I and II, hypnosis was used to treat shell shock, (now referred to as posttraumatic stress disorder), but it was not until its 1958 acceptance by the AMA that hypnosis finally achieved its long-sought respect from the medical profession. Presently, in addition to its wide-ranging use in therapy, hypnosis is being taught as an elective in many medical, dental, and nursing schools.

HOW HYPNOSIS WORKS

Although shown to be effective in tests, the exact mechanisms for the effectiveness of hypnosis are not known. Research to determine its effectiveness in pain control is ongoing, and following are some of the theories developed to date.

- ❑ Pain becomes observed rather than felt.
- ❑ When you concentrate on something else, it keeps you from becoming aware of the pain.
- ❑ The hypnotic state promotes a deep sense of relaxation that alleviates stress, which contributes to pain.
- ❑ The trance-like state, which is similar to daydreaming, makes you respond to suggestions—you become more susceptible to them when your level of awareness changes.

PAINFUL CONDITIONS THAT RESPOND WELL TO HYPNOSIS

Hypnosis is useful for managing many types of chronic pain, including those listed here.

- ❑ Back pain.
- ❑ Cluster headaches.
- ❑ Crohn's disease.
- ❑ Diverticulitis.
- ❑ Irritable bowel syndrome.
- ❑ Migraine headaches.
- ❑ Phantom pain.
- ❑ Sciatica.
- ❑ Tension headaches.
- ❑ Ulcerative colitis.

It is also helpful with such acutely painful conditions as burns, cancer (and the painful side effects of chemotherapy), and childbirth. Other conditions and areas where hypnosis can help include addictions, allergies, anxiety, bleeding control, depression, eating disorders, enhancing athletic performance, insomnia, over-coming stage fright, skin problems, stress reduction, smoking cessation, post-traumatic stress disorder, and weight loss.

Hypnotic suggestion has been used to cure warts (an example of how hypnosis may actually effect cures, not just alleviate pain). And, as noted above, hypnosis has also been useful as an anesthesia for surgical and dental procedures.

ADVANTAGES OF HYPNOSIS

❑ Hypnosis is safer and has far fewer side effects than prescribed pain medications and over-the-counter NSAIDs.

❑ Many pregnant women trained in self-hypnosis have been able to avoid epidurals during delivery.

HOW HYPNOSIS IS USED

To explain an altered state, think of a time you were reading something on a bus or train and became so immersed in it that you missed your stop. Or, after finishing an activity, you noticed you were bleeding and could not recall cutting yourself. That state of extreme concentration (or being zoned-out) is similar to what occurs under hypnosis.

Many people have a fear of being hypnotized because they believe they may lose control of themselves and behave in an embarrassing manner, reveal secrets, or not come out of the trance state. These are all misconceptions, often based on movie depictions or stage acts.

Your clinician might direct you to use particular visualization techniques, such as those described in the entry on guided imagery and visualization, while you are under hypnosis.

It is believed that hypnosis is really self-hypnosis and that the hypnotist is merely there as a guide to help access a hypnotic state. To use self-hypnosis for pain control, start by using relaxation techniques, such as deep breathing and imagining that you are on a beach or in a similarly serene place. Then concentrate on making your hand cold or numb and transfer that feeling to the painful area (this crossover into a visualization technique only points up how interrelated many mind-control techniques are).

Although it is possible to teach yourself hypnosis techniques, it is a good idea to have a practitioner guide you through the steps the first time.

CAUTIONS

Be sure your hypnotist is well trained. It is a good idea to seek a referral from your healthcare practitioner, psychologist, dentist, or any acquaintances who have had positive experiences with hypnosis.

Tapes to assist with self-hypnosis are available, but be sure to check the credentials of the person who recorded them.

(*See also* GUIDED IMAGERY and VISUALIZATION in PART 2 Treatment Section.)

CLINICAL STUDIES

Spiegel, D, Bierre, P, Rootenberg, J. "Hypnotic alteration of somatosensory perception." *The American Journal of Psychiatry*. 1989; 146(6):749–754.

In this study of twenty people, the ten who were highly hypnotizable were able to reduce or eliminate their pain with cognitive methods such as hypnosis, which suggests it has a physiological basis.

Palsson, OS, Turner, MJ, Johnson, DA, et al. "Hypnosis treatment for severe irritable bowel syndrome: investigation of mechanism and effects on symptoms." *Digestive Diseases and Sciences*. November 2002; 47(11):2605–2614.

In both studies done here, hypnosis was found to improve the painful symptoms of irritable bowel syndrome (IBS).

Simon, EP, Lewis, DM. "Medical hypnosis for temporomandibular disorders: treatment efficacy and medical utilization outcome." *Oral Surgery, Oral Medicine, Oral Pathology, Oral Radiology, and Endodontics*. July 2000; 90(1):54–63.

Twenty-eight people in this study reported a significant decrease in pain frequency, duration, and intensity with hypnosis treatments. It was concluded that medical hypnosis was an effective treatment for this disorder, in terms of reducing both symptoms and reliance on medicine.

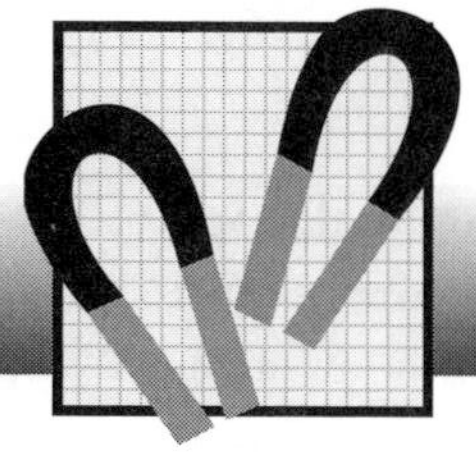

Magnet Therapy

Magnet therapy is a method of reducing pain and healing humans and animals with magnets. Considered by some to be just another new age fad, magnet therapy burst onto the contemporary scene in the early 1990s when several prominent sports figures attested to its healing powers. Golfer Jim Colbert says he wears a magnetic belt whenever he has a game to play because it relieves his back pain. Baseball great, outfielder Hank Aaron, and the former New York Yankees pitcher, Hideki Irabu, have both endorsed magnet therapy because it helps to energize and recharge them, as it does with the Miami Dolphins football team who all sit on a magnetic bench.

THE HISTORY OF MAGNET THERAPY

Actually, there is nothing new about magnetic therapy. Its curative powers were known and used far back in antiquity, in Egypt, India and China. In Greece, Hippocrates, considered "the Father of Medicine," used magnets to alleviate pain. And in the sixth century AD, magnets were used by Alexander of Talles to treat arthritis, with positive results.

The name *magnet* originated in ancient Greece when, according to legend, a shepherd named Magnes felt the iron tip of his staff being pulled by a large rock lying on the path. For some unknown reason, possibly superstition, he got the inspired idea to insert pieces of the rock into the soles of his sandals, after which, it was said, he was able to walk long distances without getting tired. Seeing how beneficial this was, the other shepherds named the powerful rock the "stone of Magnes."

Even Plato was fascinated by the phenomenon, and in the fourth century BC he performed an experiment. He suspended a line of five iron rings from a single magnet in order to prove that magnets had a powerful force that could be transmitted from ring to ring.

The French played a leading role in magnet therapy research, starting in the eighteenth century. A priest, cleric Abbé Le Noble, investigated the healing power of magnets at the request of the Royal Society of Medicine, and submitted his findings to them in 1777. The French have continued to play a leading role in investigating the healing powers of magnets to this day, as magnet research has expanded and is being conducted worldwide.

Magnet therapy has been used for treating various types of pain. The term itself was coined in the late 1870s by a researcher named Benedict who studied the pain-relieving effects of magnets, first noted a hundred years before by another French researcher, Pierre Borel.

In the 1940s, Russian army doctors used magnets to alleviate the pain suffered by amputees.

In the 1950s, Japanese researchers demonstrated that magnetic bracelets alleviated shoulder pain. In Japan today, magnets are in wide popular use, individually and in necklaces and bracelets. And more formally, the pain-relieving use of magnets in acupuncture is catching on there.

In the 1970s, magnetic necklaces and rings were used for shoulder stiffness after double-blind studies showed their effectiveness.

Work with magnets progressed rapidly in the 1980s and many research results proved their effectiveness, including studies that showed the painkilling properties of the south poles of magnets in the treatment of shoulder, and other, joint inflammation.

Magnet therapy is now being used by orthopedic surgeons to treat many painful conditions that would formerly have required surgery, and its use in sports medicine has been widely noted.

In recent years, there have been 140 million dollars worth of magnets sold annually as medical products, in the U.S. alone.

HOW MAGNET THERAPY WORKS

Magnets produce electromagnetic waves that penetrate tissue and help restore normal electrical activity to injured or diseased body areas. They promote cellular activity by speeding up electromagnetic exchanges between the interior and exterior of cells, which improves circulation to the site of pain. The electrolytes in your blood pass through the magnetic field, creating a current that can be directed by the magnet.

Magnets act to decrease pain by their direct action on the nerve fibers below the skin that transmit the pain signals to the brain. They generate electric fields in your body that help increase blood flow and stimulate nerve cells. They also increase the output of endorphins, the chemical substances produced in your brain that act as your body's natural painkillers.

The healing power in magnets is the result of their ability to restore normal polarity in diseased parts of the body. Magnets have a north and south pole with different characteristics. The north pole has a negative charge and a relaxing effect. It is this negative charge that disperses blocked energy, makes nerves less sensitive, and causes muscles to return to a normal tension level. The south pole has a positive charge and is known for its painkilling and anti-inflammatory properties.

When normal electrical activity is restored to injured or diseased body areas, the blood vessels dilate, increasing blood flow and the ability to attract more oxygen. In addition to their pain-relieving capabilities, magnets also have a positive effect on bones and joints. They change the migration of calcium ions to heal painful broken bones faster. They can move calcium away from arthritic joints and attract iron in the blood to stimulate circulation. They also relax muscles and improve capillary action.

Although there is a continuing mystery surrounding magnetism and exactly *why* magnets are such effective pain relievers and healers, we do know that they work on the cellular level. As Dr. Richard Broeringmeyer, a chiropractor and nutritionist who researches and practices magnet therapy says, "The energy of the magnet is the energy of the universe, and we can find this energy in the cells of our body." He adds, "Life is not possible without electromagnetic fields, and optimum health is not possible if the electromagnetic fields are out of balance for long periods of time. Magnetic energy is nature's energy in perfect balance."

PAINFUL CONDITIONS THAT RESPOND WELL TO MAGNET THERAPY

- ❑ Achilles tendonitis.
- ❑ Back, neck, and shoulder pain.
- ❑ Bursitis.
- ❑ Carpal tunnel syndrome.
- ❑ Cluster headache.
- ❑ Dental pain.
- ❑ Fibromyalgia.
- ❑ Migraine headaches.
- ❑ Osteoarthritis.
- ❑ Post-polio syndrome.
- ❑ Reflex sympathetic dystrophy syndrome (RSDS).
- ❑ Rheumatoid arthritis.
- ❑ Sciatica.
- ❑ Sports injuries.
- ❑ Tarsal tunnel syndrome.
- ❑ Temporomandibular joint (TMJ) pain.
- ❑ Tennis elbow.
- ❑ Tension headaches.
- ❑ Trigger finger.

Studies have also shown magnet therapy to be effective with cancer, diabetes, chest pain, fractures, postoperative pain, sprains, and wound treating and healing.

ADVANTAGES OF MAGNET THERAPY

- ❑ It is non-toxic.
- ❑ It alleviates pain and strengthens the whole body by rebalancing magnetic currents in the body.
- ❑ It reduces inflammation by helping to constrict blood vessels.
- ❑ Even though there are specific conditions listed above that respond well to magnet therapy, it can be easily used on *all parts of the body* with no discomfort.
- ❑ Magnets are non-invasive. They can be taped on, worn in your shoes, or worn as jewelry.
- ❑ Magnetic discs can be applied for long periods of time with no ill effects. (See note in Cautions.)
- ❑ Magnets do not have to be set with strict precision since the electromagnetic field affects a large area.
- ❑ Even unskilled people can treat themselves.
- ❑ Magnets can enhance other methods of treatment.
- ❑ They can reduce the amount of pain medication.
- ❑ They often alleviate pain rapidly.
- ❑ There is no problem of tolerance.
- ❑ They reduce swelling.
- ❑ They relieve pain, accelerate healing, and reduce inflammation.
- ❑ They are easily portable for emergency use in such conditions as toothaches, sprains, strains, etc.
- ❑ They are non-intrusive and unlikely to do any harm.

If your doctor or dentist isn't open to magnet therapy, you can apply magnets yourself since they don't react with other forms of treatment.

HOW TO USE MAGNETS

You can see a professional if you want to, but it is very easy to self-treat with magnets. They come in different shapes and sizes and all you have to do is place one magnet on the affected area and secure it with a velcro strap. The effect can be increased by placing more magnets over corresponding acupuncture and reflexology points.

Buy magnetic products with a rating of at least 500 gausses (the measurement of a magnet's strength, named for Carl F. Gauss, 1777–1855, a German scientist who wrote a number of important papers on magnetism and electromagnetism). You might be tempted to use refriger-

Magnets Help Save a Career

Ricard was an up-and-coming woodcarver whose work was starting to be shown in some top art galleries. Working at top speed to achieve his goal of making a living from his sculpting so he could quit his job as a furniture salesman, Ricard developed excruciating pains in his shoulder from his repetitive use of the carving tools.

Anti-inflammatories gave him some relief, but when he developed internal bleeding, he was briefly hospitalized for blood transfusions. His doctor told him he would probably need to have a shoulder replacement, but while he was undergoing preoperative testing, he was offered a major commission for a new church being built in New York. Since he couldn't pass up this once-in-a-lifetime opportunity, he asked his surgeon if it would be possible to postpone the surgery. Fortunately, the surgeon was open to alternatives and recommended that Ricard try taping magnets to his shoulder area and, at the same time, have a physical therapist observe him carving in order to determine the best way for him to hold his tools and minimize the shoulder trauma that his incorrect movements had caused.

Thanks to the combination of these two therapies, Ricard finished the commission and has been receiving more and more offers. Although not completely pain-free, he has had so much relief that he has been able to continue his woodcarving, and has postponed the surgery indefinitely.

ator magnets, but with only 10 gausses they wouldn't be much help.

CAUTIONS

It is not advisable for pregnant women to use magnetic products since it is not known what effect they may have on the fetus.

If you wear a pacemaker, there is a possibility that strong magnets could interrupt its operation.

Do not place strong magnets over your heart or aorta, near your eyes, or on your neck or head for extended periods of time because these are sensitive areas that require further studies for the use of magnet therapy.

CLINICAL STUDIES

Alfano, AP, Taylor, AG, Foresman, PA, et al. "Static magnetic fields for treatment of fibromyalgia: a randomized controlled study." *Journal of Alternative Complementary Medicine*. February 2001; 7(1):53–64.

This six-month trial of adults with fibromyalgia showed greater improvement in the pain intensity level of those exposed to magnetic fields than those in the control groups.

Brown, CS, Ling, FW, Wan, JY, et al. "Efficacy of static magnetic field therapy in chronic pelvic pain: a double-blind pilot study." *American Journal of Obstetric Gynecology*. December 2002; 187(6):1581–1587.

When applied continuously for four weeks, static magnetic field therapy improves pain disability in people with chronic pelvic pain.

In addition, placebo-controlled studies conducted in 1982 demonstrated that 84 percent of the subjects using a magnetic belt to treat lower back pain improved, as opposed to only a 38 percent improvement in the placebo group.

Double-blind studies were performed on people with post-polio syndrome. After forty-five minutes, 76 percent of those treated with magnets reported that the intensity of their pain was cut in half (this was self-rated on a pain intensity scale). In the placebo group, 19 percent of the participants reported a decrease in pain of only 12 percent.

A study at The Baylor College of Medicine showed that putting magnets over pain trigger points on the meridians gave prompt relief of pain for people with post-polio syndrome.

At Vanderbilt University Medical Center, a study reported that 80 to 90 percent of those who experienced pain from sports injuries felt relief after magnet therapy.

Clinical studies have been done on the use of magnets for tension headaches, and the National Institutes of Health is presently studying magnetic therapy.

The New York Medical College at Valhalla reported that magnets helped treat foot pain in diabetes. Their patients with foot pain from diabetes wore foot pads with low intensity magnets on one foot and a placebo pad on the other foot. After four months, almost all the participants in the study reported a decrease in pain in the foot with the pad.

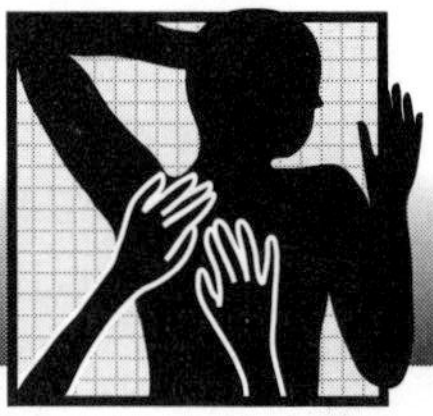

Massage

Massage therapy is a form of hands-on manipulation of the body's muscles and soft tissues. It is so highly effective for pain relief that many pain specialists are incorporating it into their programs, and some hospitals are using massage therapists in their pain-control programs. In addition to chiropractor's offices, hospitals, nursing homes, and physician's offices, massages are available at health clubs, resorts, salons, spas, and wellness centers. Besides the large number of massage locales available, many practitioners also make house calls. With such widespread use of massage therapy, it is not hard to understand the recent estimates of four to six billion dollars spent annually on massages, many of them to relieve chronic pain problems.

THE HISTORY OF MASSAGE

In ancient Greece, Hippocrates recommended massages as an aid to good health. In ancient China, Egypt, and India, scribes wrote about massage as a way to maintain health and cure disease. In the early part of the nineteenth century, Peter Henrik Ling, a Swedish athlete, developed a form of therapeutic massage, which became popular in Europe and is the reason why one type of massage is referred to as Swedish massage. At one time, a massage was considered a luxury, but it has become one of the most popular types of treatment for people with back pain or other chronic pain. Nowadays, physicians and chiropractors routinely recommend massages in the course of their treatments, and a number of insurance plans will pay for them.

HOW MASSAGE WORKS

Massage helps reduce stress, which is a contributing factor to many diseases and painful conditions. It also helps to relax contracted muscles and alleviate muscle tension in one area of the body, which can affect other areas. Massage increases blood flow, which nourishes and oxygenates the body's tissues and helps rid the cells of the lactic acid buildup that causes pain.

PAINFUL CONDITIONS THAT RESPOND WELL TO MASSAGE

- ❑ Achilles tendonitis.
- ❑ Angina.
- ❑ Back pain.
- ❑ Bursitis.
- ❑ Carpal tunnel syndrome.
- ❑ Cluster headaches.
- ❑ Crohn's disease.
- ❑ Diverticulitis.
- ❑ Endometriosis.
- ❑ Irritable bowel syndrome.
- ❑ Migraine headaches.
- ❑ Osteoarthritis.
- ❑ Pelvic floor tension myalgia.
- ❑ Postherpetic neuralgia.
- ❑ Post-polio syndrome.
- ❑ Premenstrual syndrome.
- ❑ Rheumatoid arthritis.
- ❑ Rotator cuff tendonitis.
- ❑ Sciatica.
- ❑ Tarsal tunnel syndrome.
- ❑ Tension headaches.
- ❑ Trigger finger.
- ❑ Ulcerative colitis.

In addition to the above painful conditions, massage is also beneficial for any musculoskeletal pain or neuralgia (except trigeminal neuralgia), as well as for flexibility and range of motion, improving circulation, insomnia, lowering blood pressure, reducing stress, relieving asthma, and trauma.

ADVANTAGES OF MASSAGE

- ❑ Massage is a non-invasive, non-pharmacological way to alleviate pain and stress.
- ❑ It is a pleasurable experience.
- ❑ It stimulates production of endorphins, your body's natural painkillers.
- ❑ It improves circulation.
- ❑ It relieves tension.
- ❑ It helps your body get rid of toxins.
- ❑ It is a non-threatening way of receiving the human touch that is often lacking in many people's lives.

HOW MASSAGE IS USED

There are several different massage techniques, and you might want to try different practitioners to find the type you prefer. Some techniques, such as Swedish massage, are relaxing, while others, such as Shiatsu, may be more therapeutic even if they are not quite as pleasurable. You may keep on your underwear, or take off all your clothes and have the therapist cover the parts of your body not being worked on with a sheet or towels. Experienced massage therapists adjust their treatment to the person and the ailment. Some can actually zero in on the underlying, often emotional, reason why the client's muscular system is responding adversely.

The best way to find a good massage therapist is to ask your healthcare professional for a recommendation. Friends and relatives who get massages may also be able to recommend a therapist. If you can't get to a therapist, or if you are traveling, you can self-massage with commercial devices available in body shops, sporting goods stores, catalogs, or on the Internet. Some devices pulsate, others vibrate, some are roller type, and all come in a wide variety of prices. A simple, very inexpensive way to self-massage is to put one or two tennis balls in a sock and roll your painful area over it. Of course, having a massage is much more relaxing than doing it yourself.

CAUTIONS

- ❑ If you are looking for a massage therapist on your own, either in the phone book or in advertisements, ask for references, and be sure the ads say "therapeutic massage" because some brothels advertise themselves as massage parlors.
- ❑ Massage should not be used in cases of phlebitis or thrombosis because there could be a blood clot in the area that, if disturbed, could migrate to a vital organ, such as the brain, heart, or lung.
- ❑ If you have cancer, cardiac problems, infections, or skin problems, consult with your physician before having a massage.
- ❑ Drink several glasses of water in the hours following a massage to help flush out the toxins that get released in your system during a massage.
- ❑ If your skin breaks out after a massage, it could be the type of oil the therapist uses. Ask him or her to use a different one or bring your own on the next visit.

CLINICAL STUDIES

Several studies have concluded that therapeutic massage is effective for patients with chronic low back pain.

Cherkin, DC, Eisenberg, D, et al. "Randomized Trial Comparing Traditional Chinese Medical Acupuncture, Therapeutic Massage, and Self-Care Education for Chronic Low Back Pain." *Archives of Internal Medicine.* April 23, 2001; 161(8):1081–1088.

This 2001 study concluded that massage provides lasting relief of low back pain.

Preyde, M. "Effectiveness of Massage Therapy for Subacute Low-Back Pain: A Randomized Controlled Trial." *Canadian Medical Association Journal.* June 27, 2000; 162(13):1815–1820.

This Canadian study showed that massage is effective in relieving and controlling subacute low-back pain.

MASSAGE HELPS HER STANDING

Dorothy L. had such severe pain in her thigh that she could hardly stand. Prescribed anti-inflammatories had not helped, and her doctor wanted further testing to see if back surgery was indicated. Since her massage therapist had helped her with other problems, she decided to see what massages could do for her. While performing initial relaxation techniques, the therapist asked Dorothy if she had had any unusual stress recently, and Dorothy, amazed at this acuity, replied that her stress level had indeed been unusually high due to family problems. The therapist then asked if she had ever said, "I can't stand anymore," and when Dorothy replied in the affirmative, the therapist said, "This is why you can't stand." Having this emotional pain released while her body was being relaxed helped Dorothy's thigh pain to diminish. And, once recovered, she was able to cope with further stress without becoming incapacitated.

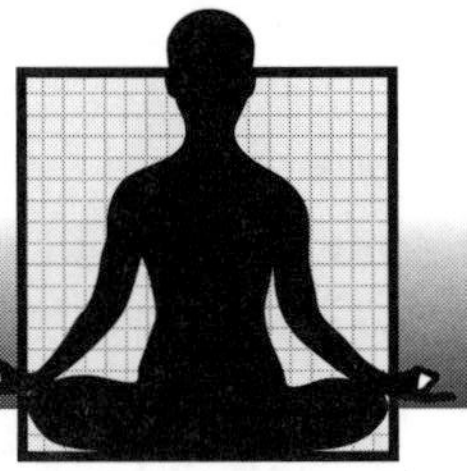

Meditation

Meditation is a method of calming your mind, relaxing it, and keeping it focused on the present. When you are meditating, your body is in an even deeper state of dreamless rest than while you are asleep, and your mind is not concerned with what has happened in the past or what may occur in the future.

THE HISTORY OF MEDITATION

Meditation has been practiced and taught since ancient times. Prophets and seers were meditators, and texts on meditation have been translated from ancient Sanskrit scriptures and the Bible. Most meditation techniques started in Asia where their primary purpose was religious. Meditation was considered a religious practice in the West as well, until the 1960s when Maharishi Mahesh Yogi brought transcendental meditation here and many movie stars and musicians became his followers. In the 1970s, Harvard researcher Dr. Herbert Benson investigated how meditation could affect health, and created a version of meditation which he called the relaxation response. Instead of using sacred Hindu Sanskrit mantras, or Western religious words, he had meditators focus on words like *one*. His book, *The Relaxation Response*, became a bestseller in the 1970s.

HOW MEDITATION WORKS

Stress contributes to all sorts of pain, and meditation can reduce stress in several ways: It reduces blood lactate, which is a marker for stress, and it reduces cortisol, the stress hormone. At the same time, meditation increases two calming hormones, melatonin and seratonin, that also relieve stress.

PAINFUL CONDITIONS THAT RESPOND WELL TO MEDITATION

All chronic pain conditions in which stress is a contributing factor respond positively to meditation. (*See* Quick Help Chart for synopsis of suggested treatments for all chronic pain conditions covered in this book.)

ADVANTAGES OF MEDITATION

- ❑ Decreased heart rate.
- ❑ Decreased muscle tension.
- ❑ Enhanced immune system.
- ❑ Increased creativity.
- ❑ Less insomnia.
- ❑ Lower blood pressure.
- ❑ Slowing of the aging process.

HOW TO USE MEDITATION

You can learn how to meditate by taking classes, listening to tapes, or reading books. Classes are listed in the yellow pages of most telephone books, or you can find them in many adult schools, holistic health centers, and increasingly, in hospital wellness centers.

Here are some basic meditative techniques to help you get started meditating on your own. They are roughly divided into two main categories, concentrative and mindfulness.

When practicing concentrative meditation, you may focus your attention on your breathing, a word, an object such as a candle flame, or a sound, to weed out distracting thoughts. Transcendental meditation, which caught on widely after its introduction in the 1960s, is a form of concentrative meditation. It is practiced by sitting in a comfortable position (the lotus works well if you do yoga), and mentally repeating a mantra. If you take a class in transcendental meditation, your instructor will give you a personalized mantra. To do concentrative meditation on your own, you can repeat a word, or even the number one, as Dr. Benson suggests. Beginning meditators often like to focus on a candle flame. Sit in a dimly lit or dark room and stare at a candle flame for a few minutes. Then close your eyes, cup your hands over them, and see the flame in your mind's eye as you continue to empty your mind of outside distractions. You can listen to a meditation tape, or even concentrate on a sound, such as a ticking clock. Another technique is to concentrate on your breathing. You can either be aware of your abdomen rising and falling, or notice how the breath feels cool entering your nose and warm as you exhale. If you have localized pain, you can meditate on it by seeing it as a colored spot, then diluting it or shrinking it and flicking it away. (Although this technique crosses over into visualization, it has been taught in meditation classes, underscoring the interdisciplinary nature of many mind-control techniques.)

Mindfulness meditation involves being aware of what is going on around you while not reacting to it, staying instead completely in the present moment. You might watch clouds or sit outside and listen to the sounds of birds, children playing, traffic, wind—all sounds of daily life. You can use an activity as mindful meditation. If you are exercising, for example, give it your complete attention. Don't read on the stairmaster. Instead, feel every sensation in your legs as you move them, and take notice how your breathing changes. If you are walking, notice how each step makes your heel and the ball of your foot feel.

If thoughts enter your mind while you are meditating, simply observe them. Just allow them to float past.

CAUTIONS

Meditation is not a substitute for medical treatment. If you are on medication, do not stop taking it until your healthcare professional agrees that you can.

If you have respiratory problems, you might want to use a technique other than breath work.

If you are under psychiatric care, check with your therapist to be sure meditation is safe for you.

CLINICAL STUDIES

Most major research on meditation has been for cardiovascular disease, high blood pressure, and immune function. But the following studies have been done specifically to determine the effects of meditation on pain.

Kabat-Zinn, J, Lipworth, L, Burney, R, et al. "Four year follow-up of a meditation-based program for the self-regulation of chronic pain: Treatment outcomes and compliance." *Clinical Journal of Pain.* 1986; 2:159–173.

This study on 225 people with chronic pain showed that training and practice in mindfulness meditation provided long-term benefits.

Kabat-Zinn, J., Lipworth, L. and Burney, R. "The clinical use of mindfulness meditation for the self-regulation of chronic pain." *Journal of Behavioral Medicine.* 1985; 8:163–190.

This study of ninety people with chronic pain showed that they were able to decrease pain-related drugs after they were trained in mindfulness meditation.

Kaplan, KH, Goldenberg, DL, and Galvin-Nadeau, M. "The impact of a meditation-based stress reduction program on fibromyalgia." *General Hospital Psychiatry.* September 1993; 15(5):284–289.

All seventy-seven people showed improvement and 51 percent showed marked improvement in this ten-week study on how mindfulness meditation can affect fibromyalgia pain.

Nutritional Therapy

While most people associate what they eat with the potential for digestive problems, heart disease, and skin problems if they eat improperly, they may not realize that food and water also affect the musculoskeletal and nervous systems. Some foods and beverages are known to lead to inflammation, a prime cause of pain in these systems, and what you eat or drink can cause or relieve this problem.

THE HISTORY OF NUTRITIONAL THERAPY

Ancient Egyptian texts refer to the use of foods for medicinal purposes. In ancient Greece, Hippocrates, the "Father of Medicine," used diet and herbs as the basis of his treatments, and the Roman naturalist, Pliny, labeled certain fruits as medicine. In 1775, English doctors advertised cod liver oil as a miracle cure for arthritis, and the claims made for the miraculous benefits of some foods, such as the antioxidant, free-radical-fighting properties of many fruits and vegetables, continue to this day.

Drinking water has been a requirement in the life of every person who has ever lived on planet earth because, without water, we would all die. Water therapy is as old as humans, and has been considered a natural medicine for centuries, used to help control and cure acute and chronic conditions, including such painful ones as migraine headaches. Hippocrates used water as a beverage to reduce fever and treat many diseases, and down through the ages water has remained a remedy for controlling high fevers. In 1797, the Scottish physician/surgeon, Dr. James Currier, wrote an important book, *The Effects of Water, Cold and Warm, as a Remedy in Fever and Other Diseases*, in which he discussed his use of cold water for its internally stimulating abilities. As water sources became more polluted in the last century, natural spring water gained favor, until today, when the use of pure bottled water has become virtually universal.

HOW NUTRITIONAL THERAPY WORKS

Nutritional therapy works mainly by helping to reduce inflammation in your body. Since inflammation is what contributes to painful (and other) conditions, including arthritis, cancer, diabetes (type II), and heart disease, and since some foods increase inflammation while others relieve it, it makes sense to consume only those foods that reduce it in order to alleviate your pain and protect your body. In some conditions, however (primarily gastrointestinal problems), food allergies may be the culprit, not inflammation.

PAINFUL CONDITIONS THAT RESPOND WELL TO NUTRITIONAL THERAPY

Nutritional therapy is beneficial for all conditions. (*See* Quick Help Chart for synopsis of suggested treatments for all chronic pain conditions covered in this book.)

ADVANTAGES OF NUTRITIONAL THERAPY

It is non-toxic and has no side effects. Proper nutritional therapy can work wonders to increase your overall health, and even retard aging.

HOW TO USE NUTRITIONAL THERAPY

Foods containing beta-carotene act as anti-inflammatories. High carotene foods include apricots, asparagus, beets, broccoli, cantaloupe, carrots, kale, papayas, parsley, peaches, red peppers, pumpkin, spinach, sweet potatoes, yellow squash, and watercress.

Foods rich in omega-3s also act as anti-inflammatories. Your body converts omega-3s into hormone-like substances that reduce inflammation. Good sources are cod liver oil and fatty fish, such as herring, mackerel, wild salmon, sardines, and lake trout (please note, though, that mackerel and lake trout are now considered toxic). Dark green leafy vegetables, such as collard greens, kale, and spinach, along with canola oil, flaxseeds, and walnuts are good sources of omega-3s. Cherries and all kinds of berries (the darker the better) contain substances that help to reduce inflammation, as do garlic and onions.

Honey can alleviate painful conditions by triggering brain chemicals that dull how you perceive pain.

Drinking six to eight glasses of pure water a day is highly recommended by almost everyone in the health field now. Water's numerous benefits include hydrating internal organs, stimulating your liver and kidneys, helping to absorb oxygen, purifying your cells, and flushing out substances that, if allowed to concentrate, could become toxic, as for example in painful arthritis. Spa physicians in Europe consider *drinking* (not just bathing in) different mineral waters, such as high calcium, high sulphur, etc., to be an important component of their water therapies for alleviating different, often painful, conditions.

To use nutritional therapy properly, you should avoid or reduce consumption of the following:

- ❑ Excessive fat from dairy and meat products;
- ❑ Food additives;

- ❑ Meat and dairy products because they contain arachidonic acid which produces leukotrienes and inflammatory prostaglandins, both precursors of inflammation;
- ❑ Processed foods, corn oil, and sunflower oil, all sources of omega-6s, which can cause inflammation; (It is important to keep omega-3s and omega-6s in balance, but most of us consume up to twenty times more omega-6s than omega-3s because of our unhealthy reliance on heavily processed foods);
- ❑ Refined flour products;
- ❑ Sugar;
- ❑ Trans fats.

Additionally, many popular sodas contain additives, caffeine, overloads of phosphorous, and too much sugar, to name a few of their disadvantages. Best to leave them on the shelves, or in the soda machines, and choose pure bottled drinking water instead.

CAUTIONS

Even if a particular food has beneficial qualities, it is not a good idea to eat it every day because repetitive dining on the same foods can lead to food allergies. Aim for variety within the lists of suggested foods.

(*See also* HYDROTHERAPY in PART 2 Treatment Section.)

CLINICAL STUDIES

Adam, O, Beringer, C, Kless, T, et al. "Anti-inflammatory effects of a low arachidonic acid diet and fish oil in patients with rheumatoid arthritis." *Rheumatology Int.* January 2, 2003; 23(1):27–36. Epub September 6, 2002.

This controlled German study divided sixty-eight people with rheumatoid arthritis into two groups, one receiving the normal Western diet, the other an anti-inflammatory diet. At the end of eight months, those on the low-arachidonic-acid diet had a significantly greater reduction in their tender, swollen joints than the control group, especially after fish oil was given to both groups in the last two months of the study. The authors of the study concluded that a diet low in arachidonic acid ameliorates signs of inflammation in people with rheumatoid arthritis and augments the beneficial effects of fish-oil supplementation.

Ornish, D, Schweritz, LW, Billings, JH, et al. "Intensive lifestyle changes for reversal of coronary heart disease." *Journal of the American Medical Asociation.* December 16, 1998; 280(23):2001–2007.

Forty-eight people with moderate to severe heart disease, including angina, were studied in this five-year, randomized, controlled, California clinical trial. After five years, the intensive lifestyle-change group (10-percent fat, whole-foods vegetarian diet, and other alternative therapies) had continuing regression of their coronary heart disease, but by contrast, coronary heart disease continued to progress in the usual-care control group which experienced more than twice as many cardiac events as the lifestyle-change group.

NITRITES A BENEFICIAL THERAPY FOR SICKLE CELL ANEMIA?

Conventional wisdom has it that nitrates and nitrites should be assiduously avoided as carcinogens, right? Well, at least with nitrite, a natural component of leafy green vegetables and a common additive in cured meats and hot dogs, that may not be the whole story.

According to the November 2003 issue of *Nature Medicine,* researchers at the National Institutes of Health, in conjunction with colleagues at the University of Alabama and Wake Forest University, found that nitrite, a common salt, can open blood vessels, greatly increasing blood flow in the body. Another author of the study, Dr. Alan N. Schecter, an expert on sickle cell anemia at the National Institute of Diabetes, Digestive, and Kidney Diseases (NIDDK), reported that this finding not only has real potential for heart and blood disease, but also for sickle cell anemia. As reported in *The New York Times,* November 3, 2003, Dr. Schecter said the results of this study, which show that nitrite helps get more blood to areas of the body that are low in oxygen, raised the possibility of using infused or inhaled nitrites as a therapy for this inherited disorder in which defective hemoglobin causes red blood cells to distort and block small blood vessels. "Nitrite therapy could be a major new, simple and nonexpensive alternative therapy for sickle cell disease," as well as other diseases of poor circulation, he said, adding the caution that it could "take years of clinical testing" before proving conclusively that the approach is beneficial. But considering the paucity of effective therapies currently available for people with this extremely painful disease, it could be very hopeful.

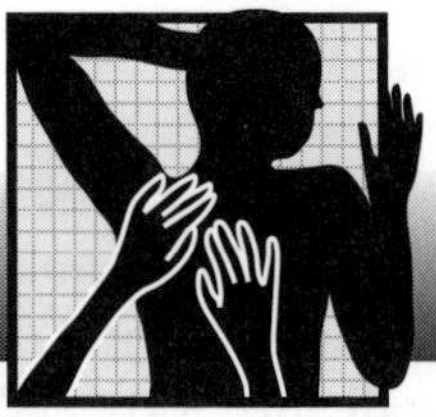

Osteopathic Manipulation

Osteopathic manipulation, one part of osteopathic medicine, is a treatment system that believes the body is entirely capable of healing itself. Understanding the body's structure and functions, with particular emphasis on the musculoskeletal system, which comprises two-thirds of the body, is the foundation of the osteopathic approach to medicine. Osteopathic practitioners use generally accepted methods of diagnosing and specialized techniques to check muscle and nerve restrictions, including osteopathic manipulative treatment (OMT), to detect and correct faulty structure and function. The osteopathic tradition has long recognized the positive effects of manipulative therapy on health, and believes that those effects go far beyond its important, but limited, use for musculoskeletal injuries in backs, joints, necks, shoulders, etc., on into rebalancing the body's whole system to lessen such illnesses as asthma, digestive disturbances, heart disease, or migraines, for example.

In recent years however, osteopathic physicians (DOs) have drawn closer to medical doctors (MDs). DOs and MDs now share offices, DOs are reimbursed by insurance just as MDs are, and not all osteopathic physicians perform osteopathic manipulation (OMT) anymore—some have put their holistic training in the background and have become almost indistinguishable from conventional doctors.

Although the four-year training of an osteopathic physician (DO) is essentially identical to that of an allopathic physician (MD), and although practitioners of osteopathy can also prescribe medicine and perform surgery, there has traditionally been a big difference between the two approaches to healing that goes back 2,400 years to Hippocrates who taught in the fourth century BC that "our natures are the physicians of our diseases." The physician, he said, should help the body recover by removing the cause of problems, and by recognizing and encouraging the body's own tendencies toward health, but should never hinder nature's own attempts toward recovery. Hippocrates also believed that doctors should study the entire patient and his environment, and he stressed the importance of focusing on the individual's health instead of the individual's diseases (the latter being the focus of a competing idea that gained prominence over time and became the foundation of the allopathic approach to treatment). Students in osteopathic colleges are trained to treat the whole person and the philosophy emphasizes preventive medicine and preventive care.

Many alternative therapies also use these wellness principles to guide them, but according to Dr. Jeffrey Perry, DO, in New York, "The key thing that is different and unique about osteopathy is that an osteopath is a physician who *cares,* so the patient has the best of all worlds. Osteopathy," he adds, "is ideal for pain treatment, because it recognizes that the entire body works together as a whole, and that disturbances in one system can impact on other functions in the body."

THE HISTORY OF OSTEOPATHY AND OSTEOPATHIC MANIPULATION

When Dr. Andrew Taylor Still, a frontier physician, lost his three children in the meningitis epidemic of 1864, he blamed their deaths on the "gross ignorance" of the medical profession and began looking for a better way of healing than with the standard (to him, barbarous) practices of the time, such as bleeding patients, handling them with dirty hands, and using leeches, potions, poisons, and toxic heavy metals on them. Dr. Still focused his studies on the structure of the human body, and by 1874 he had founded osteopathy, basing his system on Hippocratic theories and on his beliefs that the musculoskeletal system reflects and influences the condition of all the other systems in the body, and that optimum functioning depends on an unrestricted flow of blood and nerve impulses. Recognizing the power of hands-on care as a vital, less-intrusive element of diagnosis and treatment, Dr. Still believed that a mechanical disorder could be mechanically corrected by manual manipulation, and he prophetically included preventive medicine, fitness, and nutrition in his system, emphasizing their importance.

His theories were put into wide practice and, by the time of his death in 1917, 5,000 practitioners were using his osteopathic methods. In the United States today, there are approximately 47,000 DOs practicing in all fifty states and the District of Columbia (Pennsylvania, Michigan, and Ohio have the largest number of practitioners, with Florida, New York, Texas, and New Jersey close behind). Nineteen accredited colleges of osteopathic medicine graduated 2,300 students in 2000 alone, and all received a thorough scientific and academic education, as well as instruction in osteopathic principles and techniques for diagnosis and treatment. Following graduation, there is a one-year rotating internship in assorted disciplines, and possibly a residency in the specialty of choice after that (most specialists do not use OMT). Before being allowed to practice as osteopathic physicians, all students must pass a state medical board examination to receive a license in that state.

HOW OSTEOPATHIC MANIPULATION WORKS

Osteopathic physicians use their knowledge of the latest medical technology and complement it with their special hands-on treatment tool, osteopathic manipulative treatment (OMT) to diagnose, treat, even prevent, illness or injury. And when appropriate, OMT can be used in conjunction with, or in place of medication or surgery.

DOs use their eyes and hands to identify structural problems you may have, and to support the body's natural tendency toward health and self-healing, and they use their ears to listen to you and your health concerns. Then, given what they have learned, they treat you with the appropriate OMT methods and help you develop attitudes and lifestyles that don't just fight illness, but help prevent it.

PAINFUL CONDITIONS THAT RESPOND WELL TO THERAPY

- ❑ Achilles tendonitis.
- ❑ Back pains, sprains, and strains (includes disc and neck problems).
- ❑ Bursitis.
- ❑ Carpal tunnel syndrome.
- ❑ Cluster headaches.
- ❑ Dental pain.
- ❑ Endometriosis.
- ❑ Fibromyalgia.
- ❑ Frozen shoulder.
- ❑ Migraine headaches.
- ❑ Neuroma.
- ❑ Osteoarthritis.
- ❑ Pelvic floor tension myalgia.
- ❑ Peripheral neuropathy.
- ❑ Phantom pain.
- ❑ Plantar fasciitis.
- ❑ Post-polio syndrome.
- ❑ Reflex sympathetic dystrophy syndrome (RSDS).
- ❑ Rheumatoid arthritis.
- ❑ Rotator cuff tendonitis.
- ❑ Sciatica.
- ❑ Tarsal tunnel syndrome.
- ❑ Temporomandibular joint (TMJ) pain.
- ❑ Tennis elbow.
- ❑ Tension headache.
- ❑ Trigeminal neuralgia.
- ❑ Trigger finger.

In addition to the painful conditions above, Dr. Perry says that osteopathic manipulation is very useful in treating myofascial pain and other musculoskeletal problems.

ADVANTAGES OF OSTEOPATHIC MANIPULATION

Osteopathic physicians continue to be on the cutting edge of contemporary medicine. They combine today's medical technology with their caring, compassionate attitudes and their holistic approach to the body, and this enables them to provide a wide range of treatment options to their patients.

HOW OSTEOPATHIC MANIPULATION IS USED

After your medical history has been taken and any mechanical reasons for your problems have been ruled out (through blood and urine tests), the osteopathic practitioner will start a session with a structural exam to assess your posture, spine, and balance, palpating (tapping) your back, extremities, and joints to check for any

DIAGNOSIS DETERMINES CORRECT TREATMENT

Dr. Jeffrey Perry, DO, believes that one of the most important aspects of treating any painful condition is to first diagnose it correctly. When Mary came to see him, she said she was experiencing severe back pain, and even told him she knew that her L5 disc herniation was the cause of this pain. After a thorough examination, Dr. Perry decided to use OMT (osteopathic manipulative treatment) to treat her sacroiliac joint, which lies well below the lumbar spine area she had pinpointed as the obvious source of her pain. Except it wasn't that at all, as Mary found out when Dr. Perry's correct diagnosis and subsequent treatment gave her significant and long-lasting relief from her pain. If this caring osteopathic physician has any one credo, it would be to always make sure and accurately diagnose a problem before jumping in to treat a pain.

muscle or nerve restrictions and to detect any changes in tissue that could signal an injury or impairment. By touching you, the doctor establishes a connective loop; with you getting a response from the doctor's hands while the doctor is picking up messages about your body through her or his hands. Following this, your DO will apply manual forces, from holding techniques to gentle thrusts, to your body's affected areas to treat structural abnormalities, and corrective forces to relieve any joint restrictions or misalignments. The point of all this manipulation is to restore nerve and circulatory functioning and in that way help the body to heal itself.

In terms of costs, Dr. Perry says, "Since the concept is to try to let the body heal itself without interventional treatment, one may hope that the costs are less than an operation and a hospital stay, and that the number of visits to the doctor are able to be kept to a minimum."

CAUTIONS

There are no downsides to osteopathic manipulation, says Dr. Perry, only advantages. Be aware, however, that if you are seeking OMT and alternative, non-invasive, non-drug treatment, you should find out all you can about the osteopathic practitioner you plan to visit before scheduling an appointment, to make sure that OMT is a part of his/her practice.

CLINICAL STUDIES

Gamber, RG, Shores, JH, Russo, DP, et al. "Osteopathic manipulative treatment in conjunction with medication relieves pain associated with fibromyalgia syndrome: results of a randomized clinical pilot project." *Journal of the American Osteopathic Association.* June 2002; 102(6):321–325.

This study of twenty-four women favored the use of OMT for pain relief.

Knebl, JA, Shores, JH, Gamber, RG, et al. "Improving functional ability in the elderly via the Spencer technique, an osteopathic manipulative treatment: a randomized, controlled trial." *Journal of the American Osteopathic Association.* July 2002; 102(7):387–396.

Twenty-nine people with chronic shoulder pain all showed decreased pain and an increase in range of motion and after fourteen weeks of OMT.

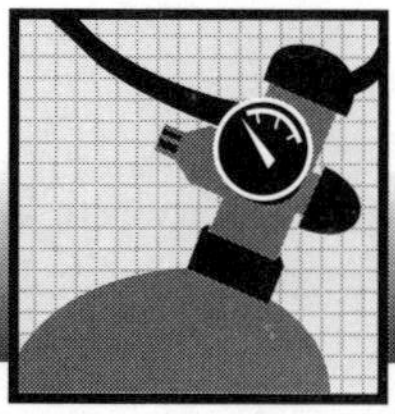

Oxygen Therapies

Oxygen comprises 21 percent of the air we breathe and is often the first line of treatment in emergencies. Although not well-known in the United States, oxygen therapies are widely used in Russia, Europe (particularly Germany and The Netherlands), China, Japan, and Cuba. There are four basic bio-oxidative therapies, of which hyperbaric oxygen therapy (HBOT), is the best known, primarily for its effective treatment of burns and the effects of smoke inhalation, decompression illness in divers, carbon monoxide poisoning, and the effects of gas gangrene due to oxygen deprivation.

According to Dr. Pavel Yutsis, a New York physician trained in oxygen therapy in his native Russia, "Hyperbaric oxygen therapy may be one of the most commonly used and yet unknown therapies in medicine today." It has a "shadow existence," he says, because the medical establishment limits its use to fifteen areas that can be treated in most hospitals, and these are the only ones assured of coverage under most medical insurance policies. To the contrary however, says Dr. Yutsis, HBOT and the related bio-oxidative therapies, hydrogen peroxide (H_2O_2), ozone therapy, and ultraviolet irradiation of blood (UVIB) have hundreds of uses for a wide-ranging list of conditions. He is encouraged because he sees the expanded innovative uses of oxygen therapies gaining a bigger foothold, and believes that, in combination with complementary/alternative holistic therapies, they will be the lynchpins of medicine in the twenty-first century.

THE HISTORY OF OXYGEN THERAPIES

Hyperbaric Oxygen Therapy (HBOT)

Three hundred years ago, according to the book, *Hyperbaric Oxygen Therapy,* by Richard Neubauer and Morton Walker, an Englishman named Joseph Henshaw used compressed air in a specially equipped room called a "domicillium" to help a test subject's digestion and respiration. The notion of oxygen as a therapy got a big boost in the eighteenth and nineteenth centuries when pressurized oxygen was used to help divers with decompression illness (the bends). By 1935, commercial uses had been developed, and to this day oxygen is used more than any other method to treat diving accidents.

Hydrogen Peroxide Therapy (H_2O_2)

Hydrogen peroxide therapy (H_2O_2), an effective oxygenator (increases oxygen in the system), along with ozone therapy (to which it is closely allied), was discovered early in the nineteenth century by both Dr. Louis-Jacques Thenard, a French chemist who called it oxygenated water, and Dr. I.N. Love, in St. Louis, Missouri, who successfully treated his patients for diphtheria, hay fever and scarlet fever, tonsillitis, and whooping cough using hydrogen peroxide diluted with water, which he inserted into their nostrils with a syringe. Until early in the twentieth century, however, commercial uses for H_2O_2 as a disinfecting and oxidizing agent overshadowed its medical uses. Then, in 1916, *The Lancet* published an article about the successful intravenous use of H_2O_2 by two British physicians, believed to be the first time hydrogen peroxide had been delivered in this manner, and several years later they published another article, about Indian troops who received successful H_2O_2 treatments for pneumonia, which reduced the then-current 80 percent mortality rate by half. In the ensuing years, a number of studies showed that H_2O_2 oxygen could be delivered into tissues simply, inexpensively, and effectively.

Dr. Charles Farr advanced the research by discovering that the fear of H_2O_2 therapy leading to increased production of harmful free radicals was groundless if no iron was present in the system, and his breakthrough has permitted the ongoing use of hydrogen peroxide therapy to this day.

Ozone Therapy

The history and use of ozone (O_3) is closely linked to hydrogen peroxide. In 1896 Nicola Tesla patented an ozone generator, and ozone was in use in the United States prior to that. In Germany in 1901, it was used to purify water, in 1915 to treat skin diseases, and in World War I to treat battle wounds and infections. In 1945, Dr. Erwin Payr injected it into his patients with circulatory problems, and over the years its scientific and technological uses have increased, particularly in Germany, which has pioneered its successful treatment for diseases, such as arthritis, cancer, hepatitis, and HIV/AIDS, by helping to destroy pathogens, plus its demonstrated ability to speed up the work of such cellular proteins as interferon and interleukin 2, both of which help to slow the growth of viruses.

Ultraviolet Irradiation of Blood (UVIB)

Early in the twentieth century, ultraviolet irradiation of blood (UVIB), also known as photoluminescence, was discovered as a preferred treatment for flu and allergies because of its demonstrated ability to almost entirely eliminate bacteria and viruses.

Although proven successful, all four of these therapies were sidelined in the 1940s and '50s when antibiotics came along, and are only now re-emerging because the harmful side effects of the so-called wonder drugs are causing more and more people to rethink their use of them and search for treatments with fewer, if any, harmful side effects.

HOW OXYGEN THERAPIES WORK

According to Dr. Yutsis, the oxygen therapies can rectify chronic degenerative conditions that develop due to three things:

- ❑ The liver becomes less and less able to detoxify;
- ❑ The body's tissues and organs develop inflammatory conditions;
- ❑ There is an increase in harmful free-radical activity.

Delivering oxygen at the cellular level, forcing it directly into the blood plasma, usually in a low-oxygen state (some believe due to a build-up of pollution), has a healing effect on the entire body for all these conditions, and without side effects. The majority of diseases damage circulation, and HBOT can override this by infusing the overall body with increased amounts of oxygen. It shows great promise, not just for its well-known uses, but also for its less-known treatment of arthritis, cerebral palsy, strokes, and HIV/AIDS, for example.

H_2O_2 and ozone are both effective in the body as immune-system enhancers, oxygenators, and oxidizers, which encourage the body's own natural utilization and production of oxygen. These active oxygen therapies can treat a large variety of chronic and acute conditions by destroying bacteria, viruses, and even some tumors.

Ultraviolet irradiation of blood (UVIB) is not technically an oxygen therapy but, by exposing the person's blood to untraviolet rays, the capacity of that blood to absorb and use oxygen is increased, and the immune defense system, as well as the body's many enzyme systems, are all stimulated to kill invading organisms, thereby acting to restore health very quickly. Also, UVIB has a great capacity to restore chemical balance in the body, and it has a cumulative effect, with each treatment enhancing the results of the previous one.

THE DISCOSAN METHOD—A BREAKTHROUGH TREATMENT FOR HERNIATED DISCS

According to the online newsletter, *Family Health News,* Dr. Cesare Varga, an orthopedic surgeon in Italy, perfected a special mixture of ozone to treat herniated discs which he has used on over 6,000 patients since first developing it in 1984. The treatment, which eliminates the need for surgery, consists of injecting a mix of ozone and oxygen into the area of the herniated disc twice a week for one to two months, generally fourteen treatments in all, depending on the patient. Dr. Varga says that his approach—soon adopted by colleagues who had previously performed surgery for the condition—has virtually zero recovery time, no side effects, no contraindications, and a 95-percent success rate. For further information on this remarkable treatment, contact *Family Health News* at the address listed in Resources in back, or go to their website *www.familyhealth news.com* to read about it.

PAINFUL CONDITIONS THAT RESPOND WELL TO OXYGEN THERAPIES

Hyperbaric Oxygen Therapy (HBOT)

- ❑ Back pain.
- ❑ Cluster headaches.
- ❑ Crohn's disease.
- ❑ Fibromyalgia.
- ❑ Migraine headaches.
- ❑ Osteoarthritis.
- ❑ Peripheral neuropathy.
- ❑ Postherpetic neuralgia,
- ❑ Post-polio syndrome.
- ❑ Reflex sympathetic dystrophy syndrome (RSDS).
- ❑ Rheumatoid arthritis.
- ❑ Tension headaches.
- ❑ Ulcerative colitis.

In addition to the painful conditions listed above, HBOT is also very effective treatment for chronic fatigue syndrome.

Hydrogen Peroxide Therapy (H_2O_2)

- ❑ Cluster headaches.
- ❑ Fibromyalgia.

Fibromyalgia Fixed by Mixed Therapies

Carol, a forty-three-year-old psychotherapist, was experiencing head-to-toe pain along her right side only. Her memory had degenerated, she had no appetite, was nauseous, depressed, tired but unable to sleep, and convinced she had Lyme disease, which is why she visited Dr. Pavel Yutsis after hearing him talk about oxygen therapies on his radio program. Following a consultation, with an examination and routine tests, plus a test for Lyme disease (which later came back negative), he gave her twenty sessions of HBOT that temporarily cleared up a number of her symptoms. But when the right-side pain returned, he started her on hydrogen peroxide therapy, along with acupuncture and a course of supplements, while continuing with her hyperbaric oxygen treatments. This combination made her feel 30 to 40 percent better after six weeks, but since her pain was ongoing, Dr. Yutsis became more and more convinced she had fibromyalgia. Further testing confirmed this and revealed that she also had many allergies and chronic fatigue syndrome, so he added chelation therapy (a process by which heavy metals are captured and eliminated through the kidneys) to the mix of treatments, and changed her diet.

The combination of all these therapies, added to the maximum amounts of oxygen that were infusing Carol's body and triggering her immune system to work better and make her stronger, did the trick. After a total of four and a half months of treatment, she never looked better, and her fibromyalgia was a thing of the past, as were her allergies and chronic fatigue syndrome. Dr. Yutsis reports that when he saw her for another, unrelated reason three years later, she was still feeling fine and told him how very grateful she was to him for solving the mystery of her debilitating illness and giving her back her life.

- ❑ Migraine headaches.
- ❑ Postherpetic neuralgia.
- ❑ Rheumatoid arthritis.
- ❑ Vascular headaches.

Ozone Therapy

- ❑ Arthritis.
- ❑ Back pain (herniated disc).
- ❑ Fibromyalgia.
- ❑ Sickle cell anemia.

Ultraviolet Irradiation of Blood (UVIB)

- ❑ Inflammatory bowel disease.
- ❑ Rheumatoid arthritis.

ADVANTAGES OF OXYGEN THERAPIES

The air we breathe and our dependence on it cannot be overemphasized because, without air (oxygen), we cannot live. And the health of a body deprived of sufficient oxygen is affected at the cellular level because microorganisms like a low-oxygen environment where they can grow and develop disease (bacteria and viruses cannot live long in active oxygen). The great advantage of using oxygen therapy is that increasing oxygen to the cells enhances their ability to kill bacteria, viruses, and the other microorganisms that cause disease in tissues. Increased oxygen in the body helps restore it to full health, eliciting few side effects in the process, and any infusion of oxygen in its active forms immediately gives the person undergoing treatment new vitality. Another advantageous side effect is that people receiving oxygen therapies have consistently noted a reduction in their pain symptoms.

The advantage of such therapies as H_2O_2, for example, is that it can be used with almost any other therapy to treat most diseases. All four therapies work well, either separately or in combination, to get the maximum amount of oxygen into the body and symbiotically balance it.

HOW OXYGEN THERAPIES ARE USED

All therapies discussed administer pure oxygen into the body at greater than normal amounts, regardless of the delivery method used or the condition being treated.

Hyperbaric Oxygen Therapy (HBOT)

With HBOT, a skilled practitioner places her/his patient in a special pressurized oxygen chamber where the person breathes in pure oxygen at greater than atmospheric pressure, thus allowing the oxygen to infuse all the body's fluids and facilitating healing because the extra oxygen carried throughout the body improves the functioning of its organs, even the most seriously deprived ones. There are a few simple procedures to follow. The clothing worn in the chamber must be 100-percent cotton, no makeup, perfume, or aftershave is permitted, nor are hairpieces, jewelry, matches, lighters, or cigarettes, and treatment is routinely postponed in case of illness. The treatment consists of three phases: ten to fifteen minutes of compression while the pressurization with pure oxygen gets to the point of equaling a diver's pressure (somewhere between sixteen to sixty feet underwater); the treatment itself, during which the person can feel free to read, watch TV, listen to music, or just relax for the amount of time specified by the doctor skilled in the application of the therapy; and the final decompression which involves the slow withdrawal of the pressure until the level is back to normal. (For more details of this and the other oxygen treatments, see Dr. Yutsis' book, *Oxygen to the Rescue.*)

Hydrogen Peroxide Therapy (H_2O_2)

According to Dr. Yutsis, the best delivery method for H_2O_2 is injections infused intravenously for forty-five minutes to an hour, generally three times a week for up to three or four months, with a possible follow-up once a week after that. These injections are, unfortunately, not covered by insurance, but the cost is worth it because the method is highly successful, much more so than hydrogen peroxide taken orally or used for bathing, and it moves the people who have undergone it from "a state of being sick to a state of being well."

Ozone Therapy

Physicians have a number of methods they can use to add ozone to our blood and tissues. The most common method is autohemotherapy, which involves taking blood from the person with a syringe (10 ml for minor autohemotherapy, and up to 250 ml for major autohemotherapy), infusing it with ozone and oxygen, then reinjecting it—into the buttocks for minor autohemotherapy, and through an IV drip for major autohemotherapy. This method, which must be given slowly because it requires the filtering organs *in* the body to process the toxins and microbes instead of having them mechanically filtered away outside the body, has been used to treat arthritis, cancer, heart disease, and HIV, and in 1951, in France, it was successfully used to prevent amputation of a person's upper thigh.

Another delivery method for this therapy is rectal insufflation to introduce oxygen and ozone into the body through the rectum, and a third method introduces these elements into the body through the skin (some who are convinced of ozone's efficacy prefer this non-invasive method). As with autohemotherapy above, it must be given slowly.

Although not as commonly used in the United States, recirculatory hemoperfusion (RHP) is a very effective method of ozone delivery, even considered by some the most effective. It consists of drawing blood and mixing the ozone with that blood outside the body, them pumping it back into the bloodstream. This method, commonly

Ozone Therapy for Sickle Cell Anemia

Sickle cell disease is a genetic disorder that affects approximately 70,000 people in the United States, primarily (though not limited to) African Americans. If your ancestors come from areas where malaria is prevalent, you could also carry the gene. If one parent has the gene, you have what is known as the sickle cell trait, but if both parents have the gene, it is likely that your offspring will have sickle cell anemia.

This is an extremely painful condition affecting the arms and legs, and the abdomen, back, and chest. What happens is that the red blood cells are forced into a crescent (sickle) shape, impeding blood flow in the small vessels. Then the tissues are injured due to the obstructed blood flow, and the amount of oxygen available to the cells is reduced. Conventional medical treatment is only symptomatic and consists of opioid analgesics for pain, aggressive antibiotic therapy for infections, and control of anemia.

However, clinical trials using ozone/oxygen therapy were conducted in Cuba with very positive results. Over fifteen sessions, fifty-five adult sickle-cell anemia patients, all suffering painful crises, were tested, and the group receiving the ozone/oxygen therapy had their crises resolved in half the time of the control group. Further, the number of crises was significantly reduced compared to the control group, both in the short-term and in a six-month follow-up, with no adverse reactions reported. Additionally, some in the treated group also showed a remarkably favorable resolution of their associated symptoms, which were also severe. Bringing more oxygen to the tissues is one of the hopeful ways that the pain of this incurable disease can be alleviated. ("Ozone Marches On." *The Family Health News.*)

practiced in Russian and Indian hospitals, can sterilize the bloodstream in a few hours.

Additionally, direct intravenous injection of 2 percent ozone and 98 percent oxygen is used in clinics all over the world. It is easy to administer (slowly also, as above) and is considered highly effective.

As with all the bio-oxidative therapies, ozone therapy is often used in conjunction with other alternative/complementary methods to increase the potential for healing.

Ultraviolet Irradiation of Blood (UVIB)

This successful approach to dealing with infections is used by many people around the world, but is almost unknown in the United States. It consists of irradiating the blood by drawing a small amount of blood (60–120 cc), exposing it to ultraviolet light, then reintroducing it into the body. This provides sufficient exposure to strengthen the immune system, and by stimulating the immune system to kill invading organisms, UVIB treatment can rapidly restore health. When properly delivered by a skilled professional, it is a very speedy method of killing bacteria and viruses that can be lifesaving in hospitals (and similar institutions) where people with compromised immune systems can be easily infected.

When you combine one bio-oxidative therapy with one or two others, you can exponentially increase the benefits of each, bringing about quicker improvements and cures, and maximizing your chances of staying healthy.

CAUTIONS

Hyperbaric Oxygen Therapy (HBOT)

Hyperbaric oxygen therapy has few side effects and those few are the result of a reaction between oxygen free radicals and cellular components, and generally occur only when the air pressure in the chamber is kept too high for too long. The pulmonary system can be affected, and rarely (one in 5,000), there can be a seizure if the person stays in too long, but it is immediately reversed as soon as the pressure is released. Some people experience changes in their eyesight (progressive reversible nearsightedness, for example), but all these conditions can be obviated by going to a practitioner skilled in the delivery of oxygen therapies.

Hydrogen Peroxide (H_2O_2) and Ozone Therapies

The primary concern of conventional medicine is that active oxygen therapies, such as hydrogen peroxide and ozone, can cause cell damage because of the possibility that these therapies can increase the production of free radicals, which are linked to the development of degenerative diseases, immune deficiencies, and aging. As previously mentioned, Dr. Charles Farr, founder of the International Oxidative Medicine Association (his widow, Skoshie Farr, is still involved with the organization), and a 1993 Nobel Prize nominee, nullified this concern when he discovered that hydrogen peroxide leads to the production of free radicals only when iron (ferrous oxide) is present. Without iron present, hydrogen peroxide converts to oxygen and becomes a benefit to the body. Although there is a positive side to free radicals—bringing energy to the cells, killing bacteria, viruses, and fungi, and regulating hormones—*too many free radicals in the body are harmful, so it is important to keep them in check.*

With these oxygen therapies, as with all complementary medicine, the objective is to maintain the balance of molecules in the body in order to repair it and prevent disease. Most healthy bodies regulate the production of free radicals to prevent an excess of them from building up, but a body fighting illness can use the extra oxygen to destroy viruses and bacteria, and to work at the cellular level. When used properly by a skilled practitioner, H_2O_2 and ozone therapies can heal faster, with fewer (if any) side effects than conventional treatments, and are nontoxic as an added plus.

Ultraviolet Irradiation of Blood (UVIB)

Few physicians know how to use the UVIB technique properly. Too much irradiation can cause depression and even lessen resistance to infections so it is important to have a fully qualified practitioner monitoring every treatment.

CLINICAL STUDIES

Di Sabato, F, Fusco, BM, Pelaia, P, et al. "Hyperbaric oxygen therapy in cluster headache." *Pain.* February 1993; 52(2):243–245.

An Italian study reported that hyperbaric oxygen (HBO) interrupted cluster headache attacks, and it indicated that HBO not only had an effect on a single attack, it also prevented the occurrence of subsequent attacks.

Pascual, J, Peralta, G, Sanchez, U. "Preventive effects of hyperbaric oxygen in cluster headache." *Headache.* May 1995; 35(5):260–261.

In a study at the University Hospital in Santander, Spain, a daily course of hyperbaric oxygen treatment showed dramatic improvement in 50 percent of the patients with chronic cluster headaches who had shown no improvement with medication. Another 25 percent showed a reduction in the frequency of the attacks.

Peach, G. "Hyperbaric oxygen and the reflex sympathetic dystrophy syndrome: a case report." *Undersea Hyperbaric Medicine.* December 1995; 22(4):407–408.

At the University of Baltimore Medical Center, a female patient with RSDS of the left foot and ankle reported a lessening of pain fifteen minutes into her first forty-five-minute hyperbaric oxygen treatment. The foot was also less cyanotic (lacking oxygen) and warmer to the touch, and subsequent treatments continued to improve her condition.

Wilson, JR, Foresman, BH, Gamber, RG, et al. "Hyperbaric oxygen in the treatment of migraine with aura." *Headache.* February 1998; 38(2):112–115.

Results of a study at the University of North Texas Health Science Center in Fort Worth showed a significant decrease in migraine headache pain following hyperbaric oxygen treatment.

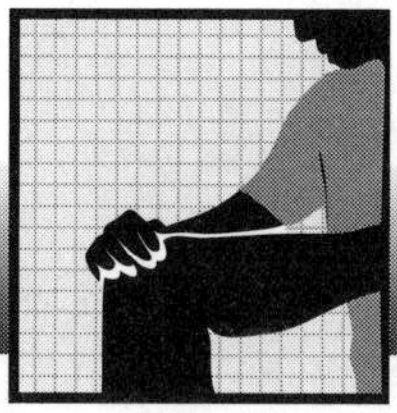

Physical Therapy

Physical therapy is a healthcare profession that evaluates, restores, and helps maintain physical function. The goal of physical therapy is to help people recover from an injury or disease and increase their independence. Physical therapists (PTs) help patients strengthen their muscles by giving them specific exercises. They teach different ways of moving, resting, and conserving energy. They may use ultrasound therapy and/or muscle-stimulating machines for pain relief, and they may recommend water therapy for joint movement. Physical therapists are required to have at least a bachelor's degree and many have master's degrees. Physical therapy was once considered alternative rehabilitation therapy, but it is now a respected medical specialty.

THE HISTORY OF PHYSICAL THERAPY

During World War I, a Reconstruction Aide Corps was formed in the United States Army to help treat the wounded. In 1916, the first department of physical therapy was formed and training programs were instituted. Physical therapy reached professional stature in 1921 with the formation of the American Physical Therapy Association. During the polio epidemics in the 1940s and '50s, physical therapists helped patients regain mobility. During World War II, its benefits were widely recognized. The field gained greater acceptance as its usefulness in rehabilitating the wounded and polio victims became apparent, and as more people were trained and techniques were expanded.

HOW PHYSICAL THERAPY WORKS

Physical therapy works by correcting and improving your body's natural healing mechanism. It increases the range of motion in the joints.

PAINFUL CONDITIONS THAT RESPOND WELL TO PHYSICAL THERAPY

- ❑ Achilles tendonitis.
- ❑ Back pain.
- ❑ Bursitis.
- ❑ Carpal tunnel syndrome (many PTs are hand specialists for CTS).
- ❑ Cluster headaches.
- ❑ Dental pain.
- ❑ Fibromyalgia.
- ❑ Frozen shoulder.
- ❑ Migraine headaches.
- ❑ Osteoarthritis.
- ❑ Phantom pain.
- ❑ Plantar fasciitis.
- ❑ Post-polio syndrome.
- ❑ Reflex sympathetic dystrophy syndrome (RSDS).
- ❑ Rheumatoid arthritis.
- ❑ Rotator cuff tendonitis.
- ❑ Sciatica.
- ❑ Sports injuries.
- ❑ Spinal stenosis.
- ❑ Tarsal tunnel syndrome.
- ❑ Temporomandibular joint (TMJ) pain.
- ❑ Tennis elbow.
- ❑ Tension headaches.
- ❑ Thoracic outlet syndrome.
- ❑ Trigger finger.

Physical therapy can also help asthma and other breathing problems, balance or bladder problems, musculoskeletal disorders, neuralgia, and posttraumatic pain, and it can be very useful in stroke rehabilitation.

ADVANTAGES OF PHYSICAL THERAPY

Physical therapists can teach you different methods of moving, resting and conserving your energy. You can learn how to listen to your body and what to do to prevent the return of symptoms. For example, if you have tennis elbow, special recommended exercises can prevent the return of any symptoms.

HOW PHYSICAL THERAPY IS USED

Physical therapy is available in health centers, hospitals, private offices, and sports facilities. It consists of:

- ❑ Exercises which may be passive, where the therapist moves the body part to increase the range of motion, or active programs, which may include stationary bikes and weightlifting equipment (passive exercises increase joint mobility, but do not strengthen the muscles, while active exercises are for strengthening);

- ❑ Hydrotherapy, including swimming; (*See* HYDROTHERAPY in PART 2 Treatment Section);
- ❑ Gait training for safety and prevention of falls;
- ❑ Massages;
- ❑ Motivation;
- ❑ Traction devices;
- ❑ Ultrasound therapy;
- ❑ Training in the use of artificial limbs, braces, and splints;
- ❑ Training in the proper use of crutches, canes, and wheelchairs.

PHYSICAL THERAPY TO THE RESCUE

Anna, a seventy-three-year-old woman with osteoarthritis in both knees, felt they were giving way when she walked, climbed stairs, or played tennis or golf. Her physical therapy program consisted of lower extremity stretching, strengthening, and endurance exercises supplemented with a variety of walking-based agility and perturbation-training techniques (perturbation refers to a small change in a physical system). At the conclusion of her twelve twice-weekly sessions, she was able to walk, climb stairs, and return to playing golf and tennis with greatly reduced pain and instability.

Fitzgerald, GK, Childs, JD, Ridge, TM, et al. "Agility and perturbation training for a physically active individual with knee osteoarthritis." *Physical Therapy.* April 2002; 82:372–382.

CAUTIONS

Physical therapists can perform an evaluation, but they cannot do the therapy until a physician recommends it. Unless they are also licensed acupuncturists, PTs should not do acupuncture, and physical therapy cannot be used to reverse peripheral neuropathy.

You should be comfortable with your physical therapist, and motivation is a part of the treatment, but remember that PTs are not psychologists.

CLINICAL STUDIES

Ekstrom, RA, Holden, K. "Examination of and intervention for a patient with chronic lateral elbow pain with signs of nerve entrapment." *Physical Therapy.* November 2002; 82:1077–1086.

A forty-three-year-old woman had right lateral elbow pain which she attributed to extensive keyboard work on a computer. Diagnosed with a mild entrapment of the deep radial nerve, she was treated fourteen times over a ten-week period with neural mobilization techniques (designed to free nerves for movement), strengthening exercises, stretching, and ultrasound. By the end of her treatment, she was pain-free, and at her four-month follow-up visit, she reported that she had resumed all her activities.

Mannerkorpi, K, Ahlmen, M, Ekdahl, C. "Six- and 24-month follow-up of pool exercise therapy and education for patients with fibromyalgia." *Scandinavian Journal of Rheumatology.* 2002; 31(5):306–310.

This Swedish study found that improvements in symptom severity, physical function, and social function were still found six and twenty-four months after the completed pool-treatment program.

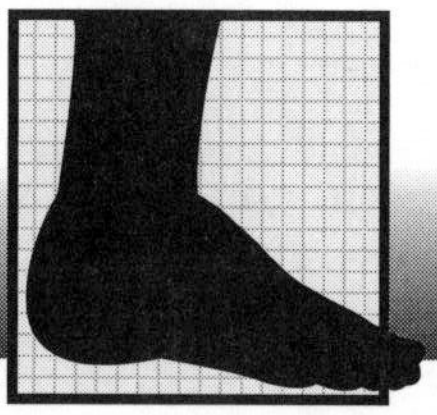

Reflexology

Reflexology is the application of pressure to specific areas (notably the foot) to help the body heal itself naturally. The basic premise is that the foot is a microcosm of the entire body and that precisely defined sections of it are connected to specific parts of the body, such as the head, neck, and the various internal organs. When pressure is applied to these specific areas, also referred to as zones, balance is restored so healing can occur naturally. Reflexology helps eliminate energy blockages, improves circulation, and relieves stress and tension. In addition to the feet, the hands and ears also have reflexes that can be used for treatment of corresponding body parts.

THE HISTORY OF REFLEXOLOGY

The practice of reflexology has been around for centuries, at least. If foot massages can be considered simple forms of reflexology, then the practice is as old as humans are, maybe even older, because some species of monkeys were known to do primitive types of foot massages. They weren't aware of its healing properties, they just did it from instinct and because it felt good.

Five thousand years ago, in India and China, the entire foot was looked upon as a mirror of the body, and Native Americans have always believed that using the feet to treat the body worked because the feet were in contact with the earth and its energy.

In ancient Egypt, the hands and the feet of sick people were used to treat their illnesses. A picture on the wall of a physician's tomb in Egypt, dating back to 2300–2500 BC, shows two men working on the feet of two other men. In a nearby inscription, the physician is responding to the patient's plea, "Don't hurt me," by saying, "I shall act so you praise me."

In the United States, in 1902, Dr. William H. Fitzgerald, an ear, nose, and throat specialist, noted that applying pressure and stroking certain reflexes in the body would result in the normal functioning of specific organs, regardless of how far they were from the area being treated. He brought his findings to the medical profession in 1913 and published a book in 1917 entitled *Zone Therapy, or Relieving Pain at Home*. Although not widely accepted by the medical profession, one colleague, Dr. Joe Shelby Riley thought the theory had merit and discussed it with a therapist in his office, Eunice Ingham, who had studied Fitzgerald's work, which concentrated mostly on the hands. While agreeing with his overall theory of reflexes, she believed that the reflexes in the feet were more sensitive than those in the hands, and she went on to develop her foot reflexology theory in the 1930s. She mapped the zones of the feet in relation to the body's organs, wrote books on the subject, and gave seminars throughout the United States. Today, most reflexologists use her method.

HOW REFLEXOLOGY WORKS

Reflexology stimulates nerve endings and reflex points in order to allow energy to flow freely through the body. When the therapist presses her or his thumbs into the different parts of the foot, if there is discomfort or pain felt in any particular area of the foot, it indicates there is an imbalance in the corresponding part of the body. When a reflexologist stimulates nerve endings and reflex points, and the energy is allowed to flow more freely throughout the body, it aids in restoring balance and warding off illness.

Although reflexologists do not make diagnoses, their probing can often determine which glands or organs are not working efficiently.

PAINFUL CONDITIONS THAT RESPOND WELL TO REFLEXOLOGY

Reflexology aids relaxation, and it helps reduce muscle tension and the stress that lowers your resistance and makes you more susceptible to physical and emotional disorders. It is useful for almost all the painful conditions addressed in this book, and it can also be used to treat a long list of disorders, ranging from acne to wrist sprains and fractures, and including anxiety, asthma, bladder problems, colds, coughs, eye problems, hemorrhoids, insomnia, and liver and gallbladder problems. It has even been known to stimulate painful kidney stones to pass

COUGHING STOPPED IN ITS TRACKS

Cassandra L. had a painful cough that hung on after a bout of bronchitis. She was going to attend a concert and didn't want to annoy those around her, so her reflexologist suggested she squeeze the top joint of her middle finger. Whenever Cassandra felt a cough coming on during the concert, she squeezed the joint and held it a minute or so, which successfully stopped the dreaded cough in its tracks and allowed her to sit through the concert without experiencing pain or disturbing her fellow concertgoers.

without surgical intervention. (*See* Quick Help Chart for synopsis of suggested treatments for all chronic pain conditions covered in this book.)

ADVANTAGES OF REFLEXOLOGY

- ❏ No expensive equipment is necessary.
- ❏ Reflexology is noninvasive and has none of the side effects of drugs.
- ❏ It helps keep your body balanced, reduces stress, revitalizes energy, and helps strengthen your immune system.
- ❏ It also stimulates circulation, and helps relieve digestive disorders, insomnia, headaches, PMS, and urinary tract problems.
- ❏ It is a more holistic approach to treatment. For example, if you consulted a reflexologist because of bronchitis, he or she would treat your entire respiratory system rather than merely addressing the condition and its symptoms.
- ❏ Illness is regarded as a breakdown of your body's systems and reflexology helps your body eliminate toxins and absorb nutrients.
- ❏ Reflexologists will not tell you to stop taking your medication. When medicine is deemed necessary, the treatment can help you absorb it more effectively.
- ❏ Reflexology can also reduce high blood pressure and relieve sinus pressure.
- ❏ Although reflexology is not used as a diagnostic tool, tenderness in a particular reflex can indicate a potential problem in the area connected to the reflex. For example, if you have tenderness in the area right under the big toe or between your toes, which are the areas connected to the teeth, you might want to see your dentist in order to nip a potential problem in the bud.

SAFARI SAVED BY REFLEXOLOGY

Laura W. was in Africa on a photographic safari when she developed a very painful toothache that was in danger of becoming chronic and effectively ending her trip. There were no dentists in the bush, but fortunately, because she was familiar with the techniques of reflexology, she knew to apply pressure to the area at the bottom of her big toe where it attaches to the foot and touches the ground. The toothache evaporated on cue and she was able to continue her safari. Back home, her dentist took a look at the tooth and told her there had been an abscess there, but it had started to resolve itself.

HOW REFLEXOLOGY IS USED

You sit in a reclining chair or lie down on a treatment table with your feet raised and supported. The reflexologist does not immediately concentrate on any particular problem, but first probes your feet looking for tender areas and signs of tension. Then, treatment begins. The practitioner employs relaxation techniques to release tension by applying gentle, firm pressure to each foot's reflex zones. If one zone appears to be more tender than another, the therapist will return to that area and give it more attention. Most reflexologists start a treatment by massaging the toes first and moving gradually toward the heel.

When using the reflexes in the hand, the fingers are massaged first and movement is directed up the hand toward the wrist. Since pressure points in the hands and feet are connected to various areas of the body, think of the fingers and toes as your head, the balls of your feet and your palms as your upper body, and your heels and the area near your wrists as your lower body.

In case you are wondering why your therapist begins a session by working on your entire foot rather than just the area connected to what is ailing you, it is because she or he is attempting to stimulate circulation throughout the body in order to eliminate any toxins that may be keeping your organs and glands from functioning efficiently. As tender spots are noted, more attention will be focused on them to bring healing to the affected area of your body.

Regarding tender spots, many people ask if a foot injury can lead to health problems and, yes, it is possible that such an injury could cause a blockage in your body. For instance, an ingrown toenail may relate to headaches. At a dinner party, Dr. Fitzgerald met a singer who said she could no longer reach the upper register tones. Throat specialists were unable to determine why she had the problem. Dr. Fitzgerald asked to examine her feet and noticed a callus on her right great toe. He applied pressure to the zone in that area for a few minutes and she said the pain in her toe had disappeared. He then asked her to try the tones of her upper register and she was able to sing two notes higher than ever before.

Self-Treating with Reflexology

You can treat yourself with reflexology. Charts of the feet and hands are available from practitioners, or in health food stores and some bookstores. Books with step-by-step instructions are available. It is a good idea to have a few professional treatments first to become acquainted with the technique. Some areas of your feet may be hard for you to reach, but it is relatively easy to work on your own hands.

Here is a brief guide to help you locate some of the reflexes.

- ❑ Your left foot relates to the left side of your body, and the right foot to the right side.
- ❑ The big toe corresponds with your head.
- ❑ Your neck and throat reflexes are on the underside of the big toe, and the back of the head and neck are on the top part of the toe.
- ❑ Spinal reflexes are located on the inside of the foot, from the middle or your great toe down to the heel bone.
- ❑ Your eye and ear reflexes are just beneath the other four toes.
- ❑ Your colon is midfoot. (Unless mentioned otherwise, all reflexes mentioned refer to the bottom of foot, the part touching the ground.)
- ❑ Your sciatic nerve is where your heel pad starts.
- ❑ Sex glands are located in the anklebone areas, both on the inside and outside of the leg.

The charts can show where on the soles of the feet the other glands are located.

You don't have to know the exact location of each reflex. You can just start massaging your entire foot from toes to heel, and if you come upon a tender spot, give it a bit more attention.

Your upper body might respond better to hand treatment because your fingers are longer than your toes and there is more area to work on. Also your hands are more convenient to reach than your feet when you are treating yourself, and are not as noticeable if you are in public. The theory is the same as for your feet, the right hand is for the right side of the body, and the left hand is for the left side. The thumb corresponds to your big toe and your fingers to the other toes.

CAUTIONS

- ❑ Keep in mind that reflexology is an adjunct to medical treatment, not a substitute for it.
- ❑ Be sure your therapist has been certified in reflexology.
- ❑ If you are pregnant, consult your obstetrician before having a reflexology treatment because reflexology has been used to help induce labor.
- ❑ If you have a vascular problem in your legs, such as phlebitis or thrombosis, consult with your healthcare provider before having foot reflexology.

CLINICAL STUDIES

Oleson, Terry, Flocco, William. "Randomized Controlled Study of Premenstrual Symptoms Treated with Ear, Hand and Foot Reflexology." *Obstetrics and Gynecology.* 1993; 82:906–911.

In the United States, conventional practitioners and reflexologists are just beginning to collaborate and do research together. This study is about the benefits of reflexology for premenstrual syndrome and showed that a significantly greater decrease in symptoms was observed among women receiving true reflexology than among those in a placebo group.

Reflexology research has mainly been done in China, Denmark, and the United Kingdom. The majority of Chi-

REFLEXOLOGY FOR A STROKE

Although strokes are not chronic pain conditions, this is another example of how a simple reflexology adjustment can completely change an outcome.

At the age of fifty-nine, Rose was a remarkably beautiful woman who still worked as a model. Since she was in such good shape and excellent health, it was a major shock to everyone when she had a massive stroke. Her husband rushed her to the emergency room where the doctors tried every heroic measure they knew to save her. She had lapsed into a coma and the neurologist said to call her children in to say goodbye. When her son, a reflexologist, arrived, he pressed the pituitary point located on her big toe as hard as he could. All of a sudden, Rose sat up and screamed out, "What is going on?" The doctors stood there openmouthed and shaking their heads. They had no idea how that could have happened. But, because her son knew what to do, Rose is now seventy-five and remains in good health.

Note: If someone is having a stroke, it is crucial to get them to the emergency room immediately, but on the way you can try to press the pituitary point located deep in the center of the pad of the big toe. It might be worthwhile for emergency room doctors to add this technique to their repertoire.

nese studies have been performed by the Reflexology Society of China where foot reflexology was found to be significantly effective in treating a wide variety of disorders. The Chinese are continuing to research over 100 health conditions that can possibly be helped by reflexology.

The United Danish Reflexologist Association has hundreds of valid case studies, particularly for pain reduction during childbirth, asthma relief, chronic constipation, headaches, and migraines.

In the United Kingdom, clinical studies are done in conjunction with mainstream healthcare practitioners. Along with trained reflexologists, Australian and South African physicians have studied the usefulness of reflexology for pain caused by arthritis, headaches, and back, neck, and shoulder problems. In Switzerland, research is being done for pain relief on terminal cancer patients.

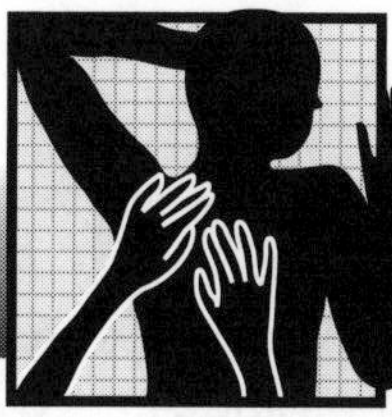

Rolfing

Rolfing, unlike some other touch therapies, does not involve a pleasurable massage. It goes much deeper, focusing on a network of connective tissue: the fascia, which surrounds the muscles; the tendons, which link muscle to the bones; and the ligaments, which join bone to bone. It is often described as painful, but is considered very effective. It is designed to place your body in balance with gravity by releasing stress patterns that keep it out of alignment. The therapy is named after Dr. Ida P. Rolf who believed that emotional, as well as physical health depends on being in proper alignment. Her method differs from chiropractic because she believed that, in addition to the spine, your head, ears, shoulders, thorax, pelvis, hips, knees, and ankles must also be properly aligned in order for you to be healthy.

THE HISTORY OF ROLFING

In the twenties, Dr. Ida P. Rolf, a biochemist, experimented with different existing therapies, including yoga and osteopathy, until she developed the holistic answer she was looking for—a system of soft-tissue manipulation and movement education that she called Structural Integration. In the sixties, she taught the technique to potential practitioners at Esalen in Big Sur, California where Rolfing became the nickname given to her technique. Today there are more than 1,000 Rolfers in private practice worldwide, and the method is also used adjunctively by chiropractors, kinesiologists, massage therapists, and others.

HOW ROLFING WORKS

Dr. Rolf noticed a relationship between muscular tension and pent-up emotions. Rolfers believe that all of us have patterns of tension that can be released by realigning our bodies. The fascia around the muscles can form adhesions in one part of our body that can negatively affect other parts of it. Breaking down tight connective tissue allows the muscles to be more flexible so the body can realign into a more functional mode. Once your body is properly aligned, it works more efficiently, with much less wear and tear. Ten Rolfing sessions can usually help you develop a more efficient movement pattern.

PAINFUL CONDITIONS THAT RESPOND WELL TO ROLFING

- ❑ Achilles tendonitis.
- ❑ Back problems, including neck pain.
- ❑ Bursitis.
- ❑ Carpal tunnel syndrome.
- ❑ Dental pain.
- ❑ Fibromyalgia.
- ❑ Frozen shoulder.
- ❑ Neuroma.
- ❑ Osteoarthritis.
- ❑ Pelvic floor tension myalgia.
- ❑ Postherpetic neuralgia.
- ❑ Post-polio syndrome.
- ❑ Reflex sympathetic dystrophy syndrome (RSDS).
- ❑ Rheumatoid arthritis.
- ❑ Rotator cuff tendonitis.
- ❑ Sciatica.
- ❑ Tarsal tunnel syndrome.
- ❑ Temporomandibular joint (TMJ) pain.
- ❑ Tennis elbow.
- ❑ Trigeminal neuralgia.
- ❑ Trigger finger.

In addition to these painful conditions, Rolfing can be very effective in treating impaired mobility, stress, and sports injuries, according to Dr. Randy Coleman, a naturopathic doctor in Pennsylvania. It can also help other conditions caused by compressed nerves.

ADVANTAGES OF ROLFING

Rolfing can have reasonably long-lasting effects in easing pain and chronic stress, and improving performance in your activities, both professional and personal. Many of those who have been Rolfed say that, in addition to having their pain relieved, they have achieved a fuller realization of their potential. Rolfing can also help to improve athletic performance, and many top athletes get Rolfed on a regular basis.

HOW ROLFING IS USED

In progressive sessions, Rolfers stretch and move the pliable connective tissue until your body is balanced along its natural axis, and gravity takes over and keeps it that way. Ten Rolfing sessions (at a cost of approximately $100 per session) is the recommended course of treatment, but most people find relief after only a few treatments, during which it is not necessary to remove any undergarments. Afterward, you will feel loose and relaxed, and you will be able to go back to work, or resume your normal activities.

CAUTIONS

Since deep pressure is applied, it is crucial to have a qualified practitioner. The Rolf Institute issues certificates to practitioners after completing two nine-week courses, and there are continuing education classes for three to five years after certification. Although the procedure can be somewhat painful while it is being performed, there should be no pain after the session is finished.

CLINICAL STUDIES

Here are several examples of the many research studies that have been performed on Structural Integration/Rolfing over the years.

Cottingham, J. "Shifts in Pelvic Inclination Angle and Parasympathetic Tone Produced by Rolfing Soft Tissue Manipulation." *Physical Therapy.* March 1988; 68:1364–1370.

The group receiving Rolfing showed positive results compared to the control group, and this provided support for the use of soft tissue pelvic manipulation for certain types of low back dysfunction and stress-related musculoskeletal disorders.

Cottingham, J, Maitland, J. "A Three-Paradigm Treatment Model Using Soft Tissue Mobilization and Guided Movement-Awareness Techniques for Patients with Chronic Back Pain: A Case Study." *The Journal of Orthopaedic and Sports Physical Therapy.* September 1997; 26(3).

Of the three methods studied, the Rolfing method of soft tissue mobilization (combined with the Alexander system of guided movement-awareness techniques) was the most successful in providing sustained improvement for the subject's chronic low back pain through a four-week follow-up.

Deutsch, JE, Derr, LL, Judd, P, et al. "Treatment of chronic pain through the use of structural integration (rolfing)." *Orthopaedic Physical Therapy Clinics of North America 2000;* 9(3):411–425.

A group of people with chronic pain benefited from structural integration (Rolfing). Their posture improved and their pain decreased, prompting the authors to recommend further controlled studies on the efficacy of S.I.

Hunt, V, Massey, W. "A Study of Structural Integration from Neuromuscular, Energy Field and Emotional Approaches." *UCLA Department of Kinesiology,* 1977.

These doctors established that Rolfing achieved its stated aims.

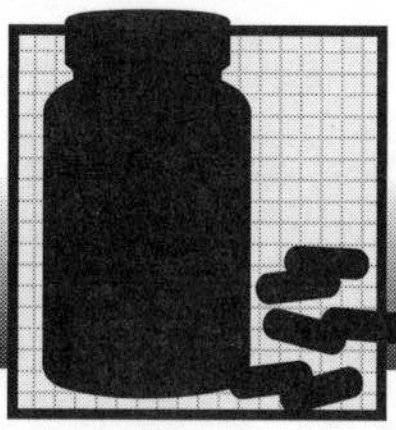

Supplement Therapy

Supplementation is often necessary because so many foods have been processed or altered that they end up lacking the proper nutrients. Vitamins, minerals, amino acids, antioxidants, enzymes and herbs (a separate entry) are all supplements, and all are beneficial for many conditions, but we are limiting the discussion here to those useful for chronic pain. You can buy supplements at health food stores, grocery stores, pharmacies, by mail, and on the Internet. They are available in many forms including capsules, geltabs, liquids, powders, and tablets.

Vitamins are substances derived from plant and animal food sources, or they may be synthetic. They are present in varying quantities in many different foods. Minerals are necessary to help your body assimilate vitamins. Soil contains minerals, which are absorbed by the fruits and vegetables you eat.

Amino acids are components of protein and act as neurotransmitters that are needed by the brain to send and receive messages. Enzymes are complex proteins produced by living plant and animal cells that help digest food, repair body tissue and aid most body functions. Antioxidants include those particular vitamins, minerals, and enzymes that protect your body from free radicals.

THE HISTORY OF SUPPLEMENT THERAPY

No one actually discovered vitamins because they were always there, present in all natural foods, but in 1880, Dr. Christian Eijkman created a vitamin deficiency in animals, then reversed the condition with an appropriate feeding regimen. Through trial and error, he discovered that removing the outer coating of rice so it would be fluffy and white caused beriberi. Dr. Eijkman published his findings about beriberi in the late nineteenth century and was ridiculed for more than twenty years, until later researchers determined that foods contained growth factors necessary to sustain life. In 1911, an enterprising European chemist, Cashmir Funk, studied Eijkman's findings. He obtained huge amounts of rice husks, concentrated them, and called the product *vitamine,* from *vita,* which means life, and from chemical substances called *amines.* Dr. Funk moved to the United States and started a vitamin business that became very successful.

Until recently, conventional medical professionals looked upon supplements only in relation to the diseases of deficiency they caused, as for example: a lack of iron caused anemia, a lack of vitamin B_1 caused beriberi, a lack of calcium caused osteoporosis, a lack of vitamin B_3 caused pellagra, a lack of vitamin C caused scurvy, and a lack of vitamin D caused rickets. Since the mid-twentieth century, however, it has been shown that supplements can have therapeutic effects, as well as preventive powers.

Linus Pauling, who won the Nobel Prize twice, once for chemistry and once for peace, believed the body's nutrient concentrations were not always adequate to nourish all its tissues and organs, and that every disease could be traced back to a mineral deficiency. He is probably best known for his research on the efficacy of vitamin C megadoses. Today, supplement therapy is widely practiced by naturopathic doctors as well as some of the more enlightened conventional practitioners.

HOW SUPPLEMENT THERAPY WORKS

Vitamins, minerals, amino acids, and enzymes work by regulating your body's metabolism. They are needed in order for your body to function normally, and are present in all natural foods. However, due to overprocessing, use of pesticides, herbicides, fungicides, foods being grown in deficient soil, and animals being medicated with hormones and antibiotics, there really is no such thing as a healthy diet today. We can no longer rely on food alone, so it is necessary to supplement our diets in order to sustain optimum health.

Unless it is a deficiency disease, such as beriberi, rickets, or scurvy, supplements cannot actually cure disease, but a growing body of evidence has shown that specific supplements can have a positive effect on particular conditions. The list is long and volumes abound on the subject, but we are limiting our discussion to those supplements that can address the painful conditions in this book.

PAINFUL CONDITIONS THAT RESPOND WELL TO SUPPLEMENT THERAPY

All conditions will benefit from therapy with supplements. Refer to individual treatment entries for specific recommendations and suggested dosages. (*See also* Quick Help Chart for synopsis of suggested treatments for all chronic pain conditions covered in this book.)

ADVANTAGES OF SUPPLEMENT THERAPY

There are no side effects. They strengthen our bodies and help them function better, making them more resistant to disease and infections.

HOW TO USE SUPPLEMENT THERAPY

According to Dr. Edward M. Wagner, it is important to take supplements in proper balance because an excess of one can cause a depletion of another. For example, he says that megadoses of zinc can deplete your body of copper and iron.

Vitamins

Some vitamins are fat-soluble and others are water-soluble. The fat-soluble vitamins are A, D, E, and K. They absorb better when taken with food. They can be stored in your body and can be toxic if too much is taken. The water-soluble vitamins, which include the Bs and Vitamin C, are not stored and are excreted within a few hours, so they should be constantly replenished. It is best to divide the dosage and take them two or three times a day.

Here is a rundown of the various vitamins and what they can do for you. Please note that they have many other benefits, but we are limiting our discussion to chronic pain control.

- ❏ Vitamin A aids tissue maintenance and repair. It acts as an antioxidant that helps protect your cells and helps protect your body against infections and inflammation.
- ❏ B_1 (thiamine) aids circulation and promotes normal muscle tone of your heart, intestines, and stomach. It aids carbohydrate metabolism, can help relieve dental pain, and is useful for treating shingles.
- ❏ B_2 (riboflavin) is beneficial for the mucous membranes in your digestive system. It also helps your body assimilate B_6 and iron. Carpal tunnel syndrome can be helped by using B_2 along with B_6. It is also useful for migraine headaches.
- ❏ B_3 (niacin) aids circulation and the digestive and nervous system. It also lowers cholesterol.
- ❏ B_5 (pantothenic acid) helps relieve stress and helps the gastrointestinal system to function normally. It also supports the adrenal glands.
- ❏ B_6 (pyridoxine) is useful for the nervous system, relieves PMS, and helps treat arthritis and carpal tunnel syndrome. It also reduces muscle spasms, neuritis, and numbness in the arms and legs. It helps your body absorb B_{12}.
- ❏ B_{12} (cyanocobalamin) helps keep the nervous system healthy and increases energy.

The B vitamins have to be kept in balance, and if you are taking therapeutic doses of one, be sure to take a supplement containing the entire range of B complex.

- ❏ Vitamin C (ascorbic acid) aids tissue repair, promotes healing, and builds collagen. It is available in a form called Ester-C, which allows better absorption.
- ❏ Vitamin E (tocopherol) accelerates healing, reduces inflammation improves circulation, and repairs tissue. It helps alleviate leg cramps and lessens heart problems.

Minerals

Minerals are also useful substances to help fight pain and they work synergistically with vitamins. It is best to take them with food. Several of the most helpful are listed below.

- ❏ Boron has been shown to alleviate osteoarthritis. It also strengthens bones and is used for menopausal problems.
- ❏ Magnesium is especially useful for headache pain and premenstrual syndrome. It acts as a muscle relaxant and antispasmodic, and has helped people with coronary heart disease, including painful angina. It works well with B_6.
- ❏ Methylsulfonylmethane (MSM), a natural sulfur compound, helps alleviate inflammation and joint pain, and promotes healing. It is available in capsule, tablet, or powder form. Take according to directions on label.
- ❏ Selenium works with vitamin E. It acts as an anti-inflammatory, helps relieve muscle pain and stiffness and aching. It is also excellent for liver problems.
- ❏ SierraSil is a composite of ninety-six minerals, including boron, calcium, chromium, copper, iron, manganese, magnesium, molybdenum, phosphorous, potassium, selenium, vanadium, and zinc. Found exclusively in the high Sierras, it is considered helpful for the pain of osteoarthritis and other joint problems.

Amino Acids

Amino acids should be taken between meals on an empty stomach.

- ❏ DL-phenylalanine (DLPA) is a natural painkiller that releases endorphins, your body's natural painkillers. It is especially useful for arthritis, back pain, migraines, and neuralgia.
- ❏ Glucosamine sulfate, a naturally occurring amino sugar, is necessary for building and maintaining connective tissues and lubricatiung fluids in the body. It is effective in alleviating the pain of arthritis, especially when taken with chondroitin sulfate.
- ❏ L-arginine helps bring energy to weak muscles.
- ❏ L-glutamine counteracts fluid retention. It helps reduce swelling and is useful for all digestive illnesses.
- ❏ L-histadine aids digestion by promoting the secretions that are needed to break down food particles so they can be properly assimilated. When food is not properly digested, it can be a contributing factor to inflammation in the bowel.
- ❏ L-proline helps rebuild joint linings, and also helps protect your coronary arteries against plaque.

- ❑ Gamma-aminobutyric acid (GABA) is a muscle relaxant.

Enzymes

When you take enzymes with food, they act as digestive aids. Between meals they act as anti-inflammatories.

- ❑ Bromelain is a natural anti-inflammatory. It is relatively inexpensive and available in a generic form.
- ❑ Multi-enzymes (combinations) are also available under various brand names.

Additional Useful Supplements

- ❑ Coenzyme Q_{10} strengthens the immune system and the heart muscle. It helps the body to generate energy and is also helpful for periodontal disease.
- ❑ Shark cartilage reduces inflammation and makes the body more alkaline.
- ❑ Evening primrose oil relieves pain and inflammation.

CAUTIONS

Vitamins may be natural or synthetic. Generally natural is better, but in some instances, such as a pollen allergy, a natural form of vitamin C might cause an allergic reaction and the synthetic form would be better.

Since megadoses of one product can cause a depletion of others, if you are going to use megadoses of supplements, it is a good idea to consult a nutritionist, a naturopathic physician, or a nutritionally savvy conventional practitioner.

(*See also* HERBAL REMEDIES, HOMEOPATHY, and NUTRITIONAL THERAPY in PART 2 Treatment Section.)

CLINICAL STUDIES

Al Faraj, S, Al Mutairi, K. "Vitamin D deficiency and chronic low back pain in Saudi Arabia." *Spine.* January 15, 2003; 28(2):177–179.

This six-year study of 360 people, ages fifteen to fifty-two, with non-specific back pain showed that vitamin-D deficiency was a major contributor to chronic low back pains, and that there was a 95-percent clinical improvement of symptoms in those treated with vitamin D supplements.

Harima, A. "The analgesic effects of L-arginine on chronic pain." *Journal of the Medical Society of Toho University* (Japan). 1997; (43)5:554–559.

Twenty-four people with various kinds of pain lasting more than six months were intravenously administered L-arginine. In all cases, they obtained moderate pain relief ten to fifteen minutes later, and an almost pain-free state thereafter, with these analgesic effects lasting between six and twenty-four hours, depending on dosage. Minimal side effects were a slight decrease in systolic blood pressure in one case, and dry mouth in several cases. Repeated doses did not build up a tolerance to the supplement, and the conclusion reached was that L-arginine-therapy is a promising choice for the management of chronic pain.

Kitade, T, Odahara, Y, Shinohara, S, et al. "Studies on the enhanced effect of acupuncture analgesia and acupuncture anesthesia by D-phenylalanine (2nd report)—schedule of administration and clinical effects in low back pain and tooth extraction." *Acupuncture Electrotherapy Res.* 1990; 15(2):121–135.

This Japanese cross-treatment study of thirty patients with low back pain who were treated with acupuncture thirty minutes after receiving oral doses of D-phenylalanine showed positive results compared to the placebo group, and showed that D-phenylalanine enhances the effect of acupuncture.

Newnham, RE. "Essentiality of boron for healthy bones and joints." *Environmental Health Perspective.* November 1994;102 Suppl 7:83–85.

This long-term, double-blind, placebo-boron-supplementation, British study of twenty people with osteoarthritis showed there was improvement in those taking daily boron supplements. It indicated that boron is an essential nutrient and that further study of its use in treatment and prevention of arthritis was warranted.

Pavelka, K, Gatterova, J, Olejarova, M, et al. "Glucosamine sulfate use and delay of progression of knee arthritis: a 3-year, randomized, placebo-controlled, double-blind study." *Archives of Internal Medicine.* October 14, 2002;162(18):2113–2123.

This Prague study of 200 people with arthritis of the knee determined that long-term treatment with glucosamine sulfate slowed the progress of arthritis of the knee, "possibly determining disease modification," according to its authors.

PHENYLALANINE—A DRUG-FREE APPROACH TO CHRONIC PAIN

There have been a number of books and studies done on the proven efficacy of D-phenylalanine in the treatment of chronic pain conditions when other painkilling methods have failed. Though it is safe, non-addictive, and non-toxic, it should be taken after meals if you have high blood pressure, and is contraindicated for pregnancy and phenylketonuria (PKU). If you want to know more about the analgesic effects of D-phenylanine, contact the Life Extension Foundation in Fort Lauderdale, FL, or go to the website *www.DoctorYourself.com* hosted by Dr. Andrew Saul.

Tai Chi, Qigong, and Yoga

Tai chi is an Eastern form of exercise that combines meditation with slow circular movements. If you watch people doing tai chi it looks as if they are performing a martial art in a slow dance form. It connects your mind and thoughts to your body and your chi, the life energy that flows through your body. The slow, even, controlled movements help you become aware of how you move your body. It is a whole-body activity that is extremely low impact and does not stress your joints or ligaments.

Qigong is a powerful self-healing method consisting of movement and meditation. Qi means life force or energy and gong means practice. There are at least 1,000 varieties of qigong, with various names, and some refer to it as the Chinese yoga. People practice qigong in large groups or by themselves. Some teachers prefer large groups because they believe more energy is present. It is a method of collecting and circulating additional energy and eliminating unbalanced or disordered energy.

The word yoga is derived from Sanskrit, an ancient language. It means to unite the body, mind, and spirit. The most popular form of yoga is hatha yoga, a combination of exercises and breath control, which has sprouted many offshoots. In the United States, yoga is usually a combination of physical and meditative practices. In the classes you will be taught the various postures, along with breathing techniques, while you stretch your body.

THE HISTORY OF TAI CHI, QIGONG, AND YOGA

Tai chi is the oldest of the martial arts. It was based on the theory of yin and yang, two energies in the universe that were described in the *I Ching*, an ancient Chinese text. The *I Ching* was originally used for meditation and predictions. Greatly simplified, yin is a retreating energy and yang is a strong, forward-moving energy. About 1,200 years ago, the philosophy of yin and yang eventually evolved from a solely mental discipline to a physical one, and in this form it became tai chi. The exercises help bring the two energies into harmony with each other. A sixteenth-century martial artist, Zhang Sanfeng, is credited with creating tai chi. He had a dream about a snake and a crane fighting each other and their graceful movements inspired him. Many Chinese practice tai chi daily and it is a common sight to see them in parks, early in the morning, going through their motions. In the early 1970s, tai chi branched out from the Chinese community and became popular with many Westerners in the United States and abroad.

Qigong, also referred to as chi kung, has been practiced since the time of the early Chinese shamans thousands of years ago. It has a martial form to enhance the strength and mindset of the warrior, and a medical gong (practice) that is used for healing purposes. In the third century AD, Hua To developed qigong exercises known as the five animal forms. In the sixth century AD, Da Mo, a monk from India, developed a combination of movement with meditation. After the Chinese revolution in 1940, qigong was labeled witchcraft and disappeared until the 1970s and '80s when it regained popularity in China and was introduced in the West.

Yoga was developed as a spiritual practice in India more than 5,000 years ago. Ancient priests, known as yogis, studied nature and observed how animals were strong and flexible and maintained their balance. From their observations, they developed a form of exercise, which they combined with their spirituality. Yoga remained strictly a Hindu practice until the twentieth century when the yogis began traveling to the West. At first, the Christian populations were better able to relate to the exercise components of the art than the spiritual, but in the mid-twentieth century, Indra Devi, known as the first lady of yoga, opened a yoga studio in Hollywood. Movie stars started to practice all elements of yoga with Devi, and she trained many teachers to carry the discipline forward. Her teacher, Krishna Macharya, also taught B. K. S. Iyengar, who founded his own school of hatha yoga that developed many followers in the United States and around the world.

HOW TAI CHI, QIGONG, AND YOGA WORK

According to Eastern philosophy, when chi flows properly through your body, your system is balanced, maintaining health. If it is disrupted, you can get sick. By practicing how to focus on the motion and control your breathing, you may eventually learn how to feel the chi and send it to any part of your body where it is needed. Tai chi works by increasing circulation and strengthening the soft tissues that support the joints.

The tai chi postures help open your joints and move your body correctly. The movements help develop muscular control rather than bulk, and people who have taken up tai chi generally have stonger abdominal muscles and better balance. Studies have shown that devel-

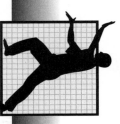

oping this balance through the practice of tai chi can help prevent falls in older people and can also reduce their blood pressure. Qigong helps the chi to flow properly, which promotes health. Both tai chi and qigong are concerned with how the chi flows to promote health, and they are considered complementary to each other rather than competitors.

Yoga postures, combined with deep breathing techniques, which nourish your body with oxygen and aid in circulating blood to your brain, help combat stress-related problems by creating a balance between your mind and body. Yoga works on the adrenals and the hormones. By toning your glands, yoga postures stimulate them to produce hormones.

Iyengar yoga, and its recent offspring, Anusara (*flowing with grace*) yoga, are ideally suited to pain relief. Both emphasize proper alignment as the starting point for a highly effective, safe yoga practice that can help you relieve your pain, while avoiding injury.

PAINFUL CONDITIONS THAT RESPOND WELL TO TAI CHI, QIGONG, AND YOGA

These treatments are especially useful for the following conditions.

- ❑ Angina.
- ❑ Back pain.
- ❑ Carpal tunnel syndrome.
- ❑ Cluster headaches.
- ❑ Crohn's disease.
- ❑ Diverticulitis.
- ❑ Endometriosis.
- ❑ Fibromyalgia.
- ❑ Gout.
- ❑ Irritable bowel syndrome.
- ❑ Migraine headaches.
- ❑ Osteoarthritis.
- ❑ Pelvic floor tension myalgia.
- ❑ Postherpetic neuralgia.
- ❑ Post-polio syndrome.
- ❑ Premenstrual syndrome.
- ❑ Sciatica.
- ❑ Tarsal tunnel syndrome.
- ❑ Tension headaches.
- ❑ Ulcerative colitis.

Since these therapies induce a profoundly relaxed state, they are beneficial for all types of painful conditions, and for health in general.

Other conditions that benefit from these Eastern movement therapies include asthma, cancer, diabetes, hypertension, and psychological problems.

ADVANTAGES OF TAI CHI, QIGONG, AND YOGA

- ❑ They do not require any special equipment.
- ❑ They help your joints stay mobile and help you to extend your range of motion.
- ❑ They aid balance, thereby helping to prevent falls, especially in older people. (The primary reason for older people ending up in nursing homes is the no-longer-manageable cascade of problems that result from falls.)
- ❑ They relieve pain by reducing stress and tension. Here is how it works: Pain causes stress, which leads to muscle tension and constriction of the blood vessels, which leads to even more pain. This sets up what is referred to as the pain cycle. With these relaxation techniques, the cycle is interrupted, the muscles and blood vessels relax, and the pain is alleviated. This is similar to the theories taught to women in natural childbirth classes.

All chronic pain conditions will benefit from these therapies. In addition, these methods will also:

- ❑ Aid your cardiovascular system;
- ❑ Help lower blood pressure;

YOGA, THE ANTI-AGING AGENT

Dr. Dharma Singh Khalsa, MD, an anesthesiologist certified in pain management, discussed what he calls "medical meditation," based on kundalini yoga (a form of hatha yoga), in an interview in the *Yoga Journal*. Answering a question related to his book, *Meditation as Medicine*, he says that medical meditation can slow down the aging process by stimulating the endocrine system. "The glands wear out as we age, producing fewer hormones," he says, adding that the yogis have a saying: *"You are as young as your spine is flexible, your hormones are active, and your nervous system is strong."* Yoga, he believes, helps all these beneficial conditions come about.

- ❑ Improve endurance, flexibility, and posture;
- ❑ Promote relaxation;
- ❑ Reduce stress;
- ❑ Strengthen bones; and
- ❑ Strengthen your muscles and organs without causing pain.

HOW TO USE TAI CHI, QIGONG, AND YOGA

Although videotapes and instructional books are available, it is a good idea to begin these Eastern movement therapies by taking classes to learn the basics and how to perform the movements correctly. Classes last about an hour and you can find them at tai chi centers, qigong centers, yoga centers, martial arts studios, YMCAs, and many health clubs. Costs range from about eight to fifteen dollars an hour and you usually have to sign up for a series of eight to ten weekly classes. You may prefer one modality, or, since they are not in conflict with each other, you may choose to practice more than one, if you desire.

Whenever you practice these methods, wear comfortable clothing, loose if you feel you are not in the best shape, but comfortable, fitted outfits with stretch lycra are considered preferable with yoga because you and your instructor can then see your body as it goes into the different postures and she/he can more easily adjust any incorrect postures that could be ineffective at best, damaging at worst, and get you going in the right direction. Make sure you are not on a slippery surface. In yoga, most people use mats and practice barefoot to more closely feel contact with the surface beneath them. Tai chi and qigong practitioners recommend loose clothing and sneakers or other soft shoes, although some prefer to practice barefoot, especially if sessions are held indoors.

NANCY'S RELIEF

For about twenty years after slipping the disc that pressed on the sciatic nerve, Nancy kept her pain at bay with daily stretching to open up her spine. The yoga posture she used, the spinal twist, kept her basically pain-free until a running injury forced her to temporarily stop the pose, leading to a return of the disc pain. Corrective treatment allowed her to resume the spinal twist and she is once again largely pain-free thanks to this vital part of her daily exercise routine.

In a tai chi class, you are taught how to position your weight properly and how to concentrate on your breathing. Exercises are performed slowly and you constantly move forward and backward, and from side to side in slow, fluid, almost meditative movements. The names of animals are used to describe these movements. You might find yourself carrying the tiger to the mountain, grasping a bird by its tail, and waving your hands like clouds. You focus on your breathing and concentrate on the area just below your navel which is believed to be the center of energy or chi flow. Practicing at home for half an hour a day is recommended. Although it is not essential, the ideal place to practice tai chi is outside on grass.

In the philosophy of qigong, there is no such thing as disease; there are only people who have imbalances of their energy. You are taught how to collect energy (chi) and how to free specific parts of your musculoskeletal system so the chi can flow freely. The exercises involve the meridian system used in acupuncture and add mind intent and breathing techniques to the physical movements, which exponentially increases their benefits.

In a yoga class, you also focus on your breathing as you perform the movements. Breathing is referred to as pranayama and the postures as asanas. You will learn that there is far more to yoga than sitting in the lotus position or cross-legged while you stare at a candle, although that too is beneficial as it promotes relaxation. You will be taught specific stretches and postures to help your body become more flexible and have an increased range of motion.

It is not within the scope of this book to give instructions for performing tai chi, qigong, or yoga. It is highly recommended that you take a series of classes with a responsible instructor. Many excellent books and videotapes are available to enhance and reinforce what you learn in a class, and daily practice will give you the best effect.

CAUTIONS

These treatments are not meant to replace medical care if you have a serious condition.

You should not feel any pain in these classes. If you do, something is wrong and you should try a different class or instructor.

Some yoga postures should not be used after age fifty. For instance, the headstand could place too much stress on the cervical vertebrae and, in older people inverted positions could be a contributing factor in strokes. If you have a serious back problem, certain postures could add to your discomfort, or even be potentially dangerous.

(*See also* ACUPUNCTURE and ACUPRESSURE, GUIDED IMAGERY and VISUALIZATION, HYPNOSIS, MASSAGE, and MEDITATION in PART 2 Treatment Section.)

CLINICAL STUDIES

Garfinkel, MS, Singhal, A, Katz, WA, et al. "Yoga-based intervention for carpal tunnel syndrome: a randomized trial." *JAMA*. June 9, 1999; 281(22):2087–2089.

This eight-week study of forty-two people with carpal tunnel syndrome showed that those doing eleven yoga postures had significant reduction in pain compared to the control group.

Garfinkel, MS, Schumacher, HR Jr, Husain, A, et al. "Evaluation of a yoga based regimen for treatment of osteoarthritis of the hands." *Journal of Rheumatology*. December 1994; 21(12):2341–2343.

In this eight-week study at the University of Pennsylvania's Rheumatology Division, the group treated with a yoga program improved significantly over the control group in terms of pain reduction and range of motion. The success in providing relief in osteoarthritis of the hands led to a recommendation for further, long-term studies.

Hain, TC, Fuller, L, Weil, L, et al. "Effects of t'ai chi on balance." *Archives of Otolaryngology-Head Neck Surgery*. November 1999; 125(11):1191–1195.

Twenty-two people with balance disorders underwent eight weeks of tai chi training at Northwestern University Medical School in Chicago and showed highly significant improvements in balance.

Kirsteins, AE, Dietz, F, Hwang, SM. "Evaluating the safety and potential use of a weight-bearing exercise, Tai-Chi Chuan, for rheumatoid arthritis patients." *American Journal of Physical and Medical Rehabilitation*. June 1991; 70(3):136-141.

There was no exacerbation of joint symptoms in this ten-week study of people with rheumatoid arthritis using this form of weight-bearing exercise, compared with the control group. Weight bearing exercises, which can stimulate bone growth and strengthen connective tissue, appear to be safe for people with rheumatoid arthritis (RA) and may serve as an alternative exercise therapy and part of a rehabilitation program. Long-term studies were recommended.

Ross, MC, Bohannon, AS, Davis, DC, et al. "The effects of a short-term exercise program on movement, pain, and mood in the elderly. Results of a pilot study." *Journal of Holistic Nursing*. June 1999; 17(2):139–147.

The measured effects of a short-term tai chi exercise program for eleven older women in Alabama included improved balance and range of motion, decreased pain, and improvement in mood, with lessened anxiety. It was concluded that these improvements could have a profound effect on the incidence of falls, injuries, resulting disability, and overall quality of life.

Wu, WH, Bandilla, E, Ciccone, DS, et al. "Effects of qigong on late-stage complex regional pain syndrome." *Alternative Therapy Health Med*. January 1999; 5(1):45–54.

Twenty-two people with complex regional pain syndrome (RSD) had three weeks of qigong instruction at the Pain Management Center in Newark, NJ, and by the end of the program, 91 percent reported less pain, compared to 36 percent of the control group. It was concluded that qigong training resulted in reduction of pain and anxiety, and future studies were proposed.

Resources
Listed by Condition and Treatment

CONDITIONS

Achilles Tendonitis

Websites

www.foot.com
This website, self-described as "the world's most comprehensive foot health site," has information on Achilles tendon. (*See* Neuroma in this section, for full listing of this resource.)

www.ourfootdoctor.com
This website of a Chicago podiatrist has information about the Achilles tendon. There is also a page on using medical magnets for foot relief.

Angina

Organizations

American College for Advancement in Medicine
23121 Verdugo Drive, Suite 204
Laguna Hills, CA 92653
Ph: 1-800-532-3688
Fax: 1-949-455-9679
Website: www.acam.org
E-mail: info@acam.org
This organization of MDs uses nutrition and chelation approaches for heart disease and other conditions.

American Heart Association
National Center
7272 Greenville Avenue
Dallas, TX 75231
Ph: 1-800-242-8721
Website: www.americanheart.org
E-mail: inquiries@heart.org
This organization is an overall source of information on heart disease.

Preventive Medicine Research Institute
900 Ridgeway, Suite 2
Sausalito, CA 94965
Ph: 1-415-332-2525
Fax: 1-415-332-5730
Website: www.pmri.org
E-mail: pmrireception@yahoo.org
This organization promotes wellness and the reversal of heart and other chronic diseases through comprehensive and effective lifestyle changes.

Pritikin Longevity Center and Spa
19735 Turnberry Way
Aventura, FL 33180
Ph: 1-800-327-1914 or 305-935-7131
Fax: 1-305-935-7111
Website: www.pritikin.com
E-mail: info@pritikin.com
The original center for treatment of heart disease through nutritional means.

Website

www.healthyhearts.com
E-mail: ccmg@healthyhearts.com
Cardiovascular Consultants Medical Group is an educational resource designed to help people understand heart disease, the number one cause of death in the United States, and how it can be prevented, diagnosed, and treated. The site includes nutritional, supplemental, and lifestyle approaches to healthy living.

Back Pain

Organizations

North American Spine Society
22 Calendar Court, 2nd Floor
La Grange, IL 60525
Ph: 1-877-774-6337
Fax: 1-708-588-1080
Website: www.spine.org
E-mail: info@spine.org
This organization provides information on common spine conditions.

Productive Rehabilitation Institute of Dallas for Ergonomics (PRIDE)
5701 Maple Avenue, Suite 100
Dallas, TX 75235
Ph: 1-214-351-6600
Fax: 1-214-351-5046
E-mail: pride@airmail.net
Website: www.pridedallas.com
This center uses a comprehensive interdisciplinary team approach for people in need of musculoskeletal rehabilitation, including those with chronic spinal disorders.

Websites

Spine-health.com
1840 Oak Avenue, Suite 112
Evanston, IL 60201
Website: www.spine-health.com
E-mail: admin@spine-health.com
This website has in-depth information to help people understand back and neck problems.
For additional helpful organizations, refer to relevant entries in PART 2 Treatment Section for the American Chiropractic Association, the American Massage Therapy Association (AMTA), the American Osteopathic Association, the American Physical Therapy Association, and the American Yoga Association.

Bursitis

Organizations

The Arthritis Foundation lists bursitis as an arthritis condition in its website. *The Arthritis Trust of America* includes bursitis in its literature on soft-tissue arthritis. (*See* Osteoarthritis in this section, for full listing of these organizations.)

Carpal Tunnel Syndrome

Organizations

Carpal Tunnel Treatment Center (CTTC)
259 North Middletown Road
Nanuet, NY 10954
Ph: 1-845-268-2021
Fax: 1-845-268-5999
Website: www.aboutcts.com
E-mail: julie@aboutcts.com
This group tells people how to find and treat their own muscle spasms that cause pain. There is an accompanying website www.julstro.com that covers the rest of the body, including tarsal tunnel syndrome, which according to this group, has the same underlying causes as CTS.

National Institute of Neurological Disorders and Stroke
NINDS
P.O. Box 5801
Bethesda, MD 20824
Ph: 1-800-352-9424 or 1-301-496-5751
Fax: 1-301-402-2186
Website: www.ninds.nih.gov
E-mail: braininfo@ninds.nih.gov
This division of the National Institutes of Health has relevant health information on CTS/TTS in booklets, journals, and articles.

Website

www.carpal-tunnel.com/
This site has information and literature on CTS.

Cluster Headaches

Organizations

American Council for Headache Education (ACHE)
19 Mantua Road
Mount Royal, NJ 08061
Ph: 1-800-255-2243 or 1-856-423-0258
Fax: 1-856-423-0082
Website: www.achenet.org
E-mail: achehq@talley.com
This nonprofit education group affiliated with the American Headache Society provides education on the nature and treatment of headaches, and coordinates support groups.

National Headache Foundation
820 N. Orleans, Suite 217
Chicago, IL 60610
Ph: 1-888-643-5552
Fax: 1-773-525-7357
Website: www.headaches.org
E-mail: info@headaches.org
This resource has up-to-date information on the causes and treatment of headaches and gives tips on self-management to minimize their impact on the quality of life.

Crohn's Disease

Organizations

Crohn's and Colitis Foundation of America, Inc.
386 Park Avenue South, 17th Floor
New York, NY 10016
Ph: 1-800-932-2423
Fax: 1-212-799-4098
Website: www.ccfa.org
E-mail: info@ccfa.org
This is a volunteer organization focused on research to improve the quality of life for people who have Crohn's disease or ulcerative colitis. They provide information for physicians and patients and publish *Inflammatory Bowel Disease*, the first journal devoted exclusively to IBD.

International Foundation for Functional Gastrointestinal Disorders
P.O. Box 17864
Milwaukee, WI 53217-8076
Ph: 1-888-964-2001 or 1-414-964-1799
Fax: 1-414-964-7176
Website: www.iffgd.org
E-mail: iffgd@iffgd.com
This is a nonprofit education and research organization that informs, assists, and supports people affected by gastrointestinal disorders.

National Digestive Diseases Information Clearinghouse
Website: www.niddk.nih.gov
This NIH division has information on digestive disturbances. (*See* Nutritional Therapy in this section, for full listing of this resource.)

Dental Pain

Organizations

Holistic Dental Association
Complementary/Alternative Dentistry
P.O. Box 5007
Durango, CO 81301
Fax: 1-970-259-1091
Website: www.holisticdental.org
E-mail: info@holisticdental.org
This group provides information and referrals, and they publish a journal, *The Communicator.*

Diverticulitis

Organizations

International Foundation for Functional Gastrointestinal Disorders
Website: www.iffgd.org
This is a nonprofit education and research organization that informs, assists, and supports people affected by gastrointestinal disorders. (*See* Crohn's Disease in this section, for full listing of this organization.)

National Digestive Diseases Information Clearinghouse
Website: www.niddk.nih.gov
This NIH division has information on digestive disturbances. (*See* Nutritional Therapy in this section, for full listing of this resource.)

Endometriosis

Organizations

The International Pelvic Pain Society
Dr. C. Paul Perry, MD, Chairman
2006 Brookwood Medical Center Drive
Suite 402, Women's Medical Plaza
Birmingham, AL 35209
Ph: 1-800-624-9676 (U.S.) or 1-205-877-2950
Fax: 1-205-877-2973
Website: www.pelvicpain.org
E-mail: pelvicpain@aol.com
This group publishes a booklet, and provides education to raise awareness about pelvic pain problems.

Websites

www.endometriosis.org
This website has research articles, case histories, and a video on endometriosis, which they refer to as "the most common cause of pelvic pain there is."

www.nlm.nih.gov/medlineplus/menstruationandpremenstrualsyndrome.html
The National Library of Medicine (NLM) and the National Institutes of Health (NIH) publish information through MedlinePlus.

Fibromyalgia

Organizations

The Fibromyalgia Network
P.O. Box 31750
Tucson, AZ 85751-1750
Ph: 1-800-853-2929
Fax: 1-520-290-5550
Website: www.fmnetnews.com
E-mail: info@fmnetnews.com
This organization provides information and education on fibromyalgia and publishes a quarterly newsletter, *Fibromyalgia Network.*

The Fibromyalgia Treatment Center, Inc.
P.O. Box 7223
Santa Monica, CA 90406
Ph: 1-310-577-7510
Fax: 1-310-821-0664
Website: www.guaidoc.com
E-mail: fmsnurse@aol.com
Dr. St. Armand's center has treatment and information about guaifenesin.

Frozen Shoulder

Website

www.nlm.nih.gov/medlineplus/shoulderinjuriesanddisorders.html
This MedlinePlus site, a service of the National Library of Medicine and the National Institutes of Health, has links to information about frozen shoulder. One link, to The American Academy of Orthopaedic Surgeons, has illustrated exercises for frozen shoulder.

Gout

Organizations

American College of Rheumatology
1800 Century Place, Suite 250
Atlanta, GA 30345
Ph: 1-404-633-3777
Fax: 1-404-633-1870
Website: www.rheumatology.org
E-mail: acr@rheumatology.org
This organization of rheumatologists (specialists in arthritis and other diseases of the joints, muscles, and bones) has a fact sheet on gout and a geographic directory of ACR members. They also publish a journal, *Arthritis and Rheumatism.*

National Institute of Arthritis and Musculoskeletal and Skin Diseases
This NIH division has information in booklets, journals, and articles. The NIAMS publication on gout is NIH publication 02-5027. (*See* Osteoarthritis in this section, for full listing of this resource.)

Website

www.healthy.net has a page on gout and a link to alternative medicine.

Irritable Bowel Syndrome (IBS)

Organizations

International Foundation for Functional Gastrointestinal Disorders
Website: www.iffgd.org
This is a nonprofit education and research organization that informs, assists, and supports people affected by gastrointestinal disorders. (*See* Crohn's Disease in this section, for full listing of this organization.)

Irritable Bowel Syndrome Association
IBS Self-Help Group
1440 Whalley Avenue #145
New Haven, CT 06515
Ph: 1-416-932-3311
Fax: 1-416-932-8909
Websites: www.ibsassociation.org and www.ibsgroup.org
E-mail: ibsa@ibsassociation.org
This organization is dedicated to helping people with IBS through support groups, treatment, and education.

National Digestive Diseases Information Clearinghouse
Website: www.niddk.nih.gov
This NIH division has information on digestive disturbances. (*See* Nutritional Therapy in this section, for full listing of this resource.)

Migraine Headaches

Organizations

American Council for Headache Education (ACHE)
Website: www.achenet.org
This nonprofit education group affiliated with the American Headache Society provides education on the nature and treatment of headaches, and coordinates support groups.

National Headache Foundation
Website: www.headaches.org
This resource has up-to-date information on the causes and treatment of headaches and gives tips on self-management to minimize their impact on the quality of life.
(*See* Cluster Headaches in this section, for full listing of these organizations.)

The National Migraine Association
113 South Saint Asaph Street, Suite 100
Alexandria, VA 22314
Ph: 1-703-739-9384
Fax: 1-703-739-2432
Website: www.migraines.org
E-mail: magnumnonprofit@hotmail.com
This migraine awareness group was created to educate, assist, and improve the quality of life for people with migraines.

Neuroma

Organizations

The American College of Foot and Ankle Surgeons
515 Busse Highway
Park Ridge, IL 60068-3150
Ph: 1-888-843-3338
Fax: 1-847-292-2022
This organization provides informational brochures on request.

Websites

Foot.Com
414 Alfred Avenue
Teaneck, NJ 07666
Ph: 1-800-526-2739
Fax: 1-800-526-0073
Website: www.foot.com
E-mail: info@foot.com
This website, self-described as "the world's most comprehensive foot health site," has an informative link to Morton's neuroma.

Podiatrychannel.com
Div. Healthcommunities.com, Inc.
136 West Street
Northampton, MA 01060
Ph: 1-888-950-0808
Fax: 1-413-587-0387
Website: www.podiatrychannel.com
E-mail: info@healthcommunities.com
There is a link to information about Morton's neuroma on this medical-specialty website, a division of Healthcommunications.com, Inc.

Osteoarthritis

Organizations

Arthritis Foundation
1330 West Peachtree Street, NW
Atlanta, GA 30357-0669
Ph: 1-800-283-7800 Option 5
Fax: 1-204-480-4774
Website: www.arthritis.org
E-mail: help@arthritis.org
This foundation offers education, support, and activities for people with arthritis, their families and friends. They have self-help instruction programs, land and water exercises, and a bimonthly magazine.

National Institute of Arthritis and Musculoskeletal and Skin Diseases Information Clearinghouse (NIAMS)
National Institutes of Health
Department of Health and Human Services
1 AMS Circle
Bethesda, MD 20892-2675
Ph: 1-877-226-4267 or 1-301-495-4884
Fax: 1-301-718-6336
Website: www.niams.nih.gov
E-mail: niamsinfo@mail.nih.gov
This division has relevant health information in booklets, journals, and articles on arthritis.

The Arthritis Trust of America
7376 Walker Road
Fairview, TN 37062-8141
Ph/Fax: 1-615-799-1002
Website: arthritistrust.org
E-mail: admin@arthritistrust.org
This group informs people as to what works for arthritis and the rheumatoid diseases through its website, its helpful links, and its list of practitioners.

Pelvic Floor Tension Myalgia

Organizations

The International Pelvic Pain Society
Website: www.pelvicpain.org
This group publishes a booklet, and provides education to raise awareness about pelvic pain problems. (*See* Endometriosis in this section, for full listing of this organization.)

The National Library of Medicine (NLM) and the National Institutes of Health (NIH) publish information on pelvic pain through MedlinePlus.

Peripheral Neuropathy

Organizations

American Diabetes Association
1701 North Beauregard Street
Alexandria, VA 22311
Ph: 800-232-3472
Website: www.diabetes.org
E-mail: askADA@diabetes.org
This large group, which provides information, support, and a weekly newsletter, lists neuropathy as one of the most common complications of diabetes.

National Diabetes Educational Program (NDEP)
1 Diabetes Way
Bethesda, MD 20892-3560
Ph: 1-800-438-5383

Fax: 1-301-907-8906
Website: http://ndep.nih.gov
E-mail: ndic@info.niddk.nih.gov
Materials on diabetes and peripheral neuropathy can be ordered from this division of the National Diabetes Information Clearinghouse (1-800-860-8747).

Neuropathy Association
60 East 42nd Street, Suite 942
New York, NY 10165-0999
Ph: 1-800-247-6968 or 1-212-692-0662
Fax: 1-212-692-0668
Website: www.neuropathy.org
E-mail: info@neuropathy.org
Referred by NINDS, The National Institute of Neurological Disorders and Stroke, this group gives information and support for people with neuropathies. www.ninds.nih.gov/health_and_medicaldisorders/peripheralneuropathy_doc.htm is the website address for it.

Phantom Pain

Websites

www.amputee-online.com
A useful website for more information and links.

www.sncpr.org.uk/amputation
The Scottish Network for Chronic Pain Research talks about amputation and pain on this website.

Plantar Fasciitis

Website

www.foot.com
This website, self-described as "the world's most comprehensive foot health site," has an informative link to plantar fasciitis. (*See* Neuroma in this section, for full listing of this resource.)

Postherpetic Neuralgia

Organizations

VZV Research Foundation
40 East 72nd Street
New York, NY 10021
Ph: 1-212-472-3181
Fax: 1-212-861-7033
Website: www.vzvfoundation.org
E-mail: vzv@vzvfoundation.org
This organization has information on chicken pox, related to shingles, and postherpetic neuralgia, which can follow shingles.

Websites

www.aftershingles.com
www.phnpain.com
Both sites have information on PHN. The first is sponsored by a pharmaceutical company.

Post-Polio Syndrome

Organizations

Futures Unlimited
8084 Highway 50 East
Columbus, MS 39702
Ph: 1-662-327-7333
Fax: 1-662-329-4271
Website: www.futuresunlimited.com
E-mail: futures@futuresunlimited.com
This group does the *Environmentally Enhanced Physical Therapy,* as outlined by the founder, Ed Snapp, in a phone interview on September 24, 2002. The website has a link to www.polionet.org, which also has information on post-polio syndrome and a newsletter.

Premenstrual Syndrome

Organizations

The International Pelvic Pain Society
Website: www.pelvicpain.org
This group publishes a booklet, and provides education to raise awareness about pelvic pain problems. (*See* Endometriosis in this section, for full listing of this organization.)

Websites

www.nlm.nih.gov/medlineplus/menstruationandpremenstrualsyndrome.html
The National Library of Medicine (NLM) and the National Institutes of Health (NIH) publish information on these conditions through MedlinePlus.

www.goodbyepms.com
The focus of this website is natural progesterone (as opposed to drugs) for this condition, which includes headaches and backaches.

Reflex Sympathetic Dystrophy Syndrome

Organizations

American RSDHope Group
P.O. Box 475
Harrison, ME 04040-0875
Ph: 1-207-583-4589
Fax: 1-207-583-4978
Website: www.rsdhope.org

E-mail: stonehed@megalink.net
This nonprofit group for patients, parents and friends of people with RSDS supplies information about the condition through a newsletter, articles, studies, a recommended-reading list, and Internet programs.

Reflex Sympathetic Dystrophy Syndrome Association of America (RSDSA)
P.O. Box 502
Milford, CT 06460
Ph: 1-877-662-7737 or 1-203-877-3790
Fax: 1-203-882-8362
Website: www.rsds.org
E-mail: info@rsds.org
This organization will send a free packet about RSDS on request. They promote education, awareness, and research on this "underdiagnosed and undertreated syndrome."

Rheumatoid Arthritis

Organizations

Arthritis Foundation
Website: www.arthritis.org
This foundation offers education, support, and activities for people with arthritis, their families and friends. They have self-help instruction programs, land and water exercises, and a bimonthly magazine.

National Institute of Arthritis and Musculoskeletal and Skin Diseases
Website: www.niams.nih.gov
This division of the NIH has relevant health information in booklets, journals, and articles on arthritis.

The Arthritis Trust of America
Website: arthritistrust.org
This group informs people as to what works for arthritis and the rheumatoid diseases through its website, its helpful links, and its list of practitioners.
(*See* Osteoarthritis in this section, for full listing of these organizations.)

Rotator Cuff Tendonitis

Organizations

www.nlm.nih.gov/medlineplus/ency/article/000438.htm is provided by the National Library of Medicine and the National Institutes of Health. Its medical encyclopedia has information on rotator cuff tendonitis.

http://physicaltherapy.about.com/library/weekly/aa103000a.htm has a diagram of the muscles involved in rotator cuff tendonitis and links to a self-test to determine if you have a rotator-cuff injury. This site is connected to a much larger one: www.about.com.

Sciatica

Organizations

North American Spine Society
Website: www.spine.org
This organization provides information on common spine conditions.

Website

Spine-health.com
Website: www.spine-health.com
This website has information to help people understand sciatica and other back problems.
(*See* Back Pain in this section, for full listing of these resources.)

Spinal Stenosis

Organizations

North American Spine Society
Website: www.spine.org
This organization provides information on spinal stenosis and other common spine conditions.

Website

Spine-health.com
Website: www.spine-health.com
This website has information to help people understand problems connected to the spine and back.
(*See* Back Pain in this section, for full listing of these resources.)

Tarsal Tunnel Syndrome

Organizations

Carpal Tunnel Treatment Center (CTTC)
Website: www.aboutcts.com
This group tells people how to find and treat their own muscle spasms that cause pain. There is an accompanying website www.julstro.com that covers the rest of the body, including tarsal tunnel syndrome (TTS), which according to this group, has the same underlying causes as CTS.

National Institute of Neurological Disorders and Stroke
NINDS
Website: www.ninds.nih.gov
This division of the National Institutes of Health has relevant health information on TTS in booklets, journals, and articles.

(*See* Carpal Tunnel Syndrome in this section, for full listing of these resources.)

Temporomandibular Joint (TMJ) Pain

Organizations

Holistic Dental Association
Website: www.holisticdental.org
This group provides information and referrals, and they publish a journal, *The Communicator.* (*See* Dental Pain in this section, for full listing of this organization.)

The TMJ Association, Ltd
P.O. Box 26770
Milwaukee, WI 53226-0770
Ph: 1-414-259-3223
Fax: 1-414-259-8112
Website: www.tmj.org
E-mail: info@tmj.org
This group's journal, *TMJ Science,* has reports and information.

Additionally, The National Center for Complementary and Alternative Medicine (NCCAM) has information on alternative/complementary approaches to TMJ pain management. (*See* General Resources for full listing of this resource.)

Tennis Elbow

Periodical

The Physician and Sports Medicine
4530 West 77th Street
Minneapolis, MN 55435
Ph: 1-952-835-3222
Fax: 1-952-835-3460
Website: www.physsportsmed.com
E-mail: The website has individual E-mail addresses for different departments.
This peer-reviewed journal contains instructions and illustrations for tennis elbow, which can be accessed at: www.physsportsmed.com/issues/1996/05_96/nirscpa.htm

Websites

www.tenniselbow.org serves as an "advanced resource" for information on tennis elbow. Of the thirteen sites listed and rated on their web page, only three do *not* list NSAIDs as a favored treatment.
One of the three is www.drweil.com and it is the only one to list supplements as helpful to the condition. Type in *tennis elbow* on his website, and in a Q&A from June 28, 2000, he will discuss the condition and the non-invasive remedies he recommends.

Tension Headaches

Organizations

American Council for Headache Education (ACHE)
Website: www.achenet.org
This nonprofit education group affiliated with the American Headache Society provides education on the nature and treatment of headaches, and coordinates support groups.

National Headache Foundation
Website: www.headaches.org
This resource has up-to-date information on the causes and treatment of headaches and gives tips on self-management to minimize their impact on the quality of life.
(*See* Cluster Headaches in this section, for full listing of these organizations.)

Thoracic Outlet Syndrome

Websites

www.nlm.nih.gov/medlineplus/thoracicoutletsyndrome.html
Clicking on this MedlinePlus site, a service of the U.S. National Library of Medicine and the National Institutes of Health, will link you to information on this condition. One site, for The American Academy of Orthopaedic Surgeons, has a list of exercises for avoiding TOS.

www.merck.com/pubs
This is the online edition of *The Merck Manual of Medical Information.* Whitehouse Station, NJ: Merck Research Laboratories, Div. Merck & Co.

Trigeminal Neuralgia

Organizations

Trigeminal Neuralgia Association National Office
2801 SW Archer Road, Suite C
Gainesville, FL 32608
Ph: 1-352-376-9955
Fax: 1-352-376-8688
Website: www.tna-support.org
E-mail: tnanational@tna-support.org
This organization acts as an advocate for people with trigeminal neuralgia. It has information and support groups, and publishes a newsletter, *TN-Alert.*

Trigger Finger

Organization

American Society of Hand Therapists (ASHT)
401 North Michigan Avenue
Chicago, IL 60611-4267
Ph: 1-312-321-6866

Fax: 1-312-673-6670
Website: www.asht.org
E-mail: ASHT@sba.com
This organization, which educates and supports people with trigger finger, has a free pamphlet on the condition. They also publish a newsletter and a journal on hand therapy.

Ulcerative Colitis—Inflammatory Bowel Disease

Organizations

Crohn's and Colitis Foundation of America, Inc.
Website: www.ccfa.org
This is a volunteer organization focused on research to improve the quality of life for people who have Crohn's disease or ulcerative colitis. They provide information for physicians and patients and publish *Inflammatory Bowel Disease,* the first journal devoted exclusively to IBD.

International Foundation for Functional Gastrointestinal Disorders
Website: www.iffgd.org
This is a nonprofit education and research organization that informs, assists, and supports people affected by gastrointestinal disorders.
(*See* Crohn's Disease in this section, for full listing of the organizations above.)
National Digestive Diseases Information Clearinghouse
Website: www.niddk.nih.gov
This NIH division has information on digestive disturbances. (*See* Nutritional Therapy in this section, for full listing of this resource.)

TREATMENTS

Acupuncture and Acupressure

Organizations, Practitioners, and Publishers

American Association of Oriental Medicine
5530 Wisconsin Avenue, Suite 1210
Chevy Chase, MD 20815
Ph: 1-888-500-7999 or 1-301-941-1064
Fax: 1-301-986-9313
Website: www.aaom.org
E-mail: info@aaom.org
Originally an organization for acupuncture information, this group changed its name in recognition of the fact that acupuncture was just one part of the scope of Oriental medicine. The members of this group are recognized as highly qualified practitioners of Oriental medicine.

Anuthep Benja-Athon, MD, PC
210 East 36th Street
New York, NY 10016
Ph: 1-212-545-7075
Website: www.MuscleJointNerve.com
Dr. Benja-Athon can be reached by e-mail through his website.

Blue Poppy Enterprises
5441 Western Avenue #2
Boulder, CO 80301
Ph: 1-800-487-9296 or 1-303-245-8372
Fax: 1-303-245-8362
Website: www.bluepoppy.com
E-mail: info@bluepoppy.com
This establishment is the world's largest English-language publisher of books (they have over eighty titles) and educational products about Chinese medicine and acupuncture. They also have a line of internal herbal formulations and topical tinctures and ointments.

Jacques Depardieu, MS, LAc
Center for Integrative Chinese Medicine
1500 Boston Post Road
Darien, CT 06820
Ph: 1-203-232-8898
Fax: 1-203-656-9533
Website: www.integrativechinesemedicine.com
E-mail: info@integrativechinesemedicine.com

Eastland Press
1240 Activity Drive
Vista, CA 92081
Ph: 1-800-453-3278
Fax: 1-800-241-3329
Website: www.eastlandpress.com
E-mail: info@eastlandpress.com
This press is the foremost publisher of textbooks for practitioners of Chinese medicine in the United States. They also have books on osteopathy and other forms of bodywork, and their publication, *The Journal of Chinese Medicine,* is the leading periodical on TCM in the West.

The American Academy of Medical Acupuncture
4929 Wilshire Boulevard, Suite 428
Los Angeles, CA 90010
Ph: 1-323-937-5514
Fax: 1-323-937-0959
Website: www.medicalacupuncture.org
E-mail: jdowdene@prodigy.net
This national organization representing physician

acupuncturists in the United States is dedicated to offering the highest-quality healthcare to patients by combining the best of both traditional Western medicine and all the multiple systems of acupuncture, and incorporating them into safe and effective medical care. They offer education and support, publish a newsletter, and have a database of acupuncturists.

The Center for Women's Health
1500 Boston Post Road
Darien, CT 06820
Ph: 1-203-656-6635
Fax: 1-203-656-9533
Website: www.centerforwomenshealth.com
E-mail: info@centerforwomenshealth.com
The center offers an integrative approach to women's health, combining the natural orientation of holistic medicine with the most current conventional care.

Traditional Chinese Medicine World Foundation
396 Broadway, Suite 502
New York, NY 10013
Ph: 1-212-274-1079
Fax: 1-212-274-9879
Website: www.tcmworld.org
E-mail: info@tcmworld.org
The foundation is dedicated to building bridges of understanding between East and West in the areas of Traditional Chinese Medicine (which includes acupuncture), qigong, natural healing, and the internal martial arts. Its mission is to serve as the source for authentic information on health and healing with TCM for practitioners and the general public.

Applied Kinesiology

Organization and Practitioners

The International College for Applied Kinesiology
6405 Metcalf Avenue, Suite 503
Shawnee Mission, KS 66202-3929
Ph: 1-913-384-5336
Fax: 1-913-384-5112
Website: www.icakusa.com
E-mail: icak@dci-kansascity.com or info@icakusa.com
This college can provide a list of practitioners in the United States.

Dr. Linda E. Merkin, DC, PC, Certified Kinesiologist
330 West 58th Street, Suite 408
New York, NY 10019
Ph: 1-212-245-3170
Fax: 1-212-315-1126
E-mail: smerkin@nyc.rr.com
Dr. Merkin took over the practice after Dr. Avery H. Ferentz passed away. She had partnered with him in bringing the Buteyko Method to New York (this breathing method is a remarkable healing modality).

Dr. Robert Porzio, Diplomate of Applied Kinesiology
1153 West Main Street
Waterbury, CT 06708
Ph: 1-203-756-7449
Fax:1-203-597-1153
E-mail: r.porzio@ntplx.net

Aromatherapy

Organizations

Aroma Medica
900 Bethlehem Pike
Erdenheim, PA 19038
Ph: 1-215-233-5210
Fax: 1-215-836-0760
Website: www.AromaMedica.com
E-mail: AromaMedica@yahoo.com
Founded by Geraldine DePaula, MD, this company has successfully used *Arthritis Formula* on patients to ease the pain of arthritis in the knees and elsewhere.

Websites

www.aromaweb.com
This website is useful for learning more about aromatherapy and specific essential oils.

Bee Venom Therapy

Organizations and Practitioners

American Academy of Neural Therapy, Inc.
P.O. Box 5023
Bellevue, WA 98008
Ph: 1-425-462-1777
Fax: 1-425-453-7015
Website: www.neuraltherapy.com
E-mail: aant@neuraltherapy.com
This organization can supply manuals and videos on bee venom therapy, answer questions about its benefits and costs, and help you locate a BVT practitioner in your area.

American Apitherapy Society
1209 Post Road
Scarsdale, NY 10583
Ph: 1-914-725-7944
Fax: 1-914-723-0920
Website: www.apitherapy.org
E-mail: aasoffice@apitherapy.org

This membership organization is devoted to promoting the use of honeybee products to treat a variety of conditions and further good health. They have a journal available by subscription and can help in finding BVT practitioners.

Apitronic Services
9611 No. 4 Rd.
Richmond, BC
Canada V7A 2Z1
Ph/Fax: 1-604-271-9414
Website: www.beevenom.com
E-mail: msimics@direct.ca
This supplier provides bee venom products and therapy-related books, literature, and the Apitherapy Education Service, which has papers and information on the therapy. He has many years of experience in this field and is very knowledgeable and informative on the subject.

Dr. Larry Cohen
Advanced Pain Care
100 Mill Plain Road
Danbury, CT 06811
Ph: 1-203-791-3940
Fax: 1-203-791-3966
Website: www.imaginelifewithoutpain.com
E-mail: l.d.cohen@worldnet.att.net
In addition to bee venom therapy, Dr. Cohen practices prolotherapy and neural therapy (needle therapies for pain relief) and frequently lectures to medical personnel on these subjects.

Dr. Andrew Kochan
5535 Balboa Boulevard, Suite 225
Encino, CA 91316
Ph: 1-818-995-9331
Fax: 1-818-995-9334
Website: www.healingartsresearch.org
E-mail: akochan@healingartsresearch.org

Biofeedback

Organizations

Association for Applied Psychophysiology and Biofeedback
10200 West 44th Avenue, Suite 203
Wheat Ridge, CO 80033
Ph: 1-303-422-8436
Fax: 1-303-422-8894
Website: www.aapb.org
E-mail: aapb@resourcecenter.com
This group has a newsletter and information about the treatment. At the same address, The Biofeedback Certification Institute of America can refer you to certified practitioners. Their website address is: www.bcia.org.

The Biofeedback Network
125 Prospect Street
Phoenixville, PA 19460
Ph: 1-610-933-8145
Fax: 1-831-301-3397
Website: www.biofeedback.org
E-mail: info@biofeedback.net
This group has an on-line magazine, information on locating a certified professional, and links to articles on biofeedback.

Bio Research Institute
331 East Cotati Avenue
Cotati, CA 94931
Ph/Fax: 1-707-795-2460
Website: www.7hz.com
E-mail: bri@7hz.com
This organization has information, articles, and training in this method.

Chiropractic

Organizations and Publication

American Chiropractic Association
1701 Clarendon Boulevard
Arlington, Virginia 22209
Ph: 1-800-896-4636 or 1-703-276-8800
Fax: 1-703-243-2593
Website: www.amerchiro.org
E-mail: memberinfo@amerchiro.org
A major source for chiropractic information. There is a monthly publication and a newsletter.

Association for Network Chiropractic Spinal Analysis
P.O. Box 7682
Longmont, Colorado 80501
Ph: 1-303-678-8086
Website: www.innateintelligence.com
Intended more for chiropractors than the general public, this group trains chiropractors, and offers referrals and support through workshops, seminars, journals, newsletters, and other means.

Dynamic Chiropractic
P.O. Box 4109
Huntington Beach, CA 92605-4109
Ph: 1-714-230-3150
Fax: 1-714-899-4273
Website: www.chiroweb.com
E-mail: listservices@mpamedia.com

This publication is an excellent resource for information and articles on chiropractic and those looking for chiropractors. The group, mpamedia, also publishes *Acupuncture Today* and *Massage Today*.

International Chiropractors Association
1110 North Glebe Road
Suite 1000
Arlington, VA 22201
Ph: 1-703-528-5000
Website: www.chiropractic.org
The original chiropractic association founded by B. J. Palmer, the son of the founder of chiropractic, Daniel David Palmer.

Compresses, Packs, and Poultices

Organization and Practitioners

The American Association of Naturopathic Physicians
3201 New Mexico Avenue, NW, Suite 350
Washington, DC 20016
Ph: 1-866-538-2267 or 1-202-895-1392
Fax: 1-202-274-1992
Website: www.naturopathic.org
E-mail: memberservices@naturopathic.org
This organization provides information, education, and support. The website lists naturopathic physicians and has pages devoted to individual practitioners, including Emily Kane, ND, quoted in the entry.

Cathy Rogers, ND
Website: www.chicospa.com
(*See* Hydrotherapy in this section, for a full listing on this naturopathic physician.)

Craniosacral Therapy

Organizations

Colorado Cranial Institute
1080 Hawthorn Ave.
Boulder, CO 80304
Ph: 1-303-443-6415
Website: www.coloradocranialinstitute.com
Although this website is in German, it is included because studies on craniosacral therapy are being performed at the Institute.

Society of Ortho-Bionomy
5875 N. Lincoln Ave.
Chicago, IL 60659
Ph: 1-800-743-4890
Fax: 1-773-506-6543
Website: www.ortho-bionomy.org
E-mail: sobioffice@aol.com
Ortho-bionomy is similar to CST, and studies on it and craniosacral therapy are being done by researchers at this organization.

Upledger Institute
11211 Prosperity Farms Road
Suite D-325
Palm Beach Gardens, FL 33410
Ph: 1-561-622-4334
Fax: 1-561-622-4771
Website: www.upledger.com
E-mail: upledger@upledger.com
This organization provides information, support and education. The website has a list of craniosacral therapists.

Cupping

Organization

New Hope Clinic
Grass Valley, CA 95945
Ph: 1-866-300-5343
Fax: 1-530-823-3443
Website: www.newhopeclinic.com
e:mail: newhope@newhopeclinic.com
This group uses cupping, as well as bioresonance and neural therapy, to treat painful conditions.

Exercise, Stretching, and Sports

Organizations

Cooper Aerobics Center
12200 Preston Road
Dallas, TX 75230
Ph: 1-800-444-5764 or 1-972-239-7223
Fax: 1-972-239-6649
Website: www.cooperaerobics.com
E-mail: info@cooperaerobics.com
The founder of this clinic, Dr. Kenneth Cooper, is the originator of the term *aerobic*. His many books on fitness and exercise are available through this center, which has a spa, a wellness center, a free newsletter and other divisions that cover many aspects of healthy living. According to the July/August 2001 *Men's Health Magazine*, the Guest Lodge at the clinic was "the best place to stay fit on the road."

National Academy of Sports Medicine
26632 Agoura Road
Calabasas, CA 91302
Ph: 1-800-460-6276 or 1-818-878-9203
Fax: 1-818-878-9203

Website: www.nasm.org
E-mail: info@nasm.org
This organization is well known for its state-of-the-art programs and products. It has a fitness-certification program, and offers more than twenty continuing-education courses in a variety of fitness disciplines.

Noll Physiological Research Center (NPRC)
The Pennsylvania State University
129 Noll Laboratory
University Park, PA 16802-6900
Ph: 1-814-865-3453
Fax: 1-814-865-4602
Website: www.noll.psu.edu
E-mail: info@noll.psu.edu
The primary missions of this center are research, teaching, service, and graduate education in the physiological sciences. The faculty, students, and staff are dedicated to investigating the benefits of physical activity and the adverse health effects of physical inactivity, and to understanding how the human body adapts to acute and chronic stress, the goal being to improve people's health all their lives. Most students at NPRC receive graduate degrees in kinesiology, physiology, or nutrition.

Guided Imagery and Visualization

Organization

Academy for Guided Imagery
P.O. Box 2070
Mill Valley, CA 94942
Ph: 1-800-726-2070
Fax: 1-415-389-9342
Website: www.interactiveimagery.com
E-mail: info@interactiveimagery.com
This academy has education and information to teach people how to access and use the power of the mind/body connection for healing. The website has a list of practitioners in guided imagery.

Heat Therapy/Cold Therapy

Websites

http://scc.u.chicago.edu/heattherapy.htm
http://scc.u.chicago.edu/icetherapy.htm
These University of Chicago websites give information on the two therapies.

www.rrca.org/publicat/ice.html
This website for the Road Runners Club of America has information on ice therapy.
Although there are thousands of websites for these two therapies, almost all are there to sell products, not dispense information or give referrals.

Herbal Remedies

Organization

Herb Research Foundation
4140 15th Street
Boulder, CO 80304
Ph: 1-303-449-2265
Fax: 1-303-449-7849
Website: www.herbs.org
E-mail: info@herbs.org
This organization is a source of science-based information, education, and research on herbal remedies. There are several publications, including one for consumers, *Herbs for Health*.

Homeopathy

Organizations

National Center for Homeopathy
801 North Fairfax Street
Alexandria, VA 22314
Ph: 1-877-624-0613 or 1-703-548-7790
Fax: 1-703-548-7792
Website: www.homeopathic.org
E-mail: info@homeopathic.org
This center refers to homeopathy as the natural medicine of the twenty-first century, and its stated aim is to promote health through homeopathy. Education, information, research, and a directory of homeopathic practitioners are provided, and there is a monthly publication, *Homeopathy Today*, available to members.

Homeopathic Educational Services
2124 Kittridge Street
Berkeley, CA 94704
Ph: 1-510-649-0294
Fax: 1-510-649-1955
Website: www.homeopathic.com
E-mail: mail@homeopathic.com
The educational services include articles, books, products, tapes, and a list of remedies. Personal consulting is also available.

Hydrotherapy

Organizations

The American Association of Naturopathic Physicians
Website: www.naturopathic.org
E-mail: memberservices@naturopathic.org
This organization provides information, education, and

support. The website lists naturopathic physicians and has pages devoted to individual practitioners. (*See* Compresses, Packs, and Poultices in this section, for full listing of this organization.)

International Society of Medical Hydrology and Climatology in Europe
Website: ismh.web.med.uni-muenchen.de
This organization has a congress in Central Europe every four years and there is a translation into English.
The American branch of this organization is:

American Society of Medical Hydrology
President: Bruce E. Becker, MD, MS
Medical Director, St. Luke's Rehabilitation Institute
Clinical Assoc Prof. University of Washington School of Medicine
711 S. Cowley, Suite 310
Spokane, WA 99202
Ph: 1-509-473-6043
Fax: 1-509-473-6020
Website: Under construction
E-mail: beckerb@st-lukes.org

Cathy Rogers, ND
Chico Water Cure Spa
6670 Chico Way NW
Bremerton, WA 98312
Ph: 1-360-692-5554
Fax: 1-360-698-7600
Website: www.chicospa.com
E-mail: Waterspa@aol.com

Hypnosis

Organization

American Society of Clinical Hypnosis
140 N. Bloomingdale Road
Bloomingdale, IL 60108-1017
Ph: 1-630-980-4740
Fax: 1-630-351-8490
Website: www.asch.net
E-mail: info@asch.net
You can obtain a list of hypnotherapists in your area by sending a stamped, self-addressed envelope to this organization.

Magnet Therapy

Organizations

Advanced Magnetic Research Institute
Eichelberger Professional Building
195 Stock Street, Suite 211B
Hanover, PA 17331
Ph: 1-717-632-0300
Fax: 1-717-632-3038
Website: www.amripa.com
E-mail: twnichol@blazenet.net
This clinic, founded by Trent W, Nichols, MD, advises on and treats many painful conditions, including fibromyalgia, herniated discs, osteoarthritis, and peripheral neuropathy.

The Bio Electro Magnetic Therapy
9541 Northwest 42nd Street
Sunrise, FL 33351
Ph: 1-866-363-3637
Fax: 1-954-578-4121
Website: www.bemt.net
E-mail: support@bemt.net
This organization provides online support and promotes natural magnetic therapy for health and the relief of many chronic pain conditions.

Biomagnetic Therapy Association
P.O. Box 394
Lyons, CO 80590
Ph: 1-303-823-0307
Website: www.biomagnetic.org
E-mail: info@biomagnetic.org
This organization provides quality education, scientific research, and professional support. There is a referral network; magnets, books, and related products are available.

Website

www.painrelief.org.uk
E-mail: alastair.lee@painrelief.org.uk
This website promotes magnetic therapy for relief of arthritis, back and neck aches, joint and muscle pain, and shoulder pain, among other painful conditions.

Massage

Organization

American Massage Therapy Association (AMTA)
820 Davis Street, Suite 100
Evanston, IL 60201-4444
Ph: 1-888-843-2682
Fax: 1-847-864-1178
Website: www.amtamassage.org
E-mail: info@amtamassage.org
This site has several interesting links and can also help you find practitioners in your area.

Meditation

Organization

Centerpointe Research Institute
1700 NW 167th Place, Suite 220
Beaverton, OR 97006-4872
Ph: 1-800-945-2741
Fax: 1-503-643-3114
Website: www.centerpointe.com
E-mail: support@centerpointe.com
This Institute has a meditation program and you can listen to a CD online.

Website

www.learningmeditation.com
Patsy Grey
1555 Hazel Lane
Winnetka, IL 60093
Ph: 1-847-441-7017
This website offers you a meditation room providing fifteen free meditations accompanied by music, and an online shop where you can purchase a number of meditation-related products, including tapes and CDs on breathing, meditations, and stress management.

Nutritional Therapy

Organizations

Feingold Association of the United States
127 East Main Street, #106
Riverhead, NY 11901
Ph: 1-800-321-3287 or 1-631-369-9340
Fax: 1-631-369-2988
Website: www.feingold.org
E-mail: Help@feingold.org
This group has information on food and food additives and their effect on health.

National Digestive Diseases Information Clearinghouse
2 Information Way
Bethesda, MD 20892-3570
Ph: 1-800-891-5389 or 1-301-654-3810
Fax: 1-301-907-8906
Website: www.niddk.nih.gov/health/digest/nddic.htm
E-mail: nddic@info.niddk.nih.gov
This division of the National Institutes of Health is concerned with digestive problems.

Retail Outlets

The Country Hen
P.O. Box 333
Hubbardston, MA 01452
Ph: 1-978-928-5333
Fax: 1-978-928-5414
Website: www.countryhen.com
E-mail: countryhen@net1plus.com
Great tasting organic omega-3 eggs are the specialty of this farm in North Central Massachusetts. They take their role as purveyors of a superior product very seriously. If you live in the Northeast, call to find out where their eggs are available. Otherwise, look for local brands of organic eggs with omega-3s in upmarket grocery stores or health food stores in your area.

Whole Foods Markets
601 North Lamar Boulevard, Suite 300
Austin, TX 78703
Ph: 1-512-476-1206
Fax: 1-512-476-5704
Website: www.wholefoods.com
E-mail: info@wholefoods.com
This premier organic foods chain originated in Austin, Texas where the national corporate office is, but it now has branches all over the United States which are excellent sources for organic foods, supplements, and natural care products. Many of their stores also have superb baked goods, deli counters, hot and cold prepared foods, juice bars, salad bars, and tables where you can eat what you have purchased.

Osteopathic Manipulation

Organizations and Practitioner

American Academy of Osteopathy
3500 DePauw Blvd., Suite 1080
Indianapolis, IN 46268
Ph: 1-317-879-1881
Fax: 1-317-879-0563
Website: www.academyofosteopathy.org
E-mail: snoone@academyofosteopathy.org
This professional organization for over 48,000 DOs teaches, advocates, and researches the science, art, and philosophy of osteopathic medicine.

American Osteopathic Association
142 E. Ontario Street
Chicago, IL 60611
Ph: 1-800-621-1773
Fax: 1-312-202-8200
Website: www.aoa-net.org
E-mail: info@aoa-net.org
This is a national organization for over 48,000 DOs in the United States and has a listing of doctors by state.

Dr. Jeffrey Perry, DO
The Hospital for Joint Diseases
Spine Center
303 Second Avenue, Suite 21
New York, NY 10003
Ph: 1-212-598-6625
Fax: 1-212-598-6195
E-mail: Drjeperry@aol.com

Oxygen Therapies

Organizations, Practitioner, and Publication

International Bio-Oxidative Medicine Foundation (IBOMF)
Suzanne Moore, Director
P.O. Box 30006
Edmond, OK 73003
Ph: 1-541-955-3372

The American College of Hyperbaric Medicine
4001 Ocean Drive
Lauderdale-by-the-Sea, FL 33308
Ph: 1-954-771-4000
Fax: 1-954-776-0670
Website: www.oceanhbo.com
E-mail: info@oceanhbo.com
This organization provides information, worldwide referrals, and videos of case studies. All treatments at their center are physician-supervised.

The Family Health News
John Taggert, Editor
9845 NE 2nd Avenue
Miami Shores, FL 33138
Ph: 1-800-284-6263
Fax: 1-800-284-6261
Website: www.familyhealthnews.com
E-mail: johnnyt@gate.net
A source for news and information on oxygen therapies.

The Foundation for Light Therapy
21218 St. Andrews Blvd. #223
Boca Raton, FL 33433
Ph: 1-561-274-7078
Fax: 1-561-488-0155
Website: www.FFLT.org
E-mail: fflt@earthlink.net
The foundation is involved in research and provides light treatments. There is a referral list for doctors in the United States and abroad.

The International Ozone Association, Inc.
Pan American Group
31 Strawberry Hill Avenue
Stamford, CT 06902
Ph: 1-203-348-3542
Fax: 1-203-967-4845
Website: www.int-ozone-assoc.org/
E-mail: mistok@int-ozone-assoc.org
This nonprofit group serves as a worldwide gathering point for ozone information and dissemination through publications, seminars, and symposia.

The Undersea Hyperbaric Medical Society
10531 Metropolitan Avenue
Kensington, MD 20895
Ph: 1-301-942-2980
Fax: 1-301-942-7804
Website: www.uhms.org
E-mail: uhms@uhms.org
This nonprofit group is the primary source of information on diving and hyperbaric medicine worldwide. They serve members in fifty countries around the world.

Dr. Pavel Yutsis
Executive Health Medical Group
1309 West 7th Street
Brooklyn, NY 11204
Ph: 1-718-259-2122
Fax: 1-718-259-3933
Dr. Yutsis regularly uses all the oxygen therapies discussed here in his alternative/complementary practice. He can also be heard on his weekly radio program, *From Allergies to Aging*, by tuning in to WEVD in Manhattan (their signal spans the East Coast).

Websites

www.oxygenhealingtherapies.com
This website provides information and education on ozone therapy, UVB therapy, oxygen chambers, and other therapies. There is a newsletter, and they can be contacted at *oxygenhealingtherapies@telus.net*.

www.oxygenhealth.com
This website is hosted by Mr. Oxygen, as author Ed McCabe, a pioneer in oxygen therapy, is dubbed. It provides information, education, and a newsletter, and contains hundreds of published reports on oxygen from all over the world. The toll-free number is 1-800-247-6553.

Physical Therapy

Organizations

American Physical Therapy Association
1111 North Fairfax Street
Alexandria, VA 22314-1488
Ph: 1-800-999-2782 or 1-703-684-2782
Fax: 1-703-684-7343
Website: www.apta.org
E-mail: svcctr@apta.org or public-relations@apta.org
The primary journal for this organization, *Physical Therapy,* contains articles and studies which contribute to the body of knowledge about physical therapy and are intended for the professional and the lay reader.

Aquatic Physical Therapy Section of the American Physical Therapy Assoc.
7853 East Arapahoe Court, Suite 2100
Centennial, CO 80112-1361
Ph: 1-303-694-4728, ext 60
Fax: 1 303-694-4869
Website: www.aquaticpt.org

Aquatic Therapy and Rehabilitation Institute
3650-A Centre Circle
Fort Mill, SC 29715
Ph: 1-803-802-5400
Fax: 1-815-371-1499
Website: www.atri.org
E-mail: ATRI@atri.org
This approach consists of physical therapists working with a client in the water; it is not water aerobics. As discussed in the *Aquatic Therapy Journal,* David Ogden, PT, has experienced success working with fibromyalgia clients in the aquatic environment.

Reflexology

Organizations

International Institute of Reflexology
P.O. Box 12642
St. Petersburg, Fl. 33733
Ph: 1-727-343-4811
Fax: 1-813-381-2807
Website: www.reflexology-usa.net
E-mail: iir@tampabay.rr.com
This sixty-year-old group was developed by Eunice Ingham who discovered that the reflexes in the feet are mirror images of different parts of the body, and is considered the originator of reflexology as it is now practiced. The institute can provide learning aids—charts, books, study guides, and video guides—and has workshops, teaching programs, and a referral service.

Reflexology Association of America
4012 S. Rainbow Blvd.
Ste. K-PMB #585
Las Vegas, NV 89103-2059
Ph:1-508-364-4234
Fax: 1-978-779-0449 Attn: RAA
Website: www.reflexology-usa.org
E-mail: inforaa@reflexology-usa.org
This nonprofit professional group promotes the advancement of reflexology and the standardization of services available to the public. There is a newsletter and a referral service available.

Reflexology Research
P.O. Box 35820
Albuquerque, NM 87176-5820
Ph: 1-505-344-9392
Fax: 1-505-344-0296
Website: www.reflexology-research.com
E-mail: footC@aol.com
This website provides research and references on reflexology.

Rolfing

Organization and Practitioner

Rolf Institute
205 Canyon Blvd.
Boulder, CO 80302
Ph: 1-800-530-8875
Fax: 1-303-449-5978
Website: www.rolf.org
E-mail: info@rolf.org

Dr. Randy Coleman, ND
2143 Locust Street
Philadelphia, PA 19103
Ph: 1-610-745-3206
Fax: 1-610-446-6274
Website: colemanfitness.com
E-mail: randy@colemanfitness.com

Supplement Therapy

Organization and Practitioner

Life Extension Foundation
1100 West Commercial Boulevard
Fort Lauderdale, FL 33309
Ph: 1-800-544-4440 or 1-954-766-8433
Fax: 1-954-202-7742 or 1-954-761-9199
Website: www.lef.org
E-mail: generalquestions@lifeextension.com
The founders of this organization have been involved in

antiaging research since the 1960s, and the aim of their nonprofit organization (founded in 1980) is to develop methods that "enable us to live in health, youth, and vigor for unlimited periods of time." They publish a magazine, *Life Extension*, and have a carefully developed list of supplements for sale.

Dr. Edward M. Wagner, ND
5150 Bingham Street
Philadelphia, PA 19120
Ph: 1-215-455-0717
Website: www.edwagnernd.com
E-mail: dred@edwagnernd.com

Website

http://dietary-supplements.info.nih.gov
This is the office of Dietary Supplements at the National Institutes of Health.

Tai Chi, Qigong, and Yoga

Organizations

American Yoga Association
P.O. Box 19986
Sarasota, FL 34276
Ph: 1-941-927-4977
Fax: 1-941-921-9844
Website: www.americanyogaassociation.org
E-mail: patricia.rockwood@americanyogaassociation.org
This nonprofit organization provides yoga instruction and educational resources to anyone interested in yoga.

Anusara Yoga
9400 Grogans Mill Road, Suite 200
The Woodlands, TX 77380
Ph: 1-888-398-9642 or 1-281-367-9763
Fax: 1-281-367-2744
Website: www.anusara.com
E-mail: oneyoga@anusara.com
Anusara yoga, an offspring of Iyengar yoga, is a highly evolved, safe form of hatha yoga founded by John Friend in 1997. Certified teachers, listed by state on the website, have had extensive training in anatomy and therapeutic yoga.

National QiGong (Chi Kung) Association
P.O. Box 540
Ely, MN 55731
Ph: 1-218-365-6330
Fax: 1-218-365-6933
Rebecca Kali, Director: nqa@citlink.net
Website: www.nqa.org
E-mail: info@nqa.org
This group maintains a list of teachers around the country on their website.

Taoist Tai Chi Society of USA
Div. International Taoist Tai Chi Society
2100 Thomasville Road
Tallahassee, FL 32308-0736
Ph/Fax: 1-850-224-5438
Website: http://taoist.org
E-mail: usa@ttcs.org
This nonprofit volunteer organization offers information on tai chi and lists its affiliates in America and around the world.

General Resources

The following resources are for overall pain conditions and natural approaches to health. Organizations and websites for individual conditions and treatments are listed above by their respective entries.

ORGANIZATIONS

American Academy of Pain Management
13947 Mono Way #A
Sonora, CA 95370
Ph: 1-209-545-0754
Fax: 1-209-533-9750
Website: www.aapainmanage.org
E-mail: aapm@aapainmanage.org
This professional group is the largest pain organization in the United States. It offers online referrals, education services, and publishes a newsletter, *American Journal of Pain Management*.

American Association of Oriental Medicine
5530 Wisconsin Avenue, Suite 1210
Chevy Chase, MD 20815
Ph: 1-888-500-7999 or 1-301-941-1064
Fax: 1-301-986-9313
Website: www.aaom.org
E-mail: info@aaom.org
Originally an organization for acupuncture information, this group changed its name in recognition of the fact that acupuncture was just one part of the scope of Oriental medicine. The members of this group are recognized as highly qualified practitioners of Oriental medicine, which has many useful pain-relief modalities.

American Chronic Pain Association (ACPA)
P.O. Box 850
Rocklin, CA 95677-0850
Ph: 1-800-533-3231 or 1-916-632-0922
Fax: 1-916-632-3208
Website: www.theacpa.org
E-mail: ACPA@pacbell.net
This organization offers support and information for people with chronic pain problems. The bias is toward orthodox establishment medicine, but there are also some alternative treatments listed.

American Holistic Heath Association
P.O. Box 17400
Anaheim, CA 92817-7400
Ph: 1-714-779-6152
Website: www.ahha.org
E-mail: mail@ahha.org
This natural health organization offers a free booklet on wellness from within, and lists practitioner members, healing centers, and alternative organizations.

American Holistic Medical Association
12101 Menaul Blvd NE, Suite C
Albuquerque, NM 87112
Ph: 1-505-292-7788
Fax: 1-505-293-758
Website: www.holisticmedicine.org
E-mail: info@holisticmedicine.org
This group is primarily for physicians who practice holistic medicine. It includes a listing of holistic physicians who take referrals and has a guide to finding a practitioner in your area.

The following four organizations are listed courtesy of The National Institute of Neurological Disorders and Stroke (NINDS), a division of the National Institutes of Health (NIH). Credit as the source is at their request, and their address is listed below.

BRAIN
NIH Neurological Institute
P.O. Box 5801
Bethesda, MD 20824

Ph: 1-800-352-9424
Fax: 1-301-402-2186
Website: www.ninds.hih.gov
E-mail: braininfo@ninds.nih.gov

American Pain Foundation
201 N. Charles Street, Suite 710
Baltimore, MD 21201-4111
Ph: 1-888-615-7246
Fax: 1-410-385-1832
Website: www.painfoundation.org
E-mail: info@painfoundation.org
This foundation offers support information, education, and resources on pain management.

National Center for Complementary and Alternative Medicine Clearinghouse
National Institutes of Health
P.O. Box 7923
Gaithersburg, MD 20898-7923
Ph: 1-888-644-6226
Fax: 1-866-464-3616
Website: http://nccam.nih.gov
E-mail: info@nccam.nih.gov
This center has information, news, and federal research initiatives on complementary and alternative medicine.

National Chronic Pain Outreach Association (NCPOA)
P.O. Box 274
Millboro, VA 24460
Ph: 1-540-862-9437
Fax: 1-540-862-9485
Website: www.chronicpain.org
E-mail: ncpoa@cfw.com
The aim of this nonprofit organization is to educate people in pain, healthcare professionals, and the public about chronic pain. Its website has an extensive list of support groups in the United States, and there is a quarterly newsletter, *Lifeline.*

National Rehabilitation Information Center (NARIC)
4200 Forbes Boulevard, Suite 202
Lanham, MD 20706-4829
Ph: 1-800-346-2742 or 1-301-562-2400
Fax: 1-301-562-2401
Website: www.naric.com
E-mail: naricinfo@heitechservices.com
This center has information on resources for disability and rehabilitation on its website. There is also a directory of related programs and products.

The Great Lakes Pain Center, Ltd.
10125 West North Avenue
Wauwautosa, WI 53226
Ph: 1-866-442-8372 or 1-414-443-6432
Fax: 1-414-443-6438
Website: www.greatlakespaincenter.com
E-mail: ssuster@aol.com
This center, headed by Stuart M. Suster, MD, specializes in the treatment of people with chronic pain who do not respond to standard methods of care. The center believes in treating the whole person without surgery or other invasive methods, and the list of chronic pain conditions they address closely mirrors the entries in this book.

The Health Resource, Inc.
933 Faulkner
Conway, AR 72034
Ph: 1-800-949-0090 or 1-501-329-5272
Fax: 1-501-329-9489
Website: www.thehealthsource.com
E-mail: moreinfo@thehealthresource.com
This medical information service provides customized research on alternative and mainstream medical options for a wide variety of conditions, and they guarantee all their reports.

WEBSITES

www.alternativemedicine.com
This website has a database of alternative medical information, and has links to the group's magazine, *Alternative Health.*

www.drweil.com
This website for Dr. Andrew Weil includes health conditions, wellness therapies, recipes, food as medicine, the herbal medicine chest, and the question and answer of the day. The "like-minded-practitioners" site lists a number of people and places in the United States and beyond who share Dr. Weil's commitment to holistic medicine.

www.holisticonline.com
E-mail: info@holisticonline.com
ICBS, Inc.
24 Canton Road
Akron, OH 44312
Ph: 1-330-733-4283
Fax: 1-733-4380
This group, primarily an online organization, has comprehensive information about health, featuring conventional, alternative, integrative, and mind-body medicine choices for health naturally.

www.drwhitaker.com
Dr. Julian Whitaker's website has health advice and solutions, and a free E-mail service, with "cutting-edge information for your most pressing health concerns." It also has links to his newsletter, *Health and Healing*, and to the Whitaker Wellness Institute in California.

www.healthnotes.com
This in-store subscription service is available in over 6500 pharmacies, supermarkets, and natural food stores. It provides credible health and lifestyle information through easy-to-use touch-screen kiosks.

www.healthy.net
This website has information on health conditions, alternative therapies, lists of practitioners, up-to-date health news, a free newsletter, and links to many healthy aspects of living.

www.MayoClinic.com
This website helps people find health information on many conditions.

www.merck.com/pubs
This is the online edition of *The Merck Manual of Medical Information.* Whitehouse Station, NJ: Merck Research Laboratories, Div. Merck & Co.

www.mercksource.com
This is another Merck website for health information to help you become more involved in your healthcare.

References
Listed by Condition and Treatment

CONDITIONS

Achilles Tendonitis

Berkow, PK, Fletcher, AJ, Beers, MH, eds. *The Merck Manual of Diagnosis and Therapy,* 16th ed. Rahway, NJ: Merck Research Laboratories; 1992:1367–1368.

Rich, Pat. "Rheumatology Update: No clear winner for tendonitis treatment." *Medical Post.* March 15, 2000; 36.

Angina

"Angina Could Be a Tip Off." *USA Today Magazine.* February 1, 1997, 125.

Wagner, Edward M, Goldfarb, Sylvia. *How to Stay Out of the Doctor's Office: An Encyclopedia for Alternative Healing.* New York, NY: Instant Improvement, Inc., 1992.

Back Pain

Duke, James A. "Healing that pain in your back (without going under the knife)." *Mother Earth News.* April 1, 2002:1111.

Fishman, Loren, Ardman, Carol. *Back Pain: How to Relieve Low Back Pain and Sciatica.* New York, NY: W.W. Norton, 1999.

Holmes, Byron, "The Lowdown on Back Pain." Saturday Evening Post March 1, 1998; 270:46.

Kolata, Gina. "With Costs Rising, Treating Back Pain Often Seems Futile." *The New York Times.* February 9, 2004, A1.

McGrath, Mike. "When Back Pain Starts in Your Head." *Prevention.* July 1, 1999; 51:135.

Murray, Michael T, Pizzorno, Joseph. *The Encyclopedia of Natural Medicine,* 2nd ed. Rocklin, CA: Prima Publishers, 1998.

Sarno, John E. *Healing Back Pain: the Mind-Body Connection.* New York, NY: Warner Books, 1991.

Smith-Fassler, Mary Elizabeth, Lopez-Bushnell, Kathy. "Acupuncture as Complementary Therapy for Back Pain." *Holistic Nursing Practice.* April 1, 2001:35

Snider, Mike. "Watch Your Back." *Ladies Home Journal.* May 1, 1994; 111:128.

Wagner, Edward M, Goldfarb, Sylvia. *How to Stay Out of the Doctor's Office: An Encyclopedia for Alternative Healing.* New York, NY: Instant Improvement, Inc., 1992.

Bursitis

"Bursitis." *The Columbia Encyclopedia,* Seventh Edition. January 1, 2002.

Munson, Marty. "Big Bursa." Medical-Care News IN: *Prevention.* May 1, 1996; 48(3):63.

Carpal Tunnel Syndrome

Bevin, Abner, Riordon, Teresa. In His Words: "Technology Can Be a Pain When it Leads to Carpal Tunnel Syndrome." *People.* May 7, 1009, 127.

"Most Carpal Tunnel Syndrome Injuries Preventable" *Online Newsletter.* February 1, 1991.

Orihill, Jack. "Are Your Feet Killing You?" *Restaurant Hospitality.* September 1, 1995 (79); 38.

"Preventing Carpal Tunnel Syndrome." *USA Today Magazine.* 125; October 1, 1996.

Wagner, Edward M, Goldfarb, Sylvia. *How To Stay Out of the Doctor's Office: An Encyclopedia for Alternative Healing.* New York, NY: Instant Improvement, Inc., 1992.

Cluster Headaches

"8 Fast Headache Cures: Home Remedies." *Men's Health.* November 1, 1996; 11:46.

Juahar, Sandeep, "Over-the-Counter Headache." *The New York Times Magazine.* January 12, 2003.

McNeil, Donald G, Jr. "Wrinkles Gone? New Uses Studied for Botox." *The New York Times.* March 2, 2003, A1.

Murray, Michael T, Pizzorno, Joseph. *The Encyclopedia of Natural Medicine,* 2nd ed. Rocklin, CA: Prima Publishers, 1998.

Nowroozi, Christine K. "Treating Serious Headaches." *Nation's Business.* September 1, 1994; 82:69.

Robbins, Lawrence, Lang, Susan S. "Finally Help for Splitting,

Aching, Throbbing Headaches." Headache Help: *Good Housekeeping*. June 1, 1995; 220(4):90.

"Stopping Persistent Headaches." *Johns Hopkins Medical Letter*, October 2001, 7.

Tague, Suzanne. "War Against Headaches." *Inside*. June 30, 1994.

Wagner, Edward M, Goldfarb, Sylvia. *How to Stay Out of the Doctor's Office: An Encyclopedia for Alternative Healing*. New York, NY: Instant Improvement, Inc., 1992.

Crohn's Disease

Digestive Disorders. *The Merck Manual*, Home Edition. Section 9, Chapter 108, 1997.

Haaf, Wendy. "Tummy Troubles." *Today's Parent*. Vol.16; August 1, 1999:23–26.

Dental Pain

Bonner, Michael. *The Oral Health Bible*. North Bergen, NJ: Basic Health Publications, 2003.

"Coping With Dental Emergencies." *Medical Update*. April 1, 2001; 2.

FDA Consumer. June 1, 1988; 22(5):6.

Stay, Flora Parsa. *The Complete Book of Dental Remedies*. Garden City Park, NY: Avery Publishing Group, 1996.

The Doctors Book of Home Remedies. Editors of Prevention Magazine Health Books. Emmaus, PA: Rodale Press, 1990.

Diverticulitis

Brown, Edwin W. "Left-sided appendicitis." *Medical Update*. Vol. 20; August 1, 1996:1(2).

Digestive Disorders. *The Merck Manual*, Home Edition. Section 9, Chapter 108, 1997.

"Diverticulosis." *The Columbia Encyclopedia*, Seventh Edition. January 1, 2002.

Haaf, Wendy. "Tummy Troubles." *Today's Parent*. Vol.16; August 1, 1999:23–26.

Endometriosis

DeMarco, Carolyn, "Natural Treatments for Endometriosis." *Contemporary Women's Issues Database*. June 1, 1994; 8:29.

Kashef, Ziba. "Coping With Endometriosis." (Health). *Essence*. February 1, 1996; 26(2):32.

Murray, Michael T, Pizzorno, Joseph. *The Encyclopedia of Natural Medicine*, 2nd ed. Rocklin, CA: Prima Publishers, 1998.

Olive, David. "Ask the Expert—Endometriosis." *National Women's Health Report*. June 1, 1998; 20:3.

"Some Facts About Endometriosis." *Contemporary Women's Issues Database*. March 1, 1999; 5.

"Tampons May Protect Against Endometriosis." *United Press International*. May 29, 2002.

Wagner, Edward M, Goldfarb, Sylvia. *How to Stay Out of the Doctor's Office: An Encyclopedia for Alternative Healing*. New York, NY: Instant Improvement, Inc. 1992.

Wallis, Claudia. Medicine: "The Career Woman's Disease? Endometriosis May Afflict as Many as 10 Million in the U.S." *Time*. April 28, 1986; 62.

Fibromyalgia

"Fibromyalgia Explained." *Health Watch News Letter*. October 3, 2001:29.

Marek, Claudia Craig. *The First Year: Fibromyalgia, An Essential Guide for the Newly Diagnosed*. New York, NY: Marlowe and Company, 2003.

Maurizio, Sandra J, Rogers, Janet L. "Recognizing and Treating Fibromyalgia." *The Nurse Practitioner*. December 1, 1997; 22(12):18.

Pearlmutter, Cathy. "The Truth About Fibromyalgia." *Prevention*. April 1, 1997 (8):86.

Sprott, H, Franki, S, Kluge, H, et al. "Pain Treatment of Fibromyalgia by Acupuncture." *Rheumatology International* 1998; 18:35–36.

St. Amand, R. Paul. *What Your Doctor May Not Tell You About Fibromyalgia*. New York, NY: Warner Books, 1999.

Wolfe, F, Ross, K, Anderson, J, et al. "Aspects of Fibromyalgia in the General Population." *Journal of Rheumatology*. 1995; 22(1):151–155.

Frozen Shoulder

Bauman, Alisa. "Relieve Frozen Shoulder Fast." *Prevention*. May 1, 2002, 164.

Burcum, Jill, "The deep freeze: a mysterious condition called frozen shoulder makes it difficult, if not impossible, to move one of the body's most complex joints. Therapy to 'thaw' the shoulder takes time." *Minneapolis Star Tribune*. March 19, 2002; 1E.

Gout

Brody, Jane E. "Gout Hobbles Plenty of Commoners, Too." *The New York Times*. April 16, 2004, F8.

Doctor's Book of Home Remedies. Emmaus, PA: Rodale Press, 1990.

Family Guide to Natural Medicine. Pleasantville, NY: The Readers Digest Association, 1993.

Murray, Michael T, Pizzorno, Joseph. *The Encyclopedia of Natural Medicine*, 2nd Ed. Rocklin, CA: Prima Publishers, 1998.

Rodale's Illustrated Encyclopedia of Herbs. Emmaus, PA: Rodale Press, 1987.

Wagner, Edward M, Goldfarb, Sylvia. *How to Stay Out of the Doctor's Office: An Encyclopedia for Alternative Healing*. New York, NY: Instant Improvement, Inc., 1992.

Irritable Bowel Syndrome

Bentley, SJ, Pearson, DJ, Rix, KJ. "Food hypersensitivity in irritable bowel syndrome." *The Lancet*. 1983; ii:295–297.

Digestive Disorders. *The Merck Manual,* Home Edition. Section 9, Chapter 108, 1997.

"Diverticulosis." *The Columbia Encyclopedia,* Seventh Edition. January 1, 2002.

Haaf, Wendy. "Tummy Troubles." *Today's Parent*. Vol.16; August 1, 1999:23–26.

Niec, AM, Frankum, B, Talley, NJ. "Are adverse food reactions linked to irritable bowel syndrome?" *American Journal of Gastroenterology*. 1998; 93:2184–2190.

Rubin, Rita, "FDA allows irritable bowel syndrome drug back on market." *USA Today*. June 10, 2002:06D.

The Associated Press. "FDA Puts Drug Back on Market." *Newsday*. June 8, 2002:A12.

Migraine Headaches

"8 Fast Headache Cures: Home Remedies." *Men's Health*. November 1, 1996; 11:46.

Juahar, Sandeep, "Over-the-Counter Headache." *The New York Times Magazine*. January 12, 2003.

Kearns, Brenda. "So Long, Migraines." *Good Housekeeping*. March, 2002, 85–91.

McNeil, Donald G, Jr. "Wrinkles Gone? New Uses Studied for Botox." *The New York Times*. March 2, 2003, A1.

Murray, Michael T, Pizzorno, Joseph. *The Encyclopedia of Natural Medicine,* 2nd ed. Rocklin, CA: Prima Publishers, 1998.

Nowroozi, Christine K. "Treating Serious Headaches." *Nation's Business*. September 1, 1994; 82:69.

Robbins, Lawrence, Lang, Susan S. "Finally Help for Splitting, Aching, Throbbing Headaches." Headache Help: *Good Housekeeping*. June 1, 1995; 220(4):90.

"Stopping Persistent Headaches." *Johns Hopkins Medical Letter,* October 2001, 7.

Tague, Suzanne. "War Against Headaches." *Inside*. June 30, 1994.

Wagner, Edward M, Goldfarb, Sylvia. *How to Stay Out of the Doctor's Office: An Encyclopedia for Alternative Healing*. New York, NY: Instant Improvement, Inc., 1992.

Neuroma

Cimons, Marlene. "Cortisone Concerns." *Runners World*. October 1, 1999; 43:42–43.

Cimons, Marlene. "Morton's neuroma (foot ailment)." *Runner's World*. October 1, 1998; 33(2):38.

The Merck Manual of Medical Information. Whitehouse Station, NJ, Merck Research Laboratories. 1997:259.

"Neuroma." The Mosby Medical Encyclopedia. October 1, 1996.

Osteoarthritis

Adler, Jerry. "Arthritis: What It Is, Why You Get It, and How to Stop the Pain." *Newsweek*. September 3, 2001:38–46.

Lemonick, Michael D. Reported by Dick Thompson, Washington, Medicine Section: "Arthritis Under Arrest. New treatments may finally succeed in putting one of the worst forms of this painful illness on ice." *Time*. September 28, 1998:75.

Meggs, William J, Svec, Carol. *The Inflammation Cure*. New York, NY: McGraw-Hill/Contemporary Books, 2003.

Murray, Michael T, Pizzorno, Joseph. *The Encyclopedia of Natural Medicine,* 2nd ed. Rocklin, CA: Prima Publishers, 1998.

Topol, Eric, MD, Chairman of the Department of Cardiovascular Medicine, Cleveland Clinic, Cleveland, Ohio.

Wagner, Edward M, Goldfarb, Sylvia. *How to Stay Out of the Doctor's Office: An Encyclopedia for Alternative Healing*. New York, NY: Instant Improvement, Inc., 1992.

Webb, Denise. "Glucosamine May Be First to Slow Arthritis Damage." *Prevention*. July 1, 2001, 71.

Pelvic Floor Tension Myalgia

Clemens, JQ, Nadler, RB, Schaffer, AJ, et al. "Biofeedback, pelvic floor re-education, and bladder training for male chronic pelvic pain syndrome." *Urology*. December 20, 2000; 56(6):951–955.

Minkin, Mary Jane. "Surprising Cause of Pelvic Pain." *Prevention*. June 1, 2002; 167.

Murray, Michael T, Pizzorno, Joseph. *The Encyclopedia of Natural Medicine,* 2nd ed. Rocklin, CA: Prima Publishers, 1998.

Peripheral Neuropathy

Bell, David. "To Hurt or Not to Hurt (Living with Diabetic Neuropathy)." *Diabetes Forecast*. June 1, 1995; 48(4):30.

"Diabetic Neuropathies: The Nerve Damage of Diabetes." National Institutes of Health (NIH) Publication No. 02-3185, May 2002.

"Pain, Pain, Go Away." *Diabetes Forecast*. February 1, 1995; 48(2):72.

Parker, James W, Parker, Philip N. The Official Patient's Sourcebook on Peripheral Neuralgia: A Revised and Updated Directory for the Internet Age. San Diego, CA: Icon Health Publications, 2002.

Phantom Pain

Brownlee, Shannon, Mitchell, Karen. "The Route of Phantom Pain." *U.S. News & World Report*. October 2, 1995; 76–78.

Clinical Study

Katz, J, Melzack, R. "Pain 'memories' in phantom limbs: review and clinical observations." *Pain*. December 1990; 43(3):319–336.

The sixty-eight people discussed in this paper all emphasized that they experienced true pain, which they described in vivid detail. It is not, they said, just a recollection of an earlier pain.

R. Melzack, who co-authored the breakthrough 1965 paper on the gate theory of pain, is frequently cited as the author of many studies on phantom pain. He co-authored the above review, which is one of more than 400 entries on the condition found on *PubMed.gov*, the National Library of Medicine's website for clinical trials and papers.

Plantar Fasciitis

Slovut, Gordon. "Low-Cost Steps Relieve Heel Pain." *Minneapolis Star Tribune*. October 24, 1996; 3E.

Clinical Study

DiGiovanni, BF, Nawoczenski, DA, Lintal, ME, et al. "Tissue-specific plantar fascia-stretching exercise enhances outcomes in patients with chronic heel pain. A prospective, randomized study." *Journal of Bone Joint Surgery—American Volume*. July 2003; 85-A(7):1270–1277.

The people who used non-weight-bearing stretching exercises for eight weeks showed a significant improvement in their pain levels over those who did not, and these findings provide an excellent alternative to the present, nonoperative treatment for chronic disabling plantar heel pain.

Postherpetic Neuralgia

Hui F, et al. "Integrative Approach to the Treatment of Postherpetic Neuralgia." *Alternative Medicine Review*. 1999; 4 (6):429–435

Kanazi, GE, Johnson, RW, Dworkin, RH. "Treatment of postherpetic neuralgia: an update." *Drugs*. May 2000; 59:1113–1126.

Post-Polio Syndrome

Castro, Janice. Medicine: "The Polio Echo: Years Later, Symptoms Return." Reported by Cheryl Crooks/Los Angeles and Joyce Leviton/Atlanta. *Time*. February 11, 1985:79.

Elmer-DeWitt, Philip. Health: "Reliving Polio: Forty Years after the Great Postwar Epidemic, The Disease is Coming Back to Haunt its Survivors." Reported by Alice Park/New York. *Time*. March 28, 1994:54.

McKenna, MAJ, Staff. "To Many who Healed Decades Ago at Warm Springs, New Pains and Problems Arise Today, as Polio Strikes Again." *The Atlanta Journal and Constitution*. June 25, 2000:A1.

"Poliomyelitis." *The Columbia Encyclopedia*, Seventh Edition. January 1, 2002.

Silver, Julie K, Halstead, Lauro S. Post-Polio Syndrome: A Guide for Polio Survivors and Their Families. Yale University Press, 2001.

Premenstrual Syndrome

Murray, Michael T, Pizzorno, Joseph. *The Encyclopedia of Natural Medicine*, 2nd ed. Rocklin, CA: Prima Publishers, 1998.

Wagner, Edward M, Goldfarb, Sylvia. *How to Stay Out of the Doctor's Office: An Encyclopedia for Alternative Healing*. New York, NY: Instant Improvement, Inc. 1992.

Reflex Sympathetic Dystrophy Syndrome (RSDS)

Arnold, Sarah. "Reflex Sympathetic Dystrophy Syndrome: How Even a Small Injury Could Change Your Life." *Accent on Living*. March 1, 1996; 40(2):102.

Moskowitz, Peter, Lang, Linda. *Living with RSDS: Your Guide to Coping with Reflex Sympathetic Dystrophy Syndrome*. Oakland, CA: New Harbinger Publications, 2003.

Peach, G. "Hyperbaric oxygen and the reflex sympathetic dystrophy syndrome: a case report." *Undersea & Hyperbaric Medicine*. 1995; 22(4):407–408.

Rheumatoid Arthritis

Adler, Jerry. "Arthritis: What It Is, Why You Get It, and How to Stop the Pain." *Newsweek*. September 3, 2001:38–46.

Lemonick, Michael D. Reported by Dick Thompson, Washington, Medicine Section: "Arthritis Under Arrest. New treatments may finally succeed in putting one of the worst forms of this painful illness on ice." *Time*. September 28, 1998:75.

Meggs, William J, Svec, Carol. *The Inflammation Cure*. New York, NY: McGraw-Hill/Contemporary Books, 2003.

Murray, Michael T, Pizzorno, Joseph. *The Encyclopedia of Natural Medicine*, 2nd ed. Rocklin, CA: Prima Publishers, 1998.

Selzer, Jed. "Merck's new drug reduces rheumatoid arthritis pain." *Reuters Business Report*. November 15, 2001.

Topol, Eric, MD, Chairman of the Department of Cardiovascular Medicine, Cleveland Clinic, Cleveland, Ohio.

Wagner, Edward M, Goldfarb, Sylvia. *How to Stay Out of the Doctor's Office: An Encyclopedia for Alternative Healing*. New York, NY: Instant Improvement, Inc., 1992.

Webb, Denise. "Glucosamine May Be First to Slow Arthritis Damage." *Prevention*. July 1, 2001, 71.

Rotator Cuff Tendonitis

Berkow, PK, Fletcher, AJ, Beers, MH, eds. *The Merck Manual of Diagnosis and Therapy*, 16th ed. Rahway, NJ: Merck Research Laboratories; 1992:1367–1368.

Kneinhenz, J, Streitberger, K, Windeler, J, et al. "Randomized clinical trials comparing the effects of acupuncture and a newly designed placebo needle in rotator cuff tendinitis." *Pain*. 1999; 83:235–241.

Rich, Pat. "Rheumatology Update: No clear winner for tendonitis treatment." *Medical Post*. March 15, 2000; 36.

Sciatica

Credit, Larry P, Hartunian, Sharon G, Nowak, Margaret J. *Relieving Sciatica*. Garden City Park, NY: Avery Publishing Group, 2000.

Doherty, Bridget. "Better than your Bed: New Therapy for Sciatic Pain." Health News: *Prevention*. August 1, 1999; (51):37.

Spinal Stenosis

Siwek, Jay. "Back Pain from a Pinched Spinal Cord." *The Washington Post*, CONSULTATION column. September 28, 1999; Z23.

The Doctor's In. "Back Pain Often Tied to Spinal Stenosis." Newsday. Column in Discovery Section. April 3, 2000; C5.

Clinical Study

Fritz, JM, Erhard, RE, Vignovic, M. "A nonsurgical approach for patients with lumbar spinal stenosis." *Physical Therapy*. September 1997; 77(9):962–973.

In this six-week trial to evaluate two patients with spinal stenosis after physical therapy, improvements were noted in all aspects of the study and larger studies with long-term follow-up were recommended.

Tarsal Tunnel Syndrome

Orihill, Jack. "Are Your Feet Killing You?" *Restaurant Hospitality.* September 1, 1995 (79); 38.

Wagner, Edward M, Goldfarb, Sylvia. *How To Stay Out of the Doctor's Office: An Encyclopedia for Alternative Healing.* New York, NY: Instant Improvement, Inc., 1992.

Temporomandibular Joint (TMJ) Pain

Bonner, Michael. *The Oral Health Bible.* North Bergen, NJ: Basic Health Publications, 2003.

"Coping With Dental Emergencies." *Medical Update.* April 1, 2001; 2.

FDA Consumer. June 1, 1988; 22(5):6.

Stay, Flora Parsa. *The Complete Book of Dental Remedies.* Garden City Park, NY: Avery Publishing Group, 1996.

The Doctors Book of Home Remedies. Editors of Prevention Magazine Health Books. Emmaus, PA: Rodale Press, 1990.

Tennis Elbow

Books

The following books are primarily for medical professionals but you may find them useful.

Hertling, Darlene, Kessler, Randolph. *Managementof Common Musculoskeletal Disorders: Physical Therapy Principles and Methods.* 2nd ed. Philadelphia, PA: J.B. Lippincott, Co., 1990.

Norkin, Cynthia C, Levangie, Pamela K. *Joint Structure and Function: A Comprehensive Analysis.* Philadelphia, PA: F.A. Davis Company, 1992.

Articles

Altshul, Sara. "Ace Elbow Pain." *Prevention.* April 1, 2001; 51.

Derrick, Henry & Staff. FITNESS Q&A: "'Tennis Elbow' Requires Careful Rehabilitation." *The Atlanta Journal and Constitution.* September 7, 2000; T10.

Donohue, Paul. "Is There Tennis After Tennis Elbow?" *St. Louis Post-Dispatch.* August 14, 1993; 02D.

Levy, Doug. "Advice To Give Injuries a Sporting Chance to Heal. Coping with Pain from Arthritis to Tennis Elbow." *USA Today.* July 19, 1996; 04D.

Nirschl, Robert P, Kraushaar, Barry S. "Keeping Tennis Elbow at Arm's Length: Simple, Effective Strengthening Exercises." *The Physician and Sports Medicine.* May 1996; 24(5).

"Using Weights Can Help Tennis Elbow." *The Washington Times.* April 7, 2002.

Tension Headaches

"8 Fast Headache Cures: Home Remedies." *Men's Health.* November 1, 1996; 11:46.

Juahar, Sandeep, "Over-the-Counter Headache." *The New York Times Magazine.* January 12, 2003.

McNeil, Donald G, Jr. "Wrinkles Gone? New Uses Studied for Botox." *The New York Times.* March 2, 2003, A1.

Murray, Michael T, Pizzorno, Joseph. *The Encyclopedia of Natural Medicine,* 2nd ed. Rocklin, CA: Prima Publishers, 1998.

Nowroozi, Christine K. "Treating Serious Headaches." *Nation's Business.* September 1, 1994; 82:69.

Robbins, Lawrence, Lang, Susan S. "Finally Help for Splitting, Aching, Throbbing Headaches." Headache Help: *Good Housekeeping.* June 1, 1995; 220(4):90.

"Stopping Persistent Headaches." *Johns Hopkins Medical Letter,* October 2001, 7.

Tague, Suzanne. "War Against Headaches." *Inside.* June 30, 1994.

Wagner, Edward M, Goldfarb, Sylvia. *How to Stay Out of the Doctor's Office: An Encyclopedia for Alternative Healing.* New York, NY: Instant Improvement, Inc., 1992.

Thoracic Outlet Syndrome

Rubin, Michael, Contributor. *Merck Manual of Medical Information.* Whitehouse Station, NJ: Merck Research Laboratories, Div. Merck & Co. 1997 ed. www.merck.com/pubs.

Clinical Study

Kenny, RA, Traynor, GB, Withington, D, et al. "Thoracic outlet syndrome: a useful exercise treatment option." *American Journal of Surgery.* February 1993; 165(2):282–284.

In this three-week Irish study of a supervised physiotherapy program, eight test subjects with severe symptoms all showed significant improvements in their symptoms, and all achieved a full range of cervical neck and shoulder movement. The authors of the study say these results confirm the efficacy of a simple treatment program for people with thoracic outlet syndrome.

Trigeminal Neuralgia

"Brain and Nerve Disorders: Trigeminal Neuralgia." Chapter 71, Section 6. *Merck Manual of Medical Information, Home Edition.* Whitehouse Station, NJ: Merck Research Laboratories, 1997.

Buchman, Dian Dincin. *The Complete Book of Water Healing.* New York, NY: Instant Improvement, Inc., 1994; 135.

Donohue, Paul. *"Trigeminal Neuralgia Causes Painful Facial Contortions." St. Louis Post-Dispatch.* July 31, 1998; E2.

Mosiman, Wendy. "Taking The Sting Out of Trigeminal Neuralgia." *Nursing.* March 1, 2001; 86.

Trigger Finger

Berkow, PK, Fletcher, AJ, Beers, MH, eds. *The Merck Manual of Diagnosis and Therapy,* 16th ed. Rahway, NJ: Merck Research Laboratories; 1992:1367–1368.

Dee, Thomas, Katz, Richard. "Trigger Fingers and Grip Go Hand in Hand." *The Tampa Tribune.* April 3, 1999; 12.

Rich, Pat. "Rheumatology Update: No clear winner for tendonitis treatment." *Medical Post.* March 15, 2000; 36.

Ulcerative Colitis

Digestive Disorders. *The Merck Manual,* Home Edition. Section 9, Chapter 108, 1997.

Haaf, Wendy. "Tummy Troubles." *Today's Parent.* Vol.16; August 1, 1999:23–26.

Halpern, Georges M. *Ulcer Free: Nature's Safe and Effective Remedy for Ulcers.* Garden City Park, NY: Square One Publishers, 2004.

TREATMENTS

Applied Kinesiology

Thie, John. *Touch for Health.* Marina del Rey, CA: DeVorss Publishers, 1973 (rev 1998).

To familiarize yourself with the diagnostic methods of applied kinesiology, you can refer to this self-help manual, written by one of the earliest practitioners of applied kinesiology. It is available through Dr. Thie's office in Malibu, CA (1-310-589-5269), or through his publisher:

DeVorss Publications

553 Constitution Avenue

Camarillo, CA 93012.

Ph: 1-805-322-9010 or 1-800-843-5743

Fax: 1-805-322-9011

Website: www.devorss.com

Website for orders: www.service@devorss.com

E-mail: service@devorss.com

Aromatherapy

Buckle, Jane. "A Review of Aromatherapy in Pain Relief." *Aromatherapy Journal.* Spring 2001; 11(1):11–12.

Lawless, Julia. *The Complete Illustrated Guide to Aromatherapy.* New York, NY: Barnes & Noble, Inc., by arrangement with Element Books, Ltd, 1997.

Bee Venom Therapy

Beck, BF. *Bee Venom Therapy—Bee Venom, Its Nature, and Its Effect on Arthritic and Rheumatoid Conditions.* New York, NY: D. Appleton-Century Co., Inc. (1935) 1997.

Broadman, J. *Bee Venom—The Natural Curative for Arthritis and Rheumatism.* Silver Spring, MD: Health Resources Press, 1997. Reprint of the original 1962 edition.

Harrar, Sari. "Desperate Measures." *The Record* (Bergen County, NJ). June 20, 1994, B01.

Hurley, Sue. "Bee-Livers Bee Stings Help Relieve Other Pain, Some Say." *St. Louis Post Dispatch,* June 26, 1997, 4.

Kegel, Maria. "Alternative Medicine's Hembing Long an Advocate of Apitherapy." *Jakarta Post* (Indonesia) June 12, 2001.

This writer has another 2001 article, "Bee Venom Therapy Takes Sting Out of Illness," in the *Jakarta Post*, an English-language paper that often does pieces on alternative health. This particular one, about a local apitherapist with clients from all over the Indonesian archipelago, was cited in *www.stopgettingsick.com*

Klinghardt, DK. "Bee Venom Therapy for Chronic Pain." *The Journal of Neurological and Orthopedic Medicine and Surgery.* 1990; 11(3):195–197.

Dr. Klinghardt, who is associated with the American Academy of Neural Therapy, describes the treatment of chronic pain with intracutaneous injections of bee venom in this article. He analyzes its effects biochemically, lists supplements that improve the effects of the therapy, discusses possible side effects (there have been very few in his practice), and concludes that bee venom appears to work extremely well, particularly in such conditions as arthitis where other methods have failed.

Kochan, Andrew, "Successful Treatment of Pain in Post-Herpetic Neuralgia with the Venom of Apis Mellifera." Presented at the Fourth International Varicella Zoster Research Foundation meeeting, March 2001.

Mraz, C. *Health and the Honeybee.* Burlington, VT: Queen City Publications, 1995:92.

Biofeedback

Alexander, CJ, Steefel, L. "Alternatives, Complementary Therapies, Biofeedback's Listen to the Body." *RN.* August 1995; 51–53.

Beiler, Pam. "Health Report: When Mind Meets Body." *Sarasota Magazine.* December 1, 1999; 22:139–140.

Bray, D. Biofeedback IN: *The Nurse's Handbook of Complementary Therapies.* Edinburgh, United Kingdom: Churchill Livingstone, 1995; 65–73.

Robbins, Jim. *A Symphony in the Brain.* New York, NY: Grove Atlantic Inc., 2001.

Most books are for biofeedback practitioners. This one above seems more geared to the public.

"Understanding Biofeedback." *Nursing.* June 1, 2002:88.

Chiropractic

Coplan-Griffiths, Michael. *Dynamic Chiropractic Today: The Complete and Authoritative Guide to this Major Therapy.* San Francisco, CA: HarperCollins, 1991. An authoritative text, combining the history, philosophy, and practice of this field of medicine, with descriptions of chiropractic treatments.

Feltman, John, ed. *Hands-On Healing.* Emmaus, PA: Rodale Press, 1989.

Martin, Raquel. *Today's Health Alternative.* Tehachapi, CA: America West Publishers, 1992. An overview with a short history of chiropractic medicine, plus anecdotes and professional training and techniques.

Palmer, Daniel David. *The Chiropractor's Adjuster.* Davenport, IA: Palmer College Press, (reprinted) 1992. This is part of, and the popular name for, *The Textbook of the Science, Art and Philosophy of Chiropractic,* an excellent book written by the father of chiropractic medicine and originally published in 1910.

Wilk, Chester. *Chiropractic Speaks Out.* Chicago, IL: Wilk Publishing Co., 1975. A clear, concise book for both patients and doctors.

To order, send $2.50 to Dr. Chester Wilk, 5130 West Belmont, Chicago, Illinois 60641, or call 1-773-725-4878.

Compresses, Packs, and Poultices

Feltman, John, ed. *Hands-On Healing*. Emmaus, PA: Rodale Press, 1989.

Green, James. *The Herbal Medicine-Maker's Handbook: a Home Manual*. Berkeley, CA: Crossing Press, div. Ten Speed Press, 2000. The entry on "Poultices and Fomentations" is very readable and very informative.

Kane, Emily. *Managing Menopause Naturally: Before, During, and Forever*. North Bergen, NJ: Basic Health Publications, 2004.

Murray, Michael T, Pizzorno, Joseph. *The Encyclopedia of Natural Medicine*, 2nd ed. Rocklin, CA: Prima Publishers, 1998.

Craniosacral Therapy

Cohen, Don. *An Introduction to CranioSacral Therapy: Anatomy, Function and Treatment*. Berkeley, CA: North Atlantic Books, 1996.

Feltman, John, ed. *Hands-On Healing*. Emmaus, PA: Rodale Press, 1989.

Milne, Hugh. *Heart of Listening: A Visionary Approach to CranioSacral Work*. Berkeley CA: North Atlantic Books, 1998.

Upledger, John E. *Your Inner Physician and You*. Berkeley, CA: North Atlantic Books, 1991.

Cupping

Chirali, Ilkay Zihni. *Traditional Chinese Medicine Cupping Therapy*. Philadelphia, PA: Churchill Livingstone, 1999.

Exercise, Stretching, and Sports

Bertrand, Amy. "Stretching Could Be The Difference Between a Good Workout and an Injury." *St. Louis Post-Dispatch;* April 7, 2003;4.

Brody, Jane E. "Start Exercising, Older Americans Urged. Inactivity Worsens Aches, Ills of Aging, Surgeons' Group Says." *Minneapolis Star Tribune*. October 20, 1996; 3E.

Kolata, Gina: Ultimate Fitness: *The Quest for Truth about Health and Exercise*. New York, NY: Farrar Straus and Giroux, 2003.

Leopold, Alison K. "Functional Fitness Means Training for Real Life." *The New York Times*. June 6, 2004.

Robertson, Sarah. "7 Easy, Feel-Good Moves." *Prevention*. November 1, 2001;134.

Tsatsouline, Pavel. *Relax into Stretch: Instant Flexibility through Mastering Muscle Tension*. St. Paul, MN: Dragon Door Publications, 2001.

Books on Pilates:

Gallagher, Sean. *The Pilates Method of Body Conditioning*. Philadelphia, PA: Trans-Atlantic Publications, 1999.

Robinson, Lynne. *Body Control*. Philadelphia, PA: Trans-Atlantic Publications, 1997.

Both books can be purchased through the publisher:

Trans-Atlantic Publications

311 Bainbridge Street

Philadelphia, PA 19147

Ph: 1-215-925-5083 or 7417

Fax: 1-215-925-1912

Website: *www.transatlanticpub.com*

E-mail: *rsmolin@ix.netcom.com*

Guided Imagery and Visualization

Bresler, David. *Free Yourself From Pain*. Topanga, CA: Alpha Books, 1997. The author is a co-founder of the Academy for Guided Imagery.

Dachman, Ken, Lyons, John. *You Can Relieve Pain*. New York, NY: HarperCollins, 1990.

Fezler, William. *Imagery for Healing, Knowledge, and Power*. New York, NY: Fireside (div. Simon and Schuster), 1990.

Rossman, Martin. *Healing Yourself, A Step by Step Program for Better Health Through Imagery*. Mill Valley, CA: Insight Publishing, 1989. The author is a co-founder of the Academy for Guided Imagery.

Silva José, Stone, Robert B. *You the Healer*. Tiburon, CA: Insight Publishing, 1989.

Simonton, O. Carl, Matthews-Simonton, Stephanie, Creighton, James. *Getting Well Again*. New York, NY: Bantam, 1992.

Heat Therapy/Cold Therapy

Cameron, MH. *Physical Agents in Rehabilitation: From Research to Practice*. Philadelphia, PA: WB Saunders Co; 1999:149–173.

Lehmann, Justus F. *Therapeutic Heat and Cold*. Philadelphia, PA: Lippincott, Williams and Wilkins, 1990.

This volume, designed for physical therapy and medical students, is out of print and has limited availability, but it is listed with Internet booksellers.

Loeser, JD. *Common Pain Problems: Guide to Practical Management*. Darien, CT: Health Communications, Inc. 1998:11–13. This booklet was referred to in the Stitik studies on hot and cold therapy cited in this entry.

Melzack, R, Wall, PD. "Pain Mechanisms: A New Theory." *Science, New Series*. November 19,1965;150(3699):971–979.

This now-famous article is the genesis of the gate theory of pain which, with modifications, is still the prevailing theory on pain.

Michlovitz, SL, ed. *Thermal Agents in Rehabilitation*. Philadelphia, PA: FA Davis Co., 1996.

Recommended for students, physical therapists, and athletic trainers.

Herbal Remedies

Duke, JA. "Using Herbal Remedies." *Mother Earth News*, December 1, 2002:92.

McCaleb, Robert S., Leigh, Evelyn, Murien, Krista. *The Encyclo-*

pedia of Popular Herbs. Boulder, CO: Herb Research Foundation, 2000.

Mindell, Earl. *Earl Mindell's Herb Bible*. New York, NY: A Fireside Book, Simon & Schuster, 1992.

Thompson, J. "Jekyll and Hyde." Health Sciences Institute, January 16, 2003. E-mail: hsiweb@agoramail.net

Tyler, VE. "Herb/Drug Interactions: The Wrong Combination Could Be Toxic." *Prevention Magazine*. September 1, 1998:93–94.

Tyler, VE. "The Truth about FDA Approval." *Prevention Magazine*. June 1, 2001:119.

Wagner, Edward M, Goldfarb, Sylvia. *How to Stay Out of the Doctor's Office: An Encyclopedia for Alternative Healing*. New York, NY: Instant Improvement, Inc., 1992.

Wagner, Edward M, Goldfarb, Sylvia. *Your Body's Most Powerful Healers*. New York, NY: Instant Improvement, Inc., 1996.

Homeopathy

Bellavite, P, Signorini, A. *Homeopathy: A Frontier in Medical Science*. Berkeley, CA: North Atlantic, 1995.

Jonas, WB, Jacobs, J. *Healing with Homeopathy*. New York, NY: Warner, 1996.

Panos, H. *Homeopathic Medicine at Home*. Los Angeles, CA: J.P. Tarcher, 1980.

Ullman, D. *The Consumer's Guide to Homeopathy*. New York, NY: Tarcher/Putnam, 1995.

Whitmarsh, TE. "When Conventional Treatment is Not Enough: A Case of Migraine without Aura Responding to Homeopathy." *The Journal of Alternative and Complementary Medicine*, 1997; 1(2):159–162.

Hydrotherapy

Batmanghelidj, F. *Your Body's Many Cries for Water*. Falls, Church, VA: Global Health Solutions, Inc., 1995. This book, about drinking water rather than bathing in it, shows how crucial a sufficient amount of water is for good health.

Buchman, Dian Dincin. *The Complete Book of Water Healing*. New York, NY: Instant Improvement, Inc. 1994.

Cameron, MH. *Physical Agents in Rehabilitation: From Research to Practice*. Philadelphia, PA: WB Saunders, Co. 1999; 149–173.

Green, James. *The Herbal Medicine-Maker's Handbook: a Home Manual*. Berkeley, CA: Crossing Press, div. Ten Speed Press, 2000. One chapter in this book, "Baths for Water Therapy," contains a very readable, accurate review of hydrotherapy.

Munson, Mary. *"Tank Heaven: Water Exercise May Unplug Pain." Prevention*. January 1, 1996; 48:40.

Reid-Campion, Margaret, ed. *Hydrotherapy: Principles and Practice*. Woburn, MA: Butterworth-Heinemann, Div. Elsevier Science/Harcourt, 1997. This book contains entries on hydrotherapy for rheumatic conditions.

Saine, Andre, Boyle, Wade. *Lectures in Naturopathic Hydrotherapy*. Sandy, OR: Eclectic Medical Publications, 1988. Explains the history, philosophy, principles, and practice of hydrotherapy.

Hypnosis

Barber, Joseph, and contributors. *Hypnosis and Suggestion in the Treatment of Pain*. New York, NY: W.W. Norton and Company, 1996.

Hilgard, Ernest R, Hilgard, Josephine R, and Editors. *Hypnosis in the Relief of Pain*. New York, NY: Brunner Mazel, 1994.

Kelly, Sean F, Kelly, Reid J. *Imagine Yourself Well: Better Health Through Self-Hypnosis*. Cambridge, MA: Perseus Publishing, 1995.

Munson, Marty, Walsh, Therese. "Smooth delivery: use your brain to control pain." (Healthy Parenting), *Prevention*. June 1, 1994; 46(2):38.

Silva, José, Stone, Robert B. *You The Healer*. Tiburon, CA: H.J. Kramer, Inc., 1989.

Magnet Therapy

Broeringmeyer, Richard. *Bioenergy Newsletter*. Murray, KY, 1986.

Burcum, Jill. "Magnetic Attraction: Magnets are being Pitched as 'Pain Relievers' for the New Millenium. Do the Claims Stick?" *Minneapolis Star Tribune*. August 25, 1999; 01E.

Dehin, Robert. *Eliminating Pain with Magnet Therapy: The Amazing Curative Powers of Magnets*. Paris, France.

Hawkins, Dana. "Take Two Magnets and Call Me Later." *US News and World Report*; 125:86.

Lore, Diana, and Staff. Healthy Living: "Magnet Pain Relief A Growing Field. Once on the Fringe, Such Therapy Now Under Serious Study." *The Atlanta Journal and Constitution*. April 17, 1999; E3.

Null, Gary. *Healing with Magnets*. New York, NY: Carroll and Graf Publ., 1998.

Park, Robert L. "America's Strange Attraction, Magnet Therapy for Pain." *The Washington Post*. September 8, 1999; H03.

Rose, Peter. *Magnet Therapy Illustrated: Natural Healing Using Magnets*. Berkeley, CA: Ulysses Press, 2001.

Massage

Fine, Judylaine. "Massage Will Help Sore Muscles Relax." *The Toronto Star*. July 31, 1998.

Hennessey, Jacqueline, Dimaline, Cherie. "The Blissful Art of Self-Massage." *Chatelaine*. July 1, 2001: 88–94.

North, Rosemarie. "Handiwork." *Waikato Times* (New Zealand). June 15, 2000: 7.

Meditation

Benson, Herbert. *The Relaxation Response*. New York, NY: Hearst Books, 1976.

Berger, KT. *Zen Driving*. New York, NY: Ballantine, 1988. The book is about being fully aware of your driving experience. It is a very good example of mindfulness meditation.

Kabat-Zinn, Jon. *Wherever You Go, There You Are*. New York, NY: Hyperion, 1994.

Kempton, Sally. *The Heart of Meditation: Pathways to a Deeper Experience*. South Fallsburg, NY: Syda Foundation, 2002.

Singh, Dharma, Stauth, Cameron. *Meditation As Medicine: Activate the Power of Your Natural Healing Force.* New York, NY: Fireside Books (Div. Simon and Schuster), 2002.

Nutritional Therapy

Barnard, Neal D. *Foods That Fight Pain.* New York, NY: Crown Publishers, 1999.

Batmanghelidj, F. *Your Body's Many Cries for Water: Don't Treat Thirst with Medications.* Falls Church, VA: Global Health Solutions, Inc., 1995.

This author considers rheumatoid arthritis to be a symptom of dehydration.

Buchman, Dian Dincin. *The Complete Book of Water Healing.* New York, NY: Instant Improvement, Inc., 1994.

Carper, Jean. *The Food Pharmacy.* New York, NY: Bantam Books, 1988.

Wagner, Edward M., Goldfarb, Sylvia. *How to Stay Out of the Doctor's Office: An Encyclopedia for Alternative Healing.* New York, NY: Instant Improvement, Inc., 1992.

Osteopathic Manipulation

Altshul, Sara. "Ease That Aching Back! See an Osteopath." *Prevention.* February 2002:50.

Chaitow, Leon. *What Is Osteopathy?* HealthWorld Online. *www.healthy.net.* Excerpted from *Osteopathy: A Complete Health Care System.*

Northrup, George W. *Osteopathic Medicine: An American Reformation.* 3rd ed. Chicago, IL: American Osteopathic Association, 1987.

Northrup, George W, ed. *Osteopathic Research: Growth and Development.* Chicago, IL: American Osteopathic Association, 1987.

Still, Andrew Taylor. *Osteopathy: Research and Practice.* Vista, CA: Eastland Press, 1992.

This is a re-publication of the 1910 book (long out of print) by the doctor who originally developed osteopathy.

Oxygen Therapies

Altman, Nathaniel. *Oxygen Healing Therapies.* Foreword by Charles H. Farr. Rochester, VT: Healing Arts Press, 1995.

McCabe, Ed. *Flood Your Body with Oxygen, Therapy for Our Polluted World.* Hallandale, FL: Energy Publications, 2003. This book has a worldwide list of practitioners who use oxygen therapies.

Neubauer, Richard A, Walker, Morton. *Hyperbaric Oxygen Therapy.* Garden City Park, NY: Avery Publishing Group, 1998.

Viebahn, Renate. *The Use of Ozone in Medicine.* 2nd American ed., transl. Andrew Lee. Heidelberg, Germany: Karl F. Haug, Publishers, 1994.

Yutsis, Pavel I. *Oxygen to the Rescue.* North Bergen, NJ: Basic Health Publications, Inc., 2003. Doctors in the United States who use oxygen therapies in their practice are listed, as well as conditions helped by oxygen therapies.

Physical Therapy

Fine, Judylaine. "Physical Therapists try to Educate Clients." *The Toronto Star.* April 10, 1998.

Ruoti, Richard, Morris, David, Cole, Andrew. *Aquatic Rehabilitation.* Philadelphia, PA: Lippincott, Williams and Wilkins, 1997.

Please note that most books on physical therapy are for therapists, not the lay reader.

Reflexology

Byers, Dwight C. *Better Health with Foot Reflexology.* Saint Petersburg, FL: Ingham Publishing, 1983 (rev. 2001). The author is the nephew of Eunice Ingham and head of the International Institute of Reflexology.

Carter, Mildred, Weber, Tammy. *Body Reflexology.* Paramus, NJ: Reward Books (Div. Parker Publishing), 1994.

Carter, Mildred. *Helping Yourself with Foot Reflexology.* West Nyack, NY: Parker Publishing, 1988.

Crane, Beryl. *Reflexology: The Definitive Practitioner's Manual.* London, England: Element Books, Ltd. (HarperCollins Imprint), 1997.

Fitzgerald, William H, Brown, Edwin. *Zone Therapy.* Mokelumne Hill, CA: Health Resources, 1917.

Feltman, John, ed. *Hands-On Healing.* Emmaus, PA: Rodale Press, 1989.

Ingham, Eunice. *Stories the Feet Can Tell.* St. Petersburg, FL: Ingham Publishing, 1938.

Ingham, Eunice. *Stories the Feet Have Told.* St Petersburg, FL: Ingham Publishing, 1948.

Kunz, Kevin and Barbara. *Hand and Foot Reflexology.* New York, NY: Fireside Books (Div. Simon & Schuster), 1992. Reflexology Research is their organization.

Kunz, Kevin and Barbara. *The Complete Guide to Foot Reflexology (Revised).* Albuquerque, NM: Kunz and Kunz, 1993.

Vennels, David F. *Reflexology for Beginners.* St Paul, MN: Llewellyn Publications, 2001.

Rolfing

Bond, Mary. *Balancing Your Body: A Self-Help Approach to Rolfing Movement.* Rochester, VT: Healing Arts Press, 1993.

Burcum, J. Roughed-Up by Rolfing. *Minneapolis Star Tribune* 1E: January 29, 2002.

Fahey, BW. *The Power of Balance: A Rolfing View of Health.* Portland, OR: Metamorphous Press, 1995.

Feltman, John, ed. *Hands-On Healing.* Emmaus, PA: Rodale Press, 1989.

Rolf, I. Rolfing: Reestablishing the Natural Alignment and Structural Integration of the Human Body for Vitality and Well-Being. Rochester, VT: Healing Arts Press, 1989.

Supplement Therapy

Mindell, Earl. *Vitamin Bible for the 21st Century.* New York, NY:Warner Books, 1999.

Murray, Michael T, Pizzorno, Joseph. *The Encyclopedia of Natural Medicine,* 2nd ed. Rocklin, CA: Prima Publishers, 1998.

Saul, Andrew. *Doctor Yourself.* North Bergen, NJ: Basic Health Publications, 2003.

Wagner, Edward M, Goldfarb, Sylvia. *How to Stay Out of the Doctor's Office: An Encyclopedia for Alternative Healing.* New York, NY: Instant Improvement, Inc., 1992.

Wagner, Edward M, Goldfarb, Sylvia. *Your Body's Most Powerful Healers.* New York, NY: Instant Improvement, Inc., 1996.

This is just a sampling. Many more books on supplements are available in bookstores and libraries, or through Internet booksellers.

Tai Chi, Qigong, and Yoga

Castleman, Michael. *Nature's Cures: From Acupuncture and Aromatherapy to Walking and Yoga, the Ultimate Guide to the Best Scientifically Proven, Drug-Free Healing Methods.* Emmaus, PA: Rodale Press, Inc., 1996.

Jahnke, Roger. *The Healing Promise of Qi.* New York, NY: Contemporary Books (Div. McGraw Hill), 2002.

Khalsa, Dharma Singh, Stauth, Cameron. *Meditation as Medicine: Activate the Power of Your Natural Healing Force.* New York, NY: Fireside Books (Div. Simon and Schuster), 2002.

Sutcliffe, Jenny. *The Complete Book of Relaxation Techniques.* Allentown, PA: The People's Medical Society, 1994.

General References

The following references are for overall pain conditions and natural approaches to health.

Catalano, Ellen M., *The Chronic Pain Control Workbook.* Oakland, CA: New Harbinger Publications, Inc., 1987.

Khalsa, Dharma Singh. *The Pain Cure.* New York, NY: Warner Books, 1999.

Loeser, JD, Melzack, R. "Pain: an overview." *The Lancet.* 1999; 353:1607–1609.

Melzack, R. "Pain: past, present and future." *Canadian Journal of Experimental Psychology.* December 1993; 47(4):615–629.

Melzack, R, Wall, PD. "Pain Mechanisms: A New Theory." *Science, New Series.* November 19,1965; 150(3699):971–979.

This now-famous article is the genesis of the gate theory of pain, which with modifications, is still the prevailing theory on pain.

Wagner, Edward M, Goldfarb, Sylvia. *How to Stay Out of the Doctor's Office: An Encyclopedia for Alternative Healing.* New York, NY: Instant Improvement, Inc., 1992.

Wall, PD, Melzak, R. eds. *Textbook of Pain,* 2nd ed. Edinburgh: Churchill Livingstone, 1989, 1–18.

About the Authors

Sylvia Goldfarb, PhD, is a writer specializing in medical topics. She has co-authored two books with Dr. Edward M. Wagner, *How To Stay Out Of The Doctor's Office: An Encyclopedia for Alternative Healing* and *Your Body's Most Powerful Healers,* both published by Instant Improvement, Inc. Her most recent book, *Allergy Relief: Effective Natural Allergy Treatments,* is published by Avery, an imprint of Penguin Putnam, Inc. Sylvia has written articles for a number of magazines, including *Focus, Natural Body and Fitness, Today's OR Nurse,* and *Veggie Times.* A graduate of Skidmore College, she belongs to the Author's Guild and serves as a faculty member and judge of the Philadelphia Writer's Conference.

Roberta W. Waddell, a graduate of Westover School and Smith College, has had more than sixteen years experience working in the alternative health field, both freelance and as the editor at a direct mail publishing house. Her more than thirty years of personal experience with chronic pain led her down many avenues of treatment, alternative and mainstream, and led her to embrace the concept of this book when it was presented to her.

Index

A

B

C

I

J

K

L

M

N

O

P

Q

R

S

T

U

V

W

Y

Z

OTHER SQUAREONE TITLES OF INTEREST

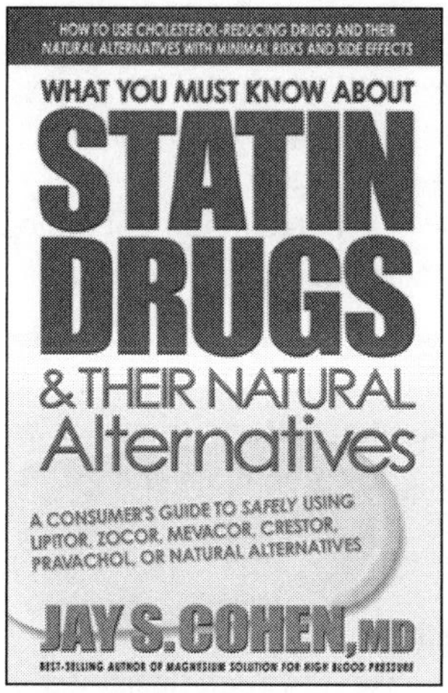

WHAT YOU MUST KNOW ABOUT STATIN DRUGS & THEIR NATURAL ALTERNATIVES

A Consumer's Guide to Safely Using Lipitor, Zocor, Pravachol, Crestor, Mevacor, or Natural Alternatives

Jay S. Cohen, MD

Written by a highly qualified researcher and physician, *What You Must Know About Statin Drugs & Their Natural Alternatives* begins by explaining elevated cholesterol and C-reactive proteins. It then examines how statins work to alleviate these problems, and discusses possible side effects. Highlighted are facts about the medications' usage, including a discussion of difficulties caused by standard dosage levels and information on safer usage. The author even explains how you can identify those who may be sensitive to statins, and offers safe and effective alternative treatments.

$15.95 US /$23.95 CAN • 204 Pages • 6 x 9-inch paperback • ISBN 0-7570-0257-9

THE MAGNESIUM SOLUTION FOR HIGH BLOOD PRESSURE

How to Use Magnesium to Help Prevent and Relieve Hypertension Naturally

Jay S. Cohen, MD

Approximately 50 percent of all Americans have hypertension, a devastating disease that can lead to hardening of the arteries, heart attack, and stroke. While many medications are available to combat this condition, these drugs come with potentially dangerous side effects. When Dr. Jay S. Cohen learned of his own vascular condition, he was well aware of the risks associated with standard treatments. Based upon his research, he selected a safer option—magnesium.

In *The Magnesium Solution for High Blood Pressure,* Dr. Cohen describes the most effective types of magnesium for treating hypertension, explores appropriate magnesium dosage, and details the use of magnesium in conjunction with hypertension meds. Here is a proven remedy for anyone looking for a safe, effective approach to the treatment of high blood pressure.

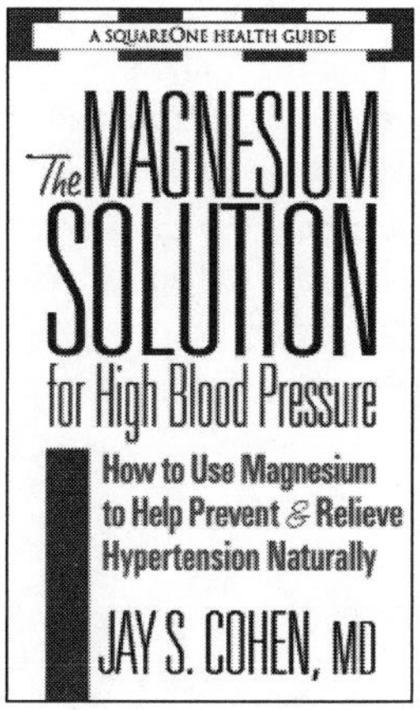

$5.95 • 96 pages • 4 x 7.5-inch mass paperback • ISBN 0-7570-0255-2

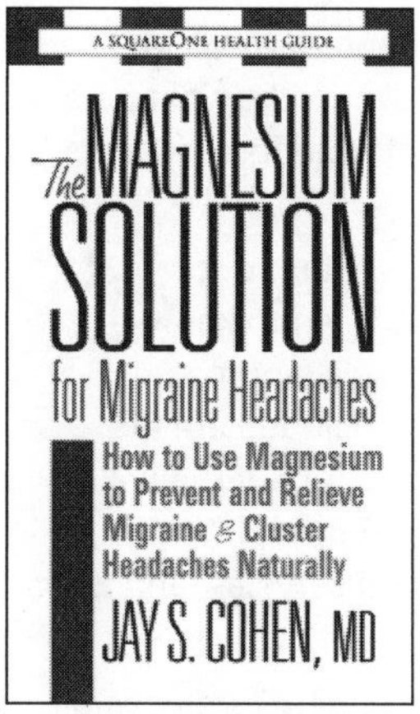

THE MAGNESIUM SOLUTION FOR MIGRAINE HEADACHES

How to Use Magnesium to Prevent and Relieve Migraine and Cluster Headaches Naturally

Jay S. Cohen, MD

More than 30 million people across North America suffer from migraine headaches. Over the years, a number of drugs have been developed to treat migraines, but these treatments don't work for everyone, and come with a high risk of side effects. Fortunately, Dr. Jay S. Cohen has discovered an alternative—magnesium.

This easy-to-understand guide explains what a migraine is, and shows how this supplement can play a key role in preventing and treating migraine headaches. It also describes what type of magnesium works best, and how much magnesium should be taken to prevent or stop migraines. For those who are looking for a safe and effective approach to the prevention and treatment of migraine and cluster headaches, Dr. Cohen prescribes a proven natural remedy in *The Magnesium Solution for Migraine Headaches.*

$5.95 • 96 pages • 4 x 7.5-inch mass paperback • ISBN 0-7570-0256-0

About the Author

Jay S. Cohen, MD, is an Associate Professor (voluntary) of Family and Preventive Medicine at the University of California, San Diego. Dr. Cohen is a widely recognized expert on prescription drugs and their natural alternatives. He has published scientific papers in leading medical journals and has written articles for *Newsweek, Bottom Line Health,* and *Life Extension Magazine.* Dr. Cohen is a highly sought-after speaker and publishes commentary for the public on current issues in health care at www.MedicationSense.com. Dr. Cohen practices preventive and integrative medicine in Del Mar, California.

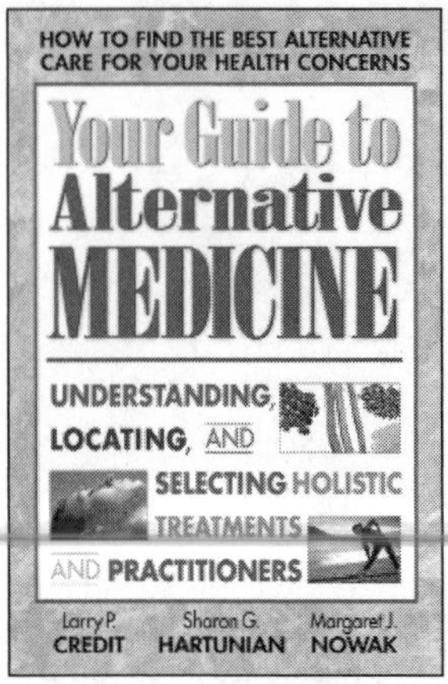

Your Guide to Alternative Medicine

Understanding, Locating, and Selecting Holistic Treatments and Practitioners

Larry P. Credit, Sharon G. Hartunian, and Margaret J. Nowak

The growing world of complementary medicine offers safe and effective solutions to many health disorders from backaches to headaches. You may already be interested in alternative care approaches, but probably also have a number of questions you'd like answered before choosing a treatment. "Will I feel the acupuncture needles?" "Does chiropractic hurt?" "What is a homeopathic remedy?" *Your Guide to Alternative Medicine* provides the fundamental facts necessary to choose an effective complementary care therapy and begin treatment.

This comprehensive reference clearly explains numerous approaches in an easy-to-read format. For every complementary care option discussed, there is a description and brief history; a list of conditions that respond; information on the cost and duration of treatment; credentials and educational background of practitioners; and more. To find those therapies most appropriate for a specific condition, there is even a unique troubleshooting chart.

Your Guide to Alternative Medicine introduces you to options that you may never have considered—techniques that enhance the body's natural healing potential and have few, if any, side effects. Here is a reference that can help you make informed decisions about all your important healthcare needs.

About the Authors

Larry P. Credit received his doctorate in Oriental medicine from SAMRA University in Los Angeles, California, and is a graduate of the New England School of Acupuncture. Dr. Credit creates complementary care programs for hospitals and schools.

Sharon G. Hartunian received a bachelor of science in psychology from Tufts University and a master of science in social work from Simmons College. She is a Licensed Independent Clinical Social Worker and a Certified Alcohol and Drug Abuse Counselor.

Margaret J. Nowak is a graduate of the New Hampshire Institute for Therapeutic Arts, and has helped develop alternative medicine and allied health programs for hospitals and colleges.

$11.95 US / $17.95 CAN • 208 pages • 6 x 9-inch paperback • ISBN 0-7570-0125-4

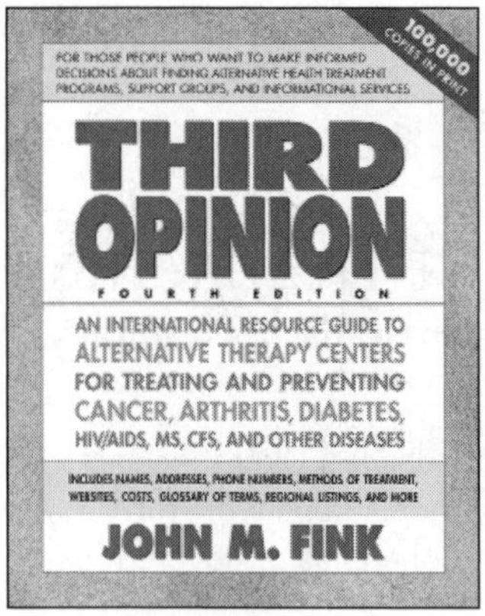

Third Opinion, Fourth Edition

An International Directory to Alternative Therapy Centers for the Treatment and Prevention of Cancer & Other Degenerative Diseases

John M. Fink

Even with the growing awareness of the value of alternative and complementary medicine, basic facts about alternative cancer treatments are hard to come by. If you don't know the right person, it may take weeks to learn even the simplest of facts. Worse, sometimes information becomes available only as a matter of chance.

Here, in this fourth revised edition, is a comprehensive guide to the growing number of alternative treatment centers located throughout the world. Everything you need to know—from addresses, phone numbers, websites, names, and prices, to philosophical approaches and methods of treatment—is provided in a clear, easy-to-use format. Also included are the educational centers, information services, and support programs that may be of interest to the person looking for alternative or adjunctive therapy. For each listing, the author has gathered all of the information necessary to make that all-important initial contact. To further help you, the author has included a glossary of terms, a regional breakdown of centers and services, and a list of informative readings.

Beyond any first and second opinions that may be offered, there are other options that you may wish to consider. *Third Opinion* offers you the opportunity to learn about these options so that you can make a truly informed decision.

About the Author

John M. Fink had been an actor for fourteen years when he lost his young daughter to cancer. Since then, he has been deeply interested in alternative adjunctive care. He has been actively involved with The International Association of Cancer Victors and Friends, and has also served as a member of the Advisory Panel for the Congressional Office of Technology Assessment's (OTA) study, Unconventional Cancer Treatments. He and his wife split their time between Southern California and Northern Michigan.

$19.95 US/$29.95 CAN • 384 pages • 7.5 x 9-inch paperback • ISBN 0-7570-0131-9

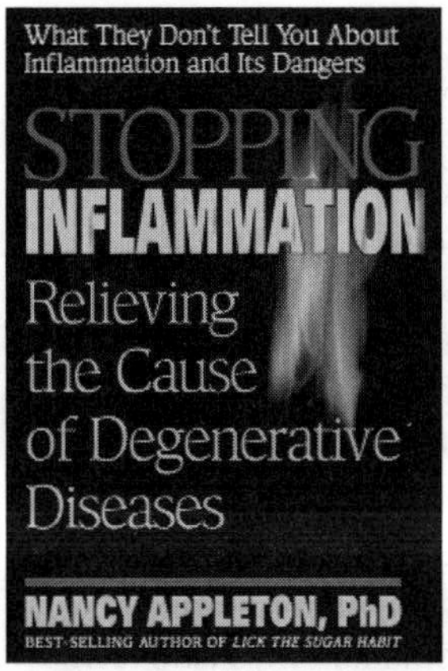

Stopping Inflammation

Relieving the Cause of Degenerative Diseases

Nancy Appleton, PhD

Inflammation is a word we hear all the time— "Your throat is inflamed," "You have some inflammation around the knee," "You have an inflamed ear." Most of us think of it as a symptom associated with an infection, irritation, or injury. Dr. Nancy Appleton, however, has discovered that it is more than just a simple reaction to a health disorder. When the body's tissues are disturbed in some manner, a series of complex reactions takes place, resulting in inflammation. In most cases, when the disorder stops, the tissue returns to its normal healthy state. At times, though, the tissue remains chronically inflamed. Dr. Appleton's early research indicated that this chronic condition is more harmful than ever suspected. Soon, she began to ask questions: What if inflammation was at the heart of various degenerative diseases? What health benefits could be gained if we could stop inflammation? *Stopping Inflammation* is the result of Dr. Appleton's ten-year quest to answer these important questions.

Drawing on the latest medical research, this book begins with a full explanation of inflammation. It then looks at inflammation's many causes, from food allergies to environmental factors to psychological stress. Next, it focuses on the various health disorders that afflict modern society—obesity, addiction, heart disease, diabetes, cancer, bowel disorders, and more—and explains the role that inflammation plays in each. Finally, the book provides a variety of nondrug treatments aimed not at controlling the problem, but at removing its cause.

About the Author

Nancy Appleton, PhD, earned her BS in clinical nutrition from UCLA and her PhD in health services from Walden University. She maintains a private practice in Santa Monica, California. An avid researcher, Dr. Appleton lecturers extensively throughout the world, and has appeared on numerous television and radio talk shows. She is the best-selling author of *Lick the Sugar Habit* and *Healthy Bones.*

$14.95 US / $22.50 CAN • 224 pages • 6 x 9-inch paperback • ISBN 0-7570-0148-3

Ulcer Free!

Nature's Safe and Effective Remedy for Ulcers

Georges M. Halpern, MD

Over four million Americans are diagnosed annually with peptic ulcer disease. Millions more go undiagnosed. For them, the resulting gastritis simply becomes a part of their daily existence, and they learn to live with heartburn, acid reflux, nausea, belching, gas, and stomach pain. For many of these people, living on over-the-counter antacids becomes a way of life. Readily available and easy-to-take, these pleasant-tasting products may stop the pain, but only temporarily. Furthermore, while the symptoms are quieted, the underlying condition can get worse. But it doesn't have to be that way. Written by a physician who himself suffered gastric pain, *Ulcer Free!* is a practical guide to understanding the causes of and effective treatments for peptic ulcer disease.

Ulcer Free! begins with a look at why we get ulcers. It examines the *Helicobacter pylori* bacterium—the newly discovered culprit behind the majority of stomach ulcers. It also discusses the growing number of ulcers caused by the overuse of NSAIDs—over-the-counter pain relievers more commonly known as aspirin, ibuprofen, naproxen, and a variety of other products. The book also details the most common signs of peptic ulcer disease, and explains the latest testing procedures for determining this condition. Next, a clear and unbiased look is given to the various treatments that can stop the symptoms and actually heal ulcers, including both conventional and alternative therapies. Finally, *Ulcer Free!* introduces the new breakthrough nutrient Zinc-Carnosine, which can be used in conjunction with other treatments or on its own.

About the Author

Georges M. Halpern, MD, attended medical school at the University of Paris, France. He subsequently received a PhD from the Faculty of Pharmacy, University of Paris XI—Chatenay Malabry. A Fellow of the American Academy of Allergy and Immunology, Dr. Halpern is board certified in internal medicine and allergy, and is Professor Emeritus of Medicine at the University of California—Davis. He is also a Distinguished Professor of Medicine at the University of Hong Kong.

$14.95 US / $22.50 CAN • 208 pages • 6 x 9-inch paperback • ISBN 0-7570-0253-6

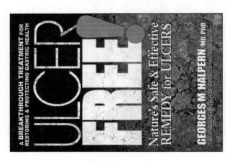

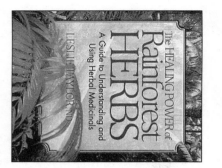

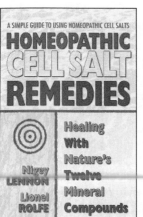